Boo
R.

£13.60

NEUROPSYCHIATRY

NEUROPSYCHIATRY

Michael R. Trimble
*Consultant Physician in Psychological Medicine
to the National Hospitals for Nervous Diseases,
Queen Square and Maida Vale, London WC1N 3BG*
and
*Senior Lecturer in Behavioural Neurology,
The Institute of Neurology, University of London*

JOHN WILEY AND SONS
Chichester · New York · Brisbane · Toronto

British Library Cataloguing in Publication Data:
Trimble, Michael R.
  Neuropsychiatry.
  1. Neuropsychiatry
  I. Title
  616.8   RC341   80-40766

  ISBN 0 471 27827 0

Phototypeset by Dobbie Typesetting Service, Plymouth, Devon, England
and printed in the United States of America

For
Denis and Peggy

Insanity being a disease, and that disease being an affection of the brain, it can therefore only be studied in a proper manner from the medical point of view.

(W. Griesinger, *Mental Pathology and Therapeutics*, London, 1857, p.9)

Acknowledgements

Although there are many physicians who, in the course of my career, have contributed to the information and ideas which are contained in this book, it is to Dr R. T. C. Pratt, my colleague and friend over the past four years, to whom I am especially grateful. We have had many hours of interesting discussion about neuropsychiatry and its problems, and throughout the writing of this book his support has been invaluable.

There are a number of people, including Dr Pratt, to whom I am most grateful for having read parts of the manuscript, and I particularly wish to acknowledge the suggestions and comments of Dr John Bates, Dr Peter Gautier-Smith, Dr Joe Herbert, Professor Ian McDonald, Dr Harold Merskey, Dr Peter Nathan, Dr Malcolm Piercy, Dr Ted Reynolds, Dr David Somekh, and Dr Jenifer Wilson–Barnett.

I would like to take this opportunity to thank Dr Bill Cobb for providing the electroencephalography records, and to Mr A. H. Prentice for his invaluable aid in producing the photographic plates.

I am indebted to my colleagues at the National Hospitals for their support in continuing to refer to the Department some of the most fascinating neuro-psychiatric problems that could ever be encountered.

I express gratitude to the nursing staff of Hughlings Jackson ward for their help and care in the management of these patients and their difficult problems.

I wish particularly to acknowledge the help of Miss M. Zietsman in the preparation of this text, since without her persistent dedication and meticulous typing, preparation of such a manuscript for publication would never have been possible.

Contents

Preface

In the course of teaching psychiatrists in training, it has become clear that many are dissatisfied with their knowledge of some basic principles of the brain and its function that underlie the behaviour disorders that they manage clinically, and many express an interest in learning more about neuropsychiatric problems which are met in practice. This book is an attempt to fulfil some of these needs, and in assessing the amount of information included, an attempt has been made to recognize that many students in psychiatry may have little or no formal neurological training, and that their more basic understanding of the neurological sciences at medical school may have been long forgotten. While this unfortunately leads, in many instances, to simplifications of complex but interesting problems, it is hoped that some will be stimulated to read further, and attempts have been made to give key references where possible.

Neurologists in training also have been taken into account, since they often express an interest in learning more about psychiatry, especially those aspects of relevance for their clinical problems. Knowledge of behaviour and its disorders is still often poorly covered in medical education, and with increased neurological training requirements many potential neurologists may complete their studies without a period of psychiatric attachment. An attempt has therefore been made to include some introductory comments about psychiatry into the book, although covering such a vast topic in a small space has, of necessity, limited discussion of many topics.

A third group of readers who may find specific interest in this book are those who wish to explore the borderlands of neurological and psychiatric disease, namely the rich field of neuropsychiatry. This term has been chosen with care and refers to disorders which, on account of their presentation and pathogenesis, do not fall neatly and clearly into one category, and require multidisciplinary ideas for their full understanding. In particular, movement disorders, epilepsy, dementia, and chronic pain have been discussed at some length because of their importance as examples of neuropsychiatric problems.

xiii

The dichotomy between neurology and psychiatry is explored in Chapter 1, where it is suggested that, partly as a reflection of historical accident, the two split apart, and that in recent years, especially since the discovery of the role of neurotransmitters in brain function and behaviour, a newer understanding of functional as opposed to structural disorders has arisen. The neurochemical correlates of several primary psychiatric illnesses have been partially unravelled, but in addition the behavioural consequences of neurological lesions and disease have become more clearly enshrined in the literature. As techniques in the measurement of abnormal neuronal activity have become sophisticated, more and more pathology is being defined in disorders where ideas of pathogenesis could not previously be entertained with conviction.

Although half a century ago neurology and psychiatry seemed to be diverging from a common purpose and standing as two stools apart, these recent advances have not only seen the stools bridged by a plank, but the whole structure has gradually come to resemble a bench, which for some seems quite comfortable. Doubtless, there are others who will find this bench disagreeable, and may wish to discard it as soon as possible, although time may not be on their side. In the early 1970s Hunter[1] commented: 'To exclude patients who have no physical signs — that is no motor or sensory deficit — from the benefit of modern scientific medicine is today perhaps the most stultifying single factor retarding psychiatric and indeed neurological progress'. The last decade has seen not only an exponential growth of knowledge in the field of the neurosciences, but also a resolution of some interdisciplinary rivalry, and laid the foundations of neuropsychiatry for at least the rest of this century.

CHAPTER 1

Historical Introduction

Psychiatry is a much older subject than neurology. Although the ancients wrote about the treatment of insanity, psychiatry as an independent discipline with its specialist practitioners, the alienists, initially developed in the seventeenth century. Around this time medicine generally was released from the shackles of Galenism and the authoritarian dogma that presided over the Middle Ages, and the study of insanity with particular reference to the mind rather than the soul became a part of this intellectual movement. The trend away from metaphysics towards a more physiological, descriptive, and empirical science was heralded by such thinkers as Johann Weyer (1515–1588), who was perhaps the first physician to take a major interest in mental illness, Francis Bacon (1561–1626), Descartes (1596–1650) and Hobbes (1588–1679). They were followed by Sydenham (1624–1689), Willis (1621–1675), who coined the term 'neurologie', and Harvey (1578–1657), who laid the foundation stones of modern medical thought.

Of most importance for neuropsychiatry are the writings of Descartes. Although, as most authors do, he was reflecting ideas current in the society in which he lived, his philosophy, so acceptable to the 'period of enlightenment', has had a profound influence on medical thought. Thus for the Christian world, labouring under the theocracy of the middle ages, any ideas regarding the 'soul', and thus the mind of man, either had to be acceptable to the religious and political views of the time, or authors were likely to be persecuted and imprisoned. Essentially the mind was not the province of either doctors or even philosophers, it was the property of the church, and had been so since the downfall of the Graeco-Roman culture. Although mental diseases were often recorded throughout the Middle Ages, no clear discussion of them by the scientists of the time are to be found. The mentally ill were regarded either as heretics or, if they were lucky, as possessed by some alien 'spirit' from the devil, and treatment was thus by burning or exorcism.

As the centuries progressed, the concept of mental illness being associated with witchcraft grew, and those afflicted became feared. Sprenger and Kraemer, two Dominican brothers, kindled these anxieties and, as part of a religious mission, set out to rid the world of witches. They formulated their ideas in a book entitled *Malleus Maleficarum — The Witches' Hammer* (1487). This was to become the mouthpiece of the Inquisition. Not only did it prove the existence of witches but also gave methods by which they could be identified. It provided fuel for the witch-hunts that followed in which thousands of mentally ill people died.

Weyer studied medicine in Paris and made mental diseases one of his special interests. He was particularly sceptical of the explanation of Sprenger and Kraemer regarding the causes of insanity, and applied himself to a methodical collection of data attempting an objective interpretation of what he saw. In 1563 he published *De Praestigiis Daemonum — The Deceptions of Demons*.

This book reviewed in detail witches, wizards, exorcism and related phenomena. It was written to affirm his belief that 'those illnesses whose origins are attributed to witches come from natural causes . . .'. At the time he was severely criticized, and was himself accused of being a wizard, so that initially his work had little impact. However, he was one of the first of a new era of physicians to take an interest in the natural causes of diseases of the mind.

Change was slow and there were still many who for various reasons were unable to shake off the metaphysical interpretation of events, not the least being their fear for their own safety. It was Descartes who provided a solution for the growing problems that were emerging in the relationship between the newly developing empirical sciences, and the more long-established theology. In his philosophy, he separated mind from body — the so-called Cartesian dualism. Thus he suggested that the laws of nature were mechanical, and the main feature which distinguished corporeal things from the mind was extension in space. What distinguished man from animals was the former's possession of a rational soul. Men's bodies could be regarded as machines and studied as such in the empiricist tradition. The soul was joined to the body by animal spirits which passed through the nerves to the mucles and 'after examining the matter with care' he concluded that the rational soul resided in the pineal gland. This dualism became so ingrained into Western thinking that it influenced the development of the neurosciences to the present day. Unfortunately it has left a legacy of confusion with regard to the mind–body problem.

Following the ideas of Descartes the stage was set for advances in the neurosciences. Given clear philosophical licence, the mind securely unexplorable and safe with theology, the body including the brain could be left unhindered for investigation. Willis, who acknowledged that man's higher functions were related to his immortal rational soul, was able to speculate about the brain and its function. Incoming sensation was received by the corpus striatum, where imagination was located, memory being related to the cortex. These were early attempts at the localization of brain functions which ultimately led to the flourishing of clinical neurology and of the clinical method of localizing abnormal pathology. These investigations were continued with the discoveries of Broca (1824–1880) in the mid-nineteenth century, and since then a host of others including Ferrier (1843–1928), Meynert (1833–1892), Wernicke (1848–1905), Derjerine (1849–1917), Liepmann (1863–1925), and Penfield (1891–1976).

An alternative direction of clinical expertise, however, was followed by a number of physicians who were primarily interested in psychiatric illness, and in particular in the nosology and neuropathology of such disorders. Thus the eighteenth century physician Cullen (1710–1790), divided all the known diseases into categories, and one of them he referred to as the 'neuroses'. This he subdivided into comata, adynamiae, spasmi and vesaniae. The latter were essentially the disorders that today are assumed under the rubric 'psychiatric'. They were disorders where judgement was impaired in the absence of pyrexia or coma, and could again be subdivided into amentia (imbecility of the judgement), melancholia (partial insanity), mania (universal insanity), and oneirodynia (inflamed or disturbed imagination during sleep) (Ref. 2, p.478). Cullen's influence was substantial. He proceeded to consider how the brain was disordered in illness, which later led Coombe (1797–1847) to subdivide disorders of the brain into two large groups, namely the organic and the functional. The latter were related to changes of brain function where local causes could not be discovered. This led to the foundation of a nosology of neuropsychiatric illness which is still in existence today.

Haslam (1764–1844), medical officer to the Bethlem Hospital, the country's oldest asylum, conducted comprehensive post-mortem examinations on the brains of insane patients. Although he failed to localize the site of insanity, it is suggested that amongst his observations was the first description of cerebral

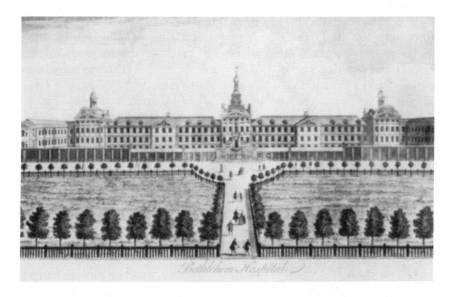

Figure 1.1. Bethlem hospital, the country's oldest asylum

syphilis. It was, however, in Germany that the most significant advances occurred. Griesinger (1817–1868), professor of psychiatry and neurology in Berlin, gave a clear lead to the idea that 'psychiatry and neuropathology are not merely two closely related fields; they are but one field in which only one language is spoken and the same laws rule (Ref. 3, p.436). For him psychiatric illness was directly related to disease of the brain. '. . . We therefore primarily, and in every case of mental disease, recognize a morbid action of that organ'. (Ref. 4, p.2). He clearly formulated the idea that normal mental processes are dependent upon the integrity of the brain, and that lesions of some parts of the brain are more likely than others to be associated wtih mental illness. He distinguished mental diseases from more transient psychic disturbances seen in well people, concluding that 'with the mental disease a change in the mental disposition of the patient and his sentiments, desires, habits, conduct and opinions . . . appears . . . his former I becomes changed . . .' (Ref. 4, p.114). The causes of insanity he divided into idiopathic — from 'influences directly on the brain — shock, injury, excessive fatigue of the brain and entire nervous system, alcoholics, narcotics, excessive mental irritation through emotion and the like' (Ref. 4, p.131), and symptomatic — which included brain dysfunction secondary to somatic illness. These of course interacted with predisposition, and the illness was finally the result of circulatory changes, 'nervous irritation of the brain' (Ref. 4, p.131), or changes in brain nutrition. Griesinger recognized the problems of classification when it was based on symptoms alone, and described sub-categories of mental illness, such as melancholia, mania, and states of mental weakness which included chronic mania, dementia and idiocy.

Griesinger's lead not only gave some coherence to a previously scattered terminology and classification of mental illness, it also drew attention to the brain as the seat of insanity, and that as such mental illnesses should be investigated in the same fashion as other illnesses. In Germany his attempts were followed by others who tried to correlate mental diseases with neuropathology, and who continued work on classification, including Erb (1840–1921) — 'the first neurologist to wield a reflex hammer'.[5] The Viennese neurologist Meynert attempted to synthetize what was then known about neurophysiology, and in particular reflex activity, with the dominant mode of psychology at the time, namely associationist psychology. Wernicke, who studied under Meynert, described polio-encephalitis superior haemorrhagica, now known as Wernicke's encephalopathy, and in his studies on the relationship of language to the cerebral cortex described sensory aphasia. Alzheimer (1864–1915) and Pick (1851–1924) attempted to correlate clinical findings with post-mortem changes and described the neuropathology of certain types of dementia. Classification was advanced by Kahlbaum (1828–1899), who described catatonia, his pupil Hecker (1843–1909), who coined the term hebephrenia, and Morel (1809–1873), who described an illness similar to hebephrenia in which mental deterioration had its onset in adolescence, and to which he gave the name 'démence précoce' (1860). The zenith of this era came with the work of Kraepelin (1856–1925). He was professor of psychiatry at Munich and Heidelberg and gathered together thousands of case studies in order to elaborate a system of classification for psychiatric illness which is still in use today. On the basis of prognosis he separated out dementia praecox from manic-depressive insanity. The former usually resulted in a picture of 'incurable mental infirmity' as opposed to the latter which was compatible with return to health between bouts of illness. Following others he divided mental illness into two groups — the endogenous and the exogenous, the former which included dementia praecox. It was left to Bonhoeffer (1865–1948) to later develop and expand the concept of the exogenous illnesses to which he gave the name 'exogenous psychic reaction types', patterns of illness which were related to external noxious substances which affected the brain.

From the above it is clear that the German neuropsychiatrists were predominantly concerning themselves with severe mental illness, in particular psychotic illness, and the abnormalities of the brain that could be associated with them. Different developments occurred in France.

Pinel (1745–1826), physician to the Bicêtre and the Salpêtrière, two large Paris asylums, and who is most famous because of his removal of the chains and shackles of patients in such institutions, had attempted a classification of disorders into melancholia, mania, dementia and idiocy. His pupil Esquirol (1772–1840) differentiated hallucinations from delusions. It was however the work of another physician from the Salpêtrière, Charcot (1825–1893) who most clearly exemplified the difference between the French and German schools. His interest was not so much with the psychoses, but with the neuroses.

The various disorders earlier characterized as 'neuroses' by Cullen were gradually broken down into entities that on neuropathological investigation could be identified with structural lesions. The concept of organic as opposed to functional disorders had progressed to lead to the independent growth of interest in the former with the expansion of neurology. Since the early speculations of Willis, Bell (1774–1842) and Magendie (1783–1855) had demonstrated that the posterior roots of the spinal cord carried sensory impulses and the anterior root motor ones. Müller (1801–1858) had pronounced his doctrine of specific energies of the nerves; Broca (1824–1880) and Wernicke had described symptoms associated with specific cerebral lesions; Griesinger's student Hitzig (1838–1907), in collaboration with Fritsch (1836–1897), further confirmed localization of brain activity using electrical stimulation of dogs' brains, which led to the later discoveries of Ferrier. Neurology as an independent discipline flourished further following the foundation in 1860 of the National Hospital for the 'Relief of Paralysis, Epilepsy, and Allied Diseases'. One of the earliest members of its staff was Hughlings Jackson (1835–1911), who made careful studies of patients with epilepsy, and by post-mortem examination attempted accurate localization of lesions. Influenced by the philosopher Spencer (1820–1903), he viewed the central nervous system as having three different levels, the highest of which resided in the frontal lobes.

6

These higher centres inhibited lower centres such that with damage 'dissolution' occurred. 'Positive' neurological symptoms were thus seen as the result of release from these lower centres, interacting with elements of the nervous system not destroyed by disease.

In this climate Charcot in 1862 was appointed Médecin de la Salpêtrière. Succeeding Pinel, he found a vast number of patients under his care who had neuropsychiatric disability. In an attempt to identify and categorize the illnesses he saw, working with such contemporaries as Marie (1853-1940), Duchenne (1806-1875) and Gilles de la Tourette (1857-1904), he gave full clinical descriptions of Parkinson's disease, which he separated from an entity which is now called multiple sclerosis, and described in detail a host of syndromes, some of which have since been rediscovered. He attempted to study the neuroses in the same fashion as other nervous disorders, namely on an anatomico-pathological basis. He examined hysterical phenomena, giving more than a third of his lecture time to the subject, and experimented with hypnotism. As one author has summed up the contributions of the Salpêtrière school: '. . . It was the first to capture for psychiatry the very last part of demonological territory . . .' (Ref. 3, p.365). With the death of Charcot however, such studies ceased and investigation of neuroses became the province of the now rapidly growing speciality of psychiatry. Exactly what influences ideas in history at any one time is unclear, but in the history of neuropsychiatry it is noted that, within certain limits, trends come and go. One historian attributed such cycles to changes in the intellectual climate, which fluctuate from Classicism to Romanticism (Ref. 6, p.289). With the former the tendency is on classification and empiricism, while the latter shows a much greater interest in introspection and individuality. At the turn of this century there was a period of 'neo-Romanticism' with increasing preoccupation in hypnotism, and interest in the unconscious. Bleuler (1857-1939) coined the term schizophrenia, extending the classification of Dementia Praecox to include a variety of acute conditions, some of which had a good prognosis, and 'many atypical melancholias and manias of other schools, especially hysterical melancholias and manias, most hallucinatory confusions, some "nervous" people and compulsive and impulsive patients, and many prison psychoses'.[7] Reflecting the growing interest in 'dynamic'* psychiatry, he developed a theory of schizophrenia blending ideas of the organicist schools with contemporary psychological explanations. His line of thinking was followed by Adolf Meyer (1866-1950), who emigrated to the United States and while professor of psychiatry at the Phipps Clinic developed his 'psychobiology' with its main emphasis on the individual, his life experiences and 'reaction types'. It is no coincidence that both Bleuler and Meyer were born in Switzerland and were students of Forel (1848-1931). However, the person

---

*The term dynamic has several meanings in the context of neuropsychiatry (Ref. 6, p.289), but in this text refers to a notion of 'psychic energy' which is usually employed as an antithesis to 'organic' in order to explain alterations of behaviour.

most associated with the development of psychiatry at this time was Freud (1856-1939). Originally interested in neuropathology, and studying under Brücke (1819-1892) and Meynert, he visited Charcot in Paris in 1885. While there he met Janet (1859-1947), who not only coined the term subconscious, but also had developed a system of psychology which emphasized the importance of unconscious mental acts in the precipitation of symptoms. On account of, or in spite of, his discussions with Janet, Freud, on returning to Vienna, collaborated with Breuer (1842-1925) in the development of new forms of treatment for the neuroses, which they referred to as 'talking therapies'. Disenchanted with hypnotism, they allowed patients to talk freely, to discharge their emotions, and noted that with such 'catharsis' patients recovered. From these early experiments Freud went on to develop the concepts of psychoanalysis, and, with an emphasis entirely on mental mechanisms, conformed completely to the dualism ushered in by Descartes. The split between neurology and psychiatry was therefore complete. The story of psychoanalysis will not be discussed further except to suggest that, as with all the ideas discussed in this chapter, the original tenets have undergone considerable change. Early dissenters such as Jung (1875-1943) and Adler (1870-1957) developed their own schools with profound modifications of Freud's ideas. Of utmost importance has been the increasing emphasis on ego mechanisms, and less emphasis on the 'id' in the control of behaviour. Freud's daughter, Anna Freud, elaborated a range of ego defence mechanisms, and writers such as Hartmann (1894-1970) concentrated on aspects of ego functioning that were concerned with adaptation of the individual to his environment, and which were 'conflict free'. The recent explosion of various ego-orientated therapies, such as Berne's (1910-1970) Transactional Analysis, are further developments of these ideas.

In spite of the dissociation between neurology and psychiatry referred to above, there have been various writers in this century who have attempted to unite developments in both fields. The French psychiatrist Ey (1900-1973), influenced by the ideas of Freud and Hughlings Jackson, developed his organodynamic psychiatry. Others have included Schilder (1886-1940), Goldstein (1878-1965), Cobb (1887-1968), Meyer, and Stengel (1902-1974). Recent developments in the fields of neurochemistry, the discovery and widespread use of a number of powerful psychotropic drugs and the elucidation of some of their possible modes of action, and the more widespread reintroduction of departments of psychiatry into general hospitals, has led once again to a clearer understanding of relationships between psychiatry and the other medical disciplines, and has indicated a way for the future development of neuropsychiatry.

CHAPTER 2

Introduction to the Nervous System

The nervous system acquires information about the world in which an organism lives, and the position of that organism in the world, by the use of sensory receptors which transmit information via afferent nerves. In order to act effectively within that environment, efferent nerves to muscles provide the final common pathway for movement. In between these afferent and efferent channels the central nervous system (CNS), composed of multiple fibre tracts and billions of cells, provides synthesis for action and decision-making. The following is not a comprehensive account of neuroanatomy and neurophysiology. It is an introduction to those aspects of the central nervous system of importance to neuropsychiatry, and as such greater attention is paid to the basal ganglia, limbic system, and certain aspects of neurochemistry. It should be emphasized that in the past, attempts to understand the CNS were based on neuroanatomical knowledge, and different nuclei were identified often only because they seemed separated by white matter. Recent neurochemical data have emphasized different functional systems within the brain, which do not conform to these earlier static views, and are leading to a different conceptualization of CNS activity, based much more on knowledge of the localization and behaviour of neurotransmitters.

AFFERENT AND EFFERENT SYSTEMS

The neurone theory, introduced in the 1890s and supported by the findings of Ramon y Cajal, implied that the nervous system consisted of individual cells, as other organs in the body were. It is the foundation of our present day concepts of nervous system function. The neurone itself consists of a soma (cell body), axon, and dendrites — fine branches which protrude from the cell body. The nerve impulse is transmitted along the axon. Individual nerves make contact with other nerves at synapses, a term originally used by Sherrington, and which denotes an area of functional contact between nerves approximately 20 nm wide. Synapses are either axo-somatic, axo-dendritic, dendro-dendritic or axo-axonic, and the 'terminal button' of the nerve cell is the commonest type of pre-synaptic structure making contact. The latter is richly provided with mitochondria, and is packed with small vesicles, 30–60 nm in diameter, called synaptic vesicles. The cell body is packed with organelles, which enable the cell to metabolize nutrients, and to provide energy for its activities, and material from it flows down the axon towards the terminal boutons. Although the precise mode of synaptic action is not clear, it is thought that with appropriate stimulation, such as electrical activity in the axon, the terminal boutons release transmitters, which have been stored in the synaptic vesicles, into the synaptic cleft. These neurotransmitters then influence the post-synaptic membrane of the cell of contact, altering the electrochemical environment of the latter, thus transmitting information from one cell to the other. This information may either be excitatory or inhibitory in terms of the alteration of potential in the post-synaptic cell. Potentials produced are therefore referred to as excitatory or inhibitory post-synaptic potentials, and they summate so that if a critical level of excitability is reached, the post-synaptic neurone will fire. Neurones within the CNS, which are capable of responding up to 100 or more times a second, are either inhibitory or excitatory but probably never both. Pre-synaptic inhibition refers to inhibition at pre-synaptic terminals (Figure 2.1). Some transmitters alter the three-dimensional shape of the post-synaptic membrane receptor proteins, which in some situations leads to changes in membrane permeability for certain ions. Other transmitters are thought to act by altering, within the cell, the activity of cyclic AMP via the enzyme adenylate cyclase. Increased production of cyclic AMP leads to increased physiological activity, and the activation of enzyme and protein production in the post-synaptic neurone.

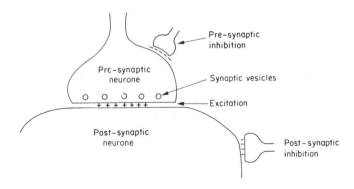

Figure 2.1. The pre- and post-synaptic neurones and the synaptic cleft

It has long been known that at the periphery there are a variety of different receptors which receive sensory information. For many years it was held, following from 'Müller's law of specific irritability' that each type of receptor was fired by a specific sensory input. Several types of receptors were described, including free nerve terminals, which end in the epithelial cells and are found all over the body, and encapsulated terminals including Pacinian corpuscles, Meissner's corpuscles, and the bulbs of Krause, with more restricted distribution. Strict specificity is now questioned, and the spatio-temporal aspects of sensory information are thought to be of more importance. There has been particular interest in receptors responsible for pain. Although it is thought that free nerve endings are of importance, it is known that pain can be elicited from areas free of such terminals, and that a variety of non-painful sensations can be felt from areas of normal skin where free nerve endings are the only type of receptor present.

Receptors are stimulated either by mechanical or chemical means, and such substances as histamine, bradykinin, serotonin and prostaglandins released from damaged tissue have been suggested as possible chemical mediators.

Impulses from receptors travel to the spinal cord along the afferent nerves. The cell bodies of these are situated in the dorsal root ganglia, or in the semilunar ganglion of the trigeminal nerve, and the fibres are of varying calibre and thickness of myelination. The myelin sheath is composed of protein and lipids, and acts to speed up the process of nerve conduction. Traditionally the afferent nerves are classified into types A, B and C, depending on their conduction velocities. The myelinated A fibres, with the fastest velocities (in the range of 75–120 metres per second) are further subdivided into alpha, beta, gamma and delta types with decreasing conduction speeds. The intensity of a stimulus is represented by variation of the rate of firing of nerve impulses, although some receptors fire only at the initiation of a stimulus, whereas others discharge continuously throughout its application.

Within the cord the nerve fibres separate, and information about different modalities is segregated as they synapse, either at or near the level of entry, or at a level distant from it. Each dorsal root contains fibres from its corresponding developmental body segment, although there is a considerable degree of overlap between adjacent regions, such that following peripheral nerve lesions the loss of sensation for pain will not exactly correspond to that for touch, and even complete lesions may not lead to clearly demarcated areas of sensory loss.

The cell bodies of the motor neurones lie in the ventral horns of the cord, and the motor nuclei of the cranial nerves. Efferent fibres leave via the anterior horn of the spinal cord and travel to the muscles. The motor neurones are classified as either alpha or gamma neurones depending on their size. They receive various inputs from the central nervous system, and an afferent feedback loop from special receptors within the muscles called muscle spindles which help adjust muscle tone.

The terminals of the alpha-motor-nerve fibres arborize and form connections with muscles at motor end-plates. The junction is similar to a synapse in the central nervous system, and the neurotransmitter involved is acetylcholine.

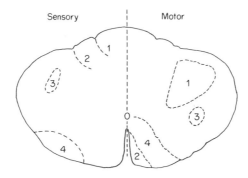

Figure 2.2. Some spinal nerve pathways, shown on a transverse section of the spinal cord, with sensory pathways shown only on the left, and motor pathways shown only on the right. Sensory pathways: 1 F. gracilis, 2 F. cuneatus, 3 Substantia gelatinosa, 4 Spinothalamic tracts. Motor pathways: 1 Lateral corticospinal tract, 2 Anterior cortico-spinal tract, 3 Rubrospinal tract, 4 Vestibulospinal tract

THE SPINAL CORD

The main sensory tracts within the spinal cord which transmit information to the thalamus and cerebral cortex are shown in Figure 2.2. Although recent evidence is leading to a reanalysis of the role of these pathways, for clinical purposes they are traditionally divided into two main groups, namely those giving information about pain, light touch and temperature, and those that provide position sense, discriminatory touch, deep pressure and vibration sense. The pain and temperature pathways first synapse in the substantia gelatinosa of the posterior grey horn, and then cross to the other side, before ascending in the spinothalamic tracts situated in the lateral and anterior white matter. Many of these fibres progress to the medulla oblongata, join with the medial lemniscus in the pons, and terminate in the ventral nuclei of the thalamus.

The exact pathways of transmission for nociceptic stimuli in the spinal cord and brainstem are unclear, but almost certainly involve more extensive pathways than these spinothalamic mechanisms. Thus the operation of anterolateral cordotomy, which theoretically would destroy pain sensation below the level of the operation, does not always do so. In addition, pain sensations, when they are lost, disappear from levels lower than the site of he section of the cord would predict, and stimulation of supposedly analgesic areas can lead to painful sensations from that area, or paradoxically to referral of pain to another area of the body.

The fibres of the posterior column ascend without crossing to the nucleus gracilis and nucleus cuneatus where they synapse, cross over and then ascend in the medial lemniscus, also to terminate in the thalamus. A similar arrangement exists for sensation from the scalp and face, the afferent fibres from the trigeminal nuclei joining the medial lemniscus after decussation in the midpons. Two essential features of these sensory systems are that the fibres are somatotopically arranged within the tracts, and that descending neuronal pathways from the cerebral cortex terminate in the nuclei of the dorsal columns, and at the origin of the neurones of the spinothalamic tracts, such that activity of the cerebral cortex, and other regions of the brain, can directly influence transmission at synapses in sensory systems.

The main descending systems include the rubrospinal, vestibulospinal, reticulospinal and pyramidal tracts. The latter, some of whose fibres originate in the 'motor' areas of the cortex, and pass through the internal capsule, continue in the pyramid of the ventral medulla oblongata, and following decussation, form the lateral corticospinal tracts which directly influence motorneurone function. The rubrospinal tract descends from the red nucleus of the mesencephalon to the same regions of the cord as the terminations of the corticospinal fibres. Afferent inputs to the red nucleus come from the cerebellum and from the cerebral cortex. The vestibulospinal tract receives fibres from the vestibular nuclei, and also influences directly activity in the alpha and gamma motorneurones. The vestibular nuclei themselves receive significant afferent connections from the cerebellum. As with the sensory system, somatotopic organization is found in these descending fibres.

THE BASAL GANGLIA AND SOME RELATED NUCLEI

Although there is no generally accepted definition of the basal ganglia, the term includes the corpus striatum (the caudate nucleus, putamen, globus pallidus and claustrum), the subthalamic nucleus, the substantia nigra, and the amygdaloid nuclear complex. The latter, however, is usually discussed in relation to the limbic system. The striatum refers to the caudate nucleus and putamen, and is the largest subcortical cell mass. The caudate nucleus, throughout its length, is closely related to the lateral ventricles, and anteriorly it is continuous with the putamen. Histochemically the caudate nucleus and the putamen are very similar, and the whole is sometimes referred to as the caudatoputamen. The nucleus accumbens is ontogenetically related to the striatum (see Figure 2.3), and has a similar cytoarchitecture, and is referred to by some as the 'limbic striatum'. It is well defined in the rat, and its homologue has been identified in the human brain. It lies ventral to the anterior horn of the lateral ventricle, and is of importance as a main projection area for dopamine neurones that arise from the ventral tegmental area of the midbrain (see below). Some fibre connections of these groups are shown in Figure 2.4.

One of the principal circuits is that which links the striatum to the cerebral cortex, globus pallidus and thalamus. Thus the whole of the neocortex sends fibres to the caudate nucleus and putamen, the projection from the sensory/

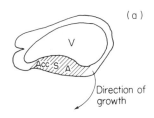

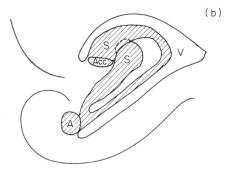

Figure 2.3. The relationship of the striatum, amygdala and nucleus accumbens (a) in embryo and (b) in adult. A, Amygdala; Acc, Accumbens; S, Striatum; V, Ventricle

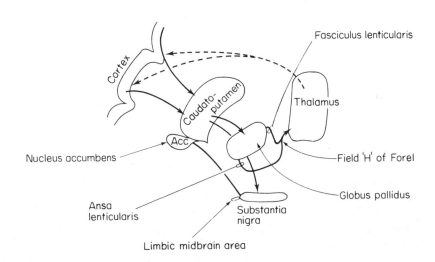

Figure 2.4. Main fibre connections of the basal ganglia

motor cortex being particularly predominant. Efferent fibres pass to the globus pallidus, although some fibres pass through this structure and terminate in the pars reticulata of the substantia nigra. These latter fibres probably contain gamma-aminobutyric acid (GABA). The main efferent projection from the globus pallidus is to the thalamus via two separate fibre bundles called the fasciculus lenticularis and the ansa lenticularis, which merge at field H of Forel. The thalamus has efferents to the cerebral cortex, thus completing the circuit. All these projections are topographically organized, and it is thought that information derived from the neocortex is processed in the basal ganglia, and fed back to the cortex, especially areas 4 and 6 (Ref. 8, p.8). Other important connections, not shown in Figure 2.3, include thalamo-striate, pallido-subthalamic and nigrostriatal fibres. The latter originate in the pars compacta of the substantia nigra, and consist of dopaminergic neurones. It is important to recognize that this collection of nuclei has significant connections with the reticular activating system and with the cerebellum. Although traditionally the basal ganglia have been considered motor in their function, recent evidence suggests not only that they are important in relation to cognitive abilities, but also stresses their relationship to sensory–motor integration and motivation.[9]

Figure 2.3 shows the development of the striatum and some of its related structures; Figure 2.3a shows the situation in embryo; and 2.3b in the adult. This indicates not only how these structures come to have their topography in the adult brain, but also the close interrelation of the striatum to the elements of the limbic system.

THE LIMBIC SYSTEM

The limbic system, originally described by Willis, was later given the name 'la grande lobe limbique' by Broca in 1878. As such it attracted relatively little attention until well into the twentieth century. It is a term used for a collection of tracts and nuclei situated mainly on the medial surface of the cerebral hemisphere. The main elements are listed in Table 2.1. It has intimate connections with the basal ganglia, especially at the amygdala and the nucleus accumbens, and with the ventral tegmental region of the mid-brain. This latter area, occupying the basomedial mid-brain area, mediodorsal to the substantia nigra, contains dopaminergic cells.

The term rhinencephalon was at one time applied to some of these structures because of their close relation to the olfactory apparatus, but their intimate connections with the hypothalamic nuclei led to the alternative name of 'visceral brain'. Papez suggested a role of some of these structures with emotion, and defined the 'Papez-circuit' of hippocampus–mamillary body–thalamus–cingulate gyrus–hippocampus. Although the term limbic system is criticized because it is increasingly difficult to segregate 'systems' that function independently within the brain, it does serve to emphasize that some areas of the brain are more related to the expression of emotion than others. From the

Table 2.1. Main elements of the limbic system

Gyri:		Nuclei:	
	Subcollosal G		Amygdaloid N
	Cingulate G		Septal N
	Parahippocampal G		
	Hippocampal formation		Hypothalamic N
	Dentate G		Epithalamic N
	Indusium griseum		Anterior thalamic N
	Subiculum		Mammillary bodies
	Entorhinal area		Habenula
	Prepiriform cortex		Raphe N
	Olfactory tubercle		Ventral tegmental area
			Dorsal tegmental nucleus
			Superior central nucleus

Pathways:	
	Fornix
	Mammillothalamic tract
	Mammillotegmental tract
	Stria terminalis
	Stria medullaris
	Cingulum
	Anterior commissure
	Medial forebrain bundle
	Lateral and medial longitudinal striae
	Dorsal longitudinal fasciculus

phylogenetic viewpoint the limbic system is composed mainly of archicortex and paleocortex, and has a relatively constant microscopic structure, in contrast to the neocortex, so highly developed in man. The situation of some of the more important elements of the limbic system within the brain and the fibre tracts connecting with them is shown schematically in Figure 2.5. It has associations not only with the surrounding neocortex, especially temporal and frontal cortex, but in addition is linked to the basal ganglia, thalamus, hypothalamus, and via the medial forebrain bundle to the midbrain. A major outflow system is the fornix carrying information to the septal region and anterior thalamic nuclei from the hippocampus. The septal region, not to be confused with the septum pellucidum, borders ventrolaterally on the nucleus accumbens and has extensive connections with it. Some of the efferent fibres from the septal area contribute to the medial forebrain bundle, which passes through the lateral hypothalamus to the tegmental area of the midbrain. This bundle contains numerous monoaminergic fibres which connect the midbrain with the prosencephalon. The septal nuclei also have connections with the stria-medullaris, which projects to the habenular nuclei, and with the stria-terminalis which links it with the amygdaloid nuclei.

THE HYPOTHALAMUS

This area, situated at the base of the brain, is composed of a variety of well-defined nuclei. The neurones of these nuclei have intimate connections with,

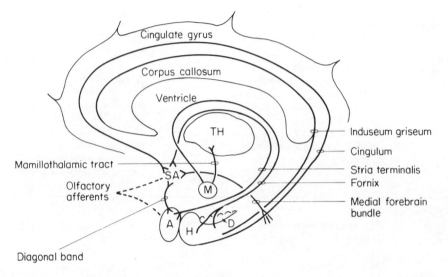

Figure 2.5. The limbic system and the fibre tracts connecting its parts. A, Amygdala; D, Dentate gyrus; H, Hippocampus; M, Mammillary body; SA, Septal/accumbens region; TH, Thalamus

and are sometimes considered part of the limbic system, but also, via neurosecretory neurones, are linked with the pituitary gland. The supraoptic and paraventricular nuclei synthesize oxytocin and vasopressin. These substances pass down the axons of the cells to the posterior pituitary gland, where they are released into the bloodstream. The nuclei of the basal hypothalamus are mainly concerned with the production of releasing hormones and inhibiting factors. These latter substances, the majority of which are peptides, regulate the output of hormones from the anterior pituitary. Efferent hypothalamic fibres terminate on capillary vessels in the pituitary stalk, the latter which feed into the hypothalamohypophysial–portal system which supplies the pars distalis of the pituitary. Releasing and inhibitory factors are thus carried in these vessels to cells in the pituitary, where hormone release is effected. In addition to providing links between the neural and endocrine systems, efferent autonomic nerves also originate from the hypothalamus, which pass down the spinal cords to innervate the symphatetic and parasympathetic nervous systems.

RETICULAR ACTIVATING SYSTEM (RAS)

Like the limbic system, this area of the neural apparatus has been recognised for many years but only recently, since the now classical observations of Moruzzi and Magoun[10] in 1949, has become an area recognized as profoundly important in neuropsychiatry. Following electrical stimulation of the brainstem, bilateral desynchronization of the electroencephalogram (EEG) occurs, which changes are thought to be mediated by neural activity passing to the cortex via the thalamus. Destruction of these brainstem areas leads to a state of 'behavioural somnolence'. These events are thought to occur because of an activating system, reticular in its appearance on account of numerous aggregations of cells separated by many fibres, which extends from the lower medulla oblongata to the midbrain, and includes various thalamic nuclei. It is surrounded by ascending and descending fibre bundles, such as the spinothalamic tract, and various nuclei, including those of some of the cranial nerves, from which it receives collateral fibres. It also receives fibres from the hypothalamic–limbic system, from the cerebral cortex and from the cerebellum. Within its substance are areas sensitive to afferent inputs from the cardiovascular and respiratory systems, and it contains groups of nuclei including the midline raphe nuclei and the nucleus coeruleus. Some of its efferent fibres pass down the spinal cord (reticulospinal tract), and influence motor neurone activity and sensory input. By means of its diffuse projections to the cerebral cortex, the RAS modulates arousal, and controls conscious activity, including sleep-wake cycles. Some tonic activity in the RAS is maintained by afferent stimuli, and of all the intpus influencing it, the most effective appear to be acoustic and pain impulses (Ref. 11, p.328).

THE CEREBRAL CORTEX

Some parts of the cortex, such as the archicortex, have already been referred to. The main feature of the human brain, compared to that of other mammals, is the increased development of the neocortex. Generally it is recognized that there are six layers to this cortex, topographically divided into various areas, based on microscopic differences, which were numbered after the system of Brodmann. Four lobes have been demarcated, and these, along with some of the important Brodmann areas, are shown in Figure 2.6. Pyramidal cells are found mainly in layer 5, and their fibres pass from the cortex, in particular area 4 (the 'motor' cortex), via the internal capsule situated between the thalamus and the globus pallidus, to the pyramidal tract. It is important to note that the latter is not only composed of fibres from area 4, but receives input from other cortical areas including area 6 (the premotor area) and areas 3, 2 and 1 (the 'sensory' cortex).

The majority of afferent fibres to the cerebral cortex come from the thalamic nuclei, project mainly to the superficial layers, and are topographically organized. Thus the thalamus transmits sensory information relayed to it to the 'sensory' cortical areas, the latter having well-developed second and fourth layers. The fact that topographical representation is found in these projections has led to the characterization of 'homunculi' on the surface of the cortex. Such diagrams emphasize not only that precise information regarding peripheral events is transmitted to the cortex, but also that the amount of cortical tissue allocated to a peripheral area is related, not to the size of that area, but to its importance as a receptor of information.

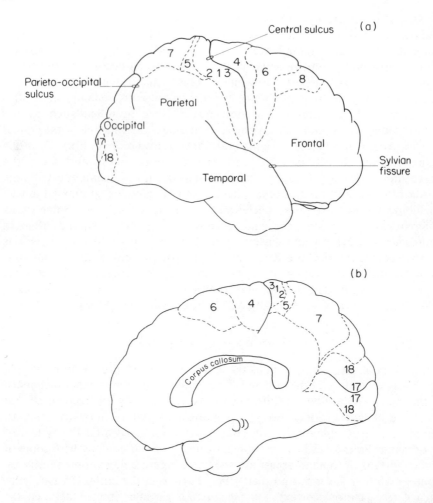

Figure 2.6. The cerebral cortex, with areas numbered after the system of Brodmann.
(a) Lateral view, (b) medial view

Other important cortical connections include the efferent fibres to the basal ganglia, limbic system, red nucleus and reticular formation. In addition there exists a large number of association fibres that link areas of the same hemisphere, and commissural fibres that link homotopic points between the two hemispheres. Cortical association areas, that is areas of cortex influenced primarily by other parts of the cortex rather than by afferents from the thalamus, are especially well-developed in man, and include parts of the frontal, temporal and parietal lobes. The largest of the commissures is the corpus callosum, and its prime function appears to be transfer of information from one hemisphere to the other. Smaller commissures exist, such as the anterior commissure, for connections between areas of the paleocortex.

It is known that the cells of the cortex have a columnar arrangement which is thought to have functional significance. Thus afferent fibres are thought to stimulate, via interneurones, multiple pyramidal cells within a column and neighbouring columns, such that many pyramidal cells can fire in unison to achieve effective movement. In addition other interneurones, with predominantly inhibitory properties, influence adjacent columns to highlight the action of the excitatory units.

NEUROCHEMICAL ASPECTS OF CNS ACTIVITY

In the same way that acetylcholine is known to be a transmitter at the neuromuscular junction, the main neurotransmitters of neuropsychiatric interest in the CNS include dopamine, noradrenaline, serotonin, acetylcholine, and GABA. In addition a variety of peptides have recently been discovered which are themselves either neurotransmitters, or neuromodulators that in some way regulate neurotransmitter activity. Following release of neurotransmitters into the synaptic cleft, they are either broken down enzymatically, or taken back by the pre-synaptic neurone for further use.

Acetylcholine

This is synthesized from choline and acetyl co-enzyme A, in a reaction catalysed by choline acetyltransferase. Choline cannot be synthesized within the brain, and is transported there from the blood. When released, acetylcholine is broken down by acetylcholinesterase. In the CNS high amounts are found in the caudate nucleus, hippocampus and cortex. There are several interconnected cholinergic pathways forming an ascending tegmental-mesencephalic–cortical system which innervates the cortex, cerebellum, limbic system, thalamus and corpus striatum.

GABA

GABA is found in the brain and spinal cord, and in particularly high concentrations in the substantia nigra, globus pallidus, hypothalamus, inferior colliculus, and periaqueductal grey regions. Lesser amounts are found in the caudate nucleus and thalamus. L-glutamate is converted into GABA by the enzyme glutamate decarboxylase, and GABA is metabolized by the enzyme GABA transaminase. GABA does not easily cross the blood–brain barrier, and within the CNS is thought to be an inhibitory neurotransmitter.

Serotonin

This substance is synthesized from tryptophan as shown in Figure 2.7. Tryptophan derives largely from the diet, and since the enzyme tryptophan hydrolase is usually not fully saturated, serum tryptophan levels influence

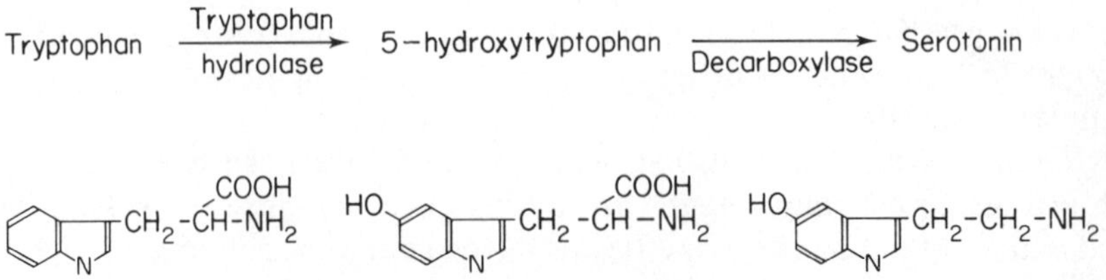

Tryptophan $\xrightarrow[\text{hydrolase}]{\text{Tryptophan}}$ 5−hydroxytryptophan $\xrightarrow[\text{Decarboxylase}]{}$ Serotonin

Figure 2.7. Biosynthesis of serotonin

CNS levels. The main enzymes involved in synthesis are tryptophan hydrolase and the amino acid decarboxylase. Serotonin is broken down into 5-hydroxyindole acetic acid (5HIAA) by a monoamine oxidase enzyme. Localization of the serotonin neurones in the CNS has recently been accomplished by special techniques. For example, in fluorescent histochemistry, conversion of parent compounds to their fluorescent derivatives is achieved by treatment with formaldehyde gas, which thus allows them to be identified. Alternatively, antibodies may be developed to specific synthesizing enzymes which, again using fluorescent histochemistry, allow precise localization and mapping of neurochemical pathways.

The majority of serotonin neurones are found in the brainstem raphe nuclei, fibres from which project both downwards to the spinal cord, and upwards to the brainstem and forebrain via the medial forebrain bundle. These pathways are shown in Figure 2.8. Stimulation of this system produces depression of neuronal firing in the amygdala, suprachiasmatic nucleus of the hypothalamus, caudate nucleus, substantia nigra, trigeminal nucleus, spinal cord interneurones and spinothalamic tract neurones. Excitatory effects are noted on cells in the reticular activating system, the pyramidal cells of the hippocampus, and the lateral geniculate cells (Ref. 12, p.172). The raphe nuclei receive a prominent input from the habenula nuclei, and maintain tonic firing rates within a relatively narrow range, except when desynchronized during sleep.

Catecholamines

The metabolic pathways for the catecholamines are shown in Figure 2.9. Tyrosine hydrolase, more fully saturated than tryptophan hydrolase, is the enzyme responsible for conversion of tyrosine to dopa. This latter substance is decarboxylated to form dopamine, which in the presence of dopamine-beta-hydrolase is converted to noradrenaline. The latter, in a few CNS neurone sites, is further converted by N-methylation to adrenaline. The breakdown of noradrenaline and dopamine utilizes two main enzyme systems. Within the neurone, monoamine oxidase (MAO) enzymes exist. There are thought to be at least two types of MAO (type A and type B) that preferentially influence different transmitters, and themselves are inhibited by different MAO inhibitors. Catechol-O-methyl transferase is the second enzyme system

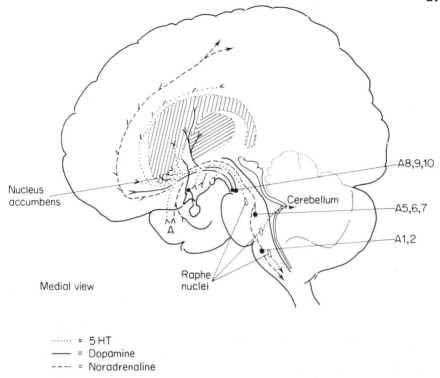

Nucleus accumbens

Cerebellum

A8,9,10

A5,6,7

A1,2

A

Raphe nuclei

Medial view

······· = 5 HT
——— = Dopamine
- - - - = Noradrenaline

Figure 2.8. Some monoamine pathways in the brain. A, Amygdala; hatched area: Caudate nucleus/putamen

involved in degradation, and appears to act on transmitter within the synaptic cleft. The major CNS metabolite of dopamine is homovanillic acid (HVA). Noradrenaline breaks down to vanillomandelic acid (VMA) and methoxyhydroxy-

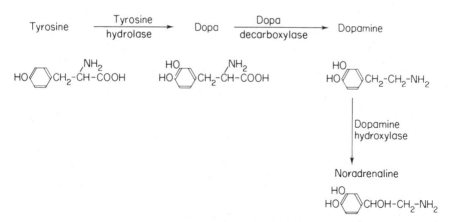

Figure 2.9 Biosynthesis of catecholamines

phenylglycol (MHPG), the main catabolite from the central nervous system being MHPG.

As with serotonin, the catecholamine neurones are found in relatively discrete areas of the CNS, although their efferent projections are widespread. On the basis of work in the rat and other mammals, catecholamine nuclei have been designated as A_1, A_2, etc., up to A_{13}.[13] It is thought that while there are differences in detail, the localization of monoamine systems in humans is similar to that of the rat.[14] Of major importance in neuropsychiatry are the neurones originating in the A_9 and A_{10} areas (the substantia nigra and adjacent ventral tegmental area). In these areas the majority of dopamine neurones supplying the corpus striatum and the limbic system arise. The A_{12} and A_{13} regions in the diencephalon give rise to dopaminergic fibres which innervate the median eminence. Using this terminology the A_5 and A_6 regions represent the locus coeruleus, from which fibres pass to innervate the hippocampus, pontine reticular formation, vagal nuclei, geniculate body and neocortex. One projection goes to the raphe nuclei and directly influences the serotonin containing neurones.

Dopamine systems within the CNS can be divided into at least four major groups: the nigrostriatal, mesolimbic, mesocortical, and tuberoinfundibular systems. The nigrostriatal neurones (A_9) are predominantly inhibitory, although they may also be excitatory.[15] The mesolimbic system consist of fibres arising from the ventral tegmental area (A_{10}), which transmit to the olfactory tubercule, nucleus accumbens, nucleus of the stria terminalis, and the amygdala. These neurones are also thought to be inhibitory. It has been suggested that the nigrostriatal and the mesolimbic systems are parallel

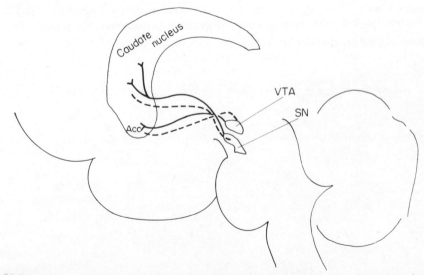

Figure 2.10. Mesolimbic and nigrostriatal dopamine systems. Acc, nucleus accumbens; SN, substantia nigra; VTA, ventral tegmental area. Heavy line, dopamine pathways; dashed line = possible GABA pathways

systems with similar feedback loops (see Figure 2.10) mediated by GABA.[16] Although there are some similarities between the two systems, including their similar embryological origin, there are also differences which include the response to some dopamine-blocking antipsychotic drugs.[17] The mesocortical dopamine system projects from the A_{10} region primarily to the cingulate gyrus the entorhinal area and the prefrontal cortex. A feature of all these pathways is a great divergence, in that one cell may synapse with many thousands of others.

The tuberoinfundibular dopamine system has gained recent importance because of the recognition that prolactin inhibitory factor is probably dopamine, and increased dopaminergic activity in these neurones leads to a decrease in serum prolactin. Dopamine is probably also involved in the control of the secretion of other anterior pituitary hormones. At least two types of dopamine receptor are now recognized, one of which is linked to the adenyl cyclase, which may be preferentially influenced by different dopamine agonist and antagonist drugs.

Peptides

The existence of some peptides, such as substance P, in the brain, has been recognized for a number of years, and the possibility that they may be involved in neurotransmission is now accepted. Many peptides influence behaviour in a variety of species including thyrotropin releasing factor, melanocyte stimulating hormone release-inhibiting factor, somatostatin (which inhibits the release of growth hormone) and luteinizing hormone releasing factor. Other CNS peptides of importance include prolactin, ACTH, vasopressin and oxytocin.

Much attention has recently been focused on naturally occurring substances within the brain that possess opiate-like activity. The 'endorphins' are a variety of peptide compounds structurally related to fragments of the pituitary hormone β-lipotropin. Some relationships of these are shown in Figure 2.11a. It can be seen that the carboxyl terminal of β-lipotropin forms β-endorphin, and the first five residues of the latter form met-encephalin (Figure 2.11b). Endorphin receptors have now been localized in the CNS, in particular in the corpus striatum, the anterior hypothalamus, and areas of the limbic system. In the brain, encephalin predominates, while the cell bodies containing β-endorphin are predominantly localized in the hypothalamic–pituitary system. The highest concentrations of endorphin receptors and encephalins occur in the region of the amygdala. It has been shown that the endorphin molecule has structural similarities with morphine, and both met-encephalin and leu-encephalin have been isolated and identified within the brain, and have been shown to possess behavioural and analgesic properties. Encephalin neurones may interact with monoamine neurones altering release of their transmitters, some possible relationships between encephalin neurones and monoamine neurones being shown diagrammatically in Figure 2.12.

(a)

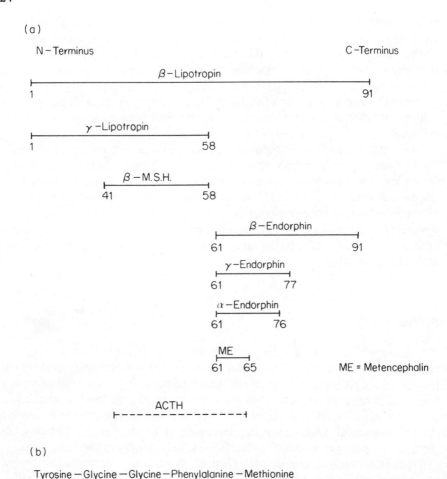

Figure 2.11. (a) β-Lipotropin and some of its peptide derivatives. (b) Amino acid sequence of metencephalin

BRAIN–BEHAVIOUR RELATIONSHIPS

Knowledge of the relationship between the brain and behaviour has primarily been developed from observations of behaviour following lesions, artificial or otherwise, and from the results of stimulation experiments. More recently changes in behaviour correlating with altered neurotransmitter function have also been evaluated.

Sensory stimuli are relayed somatotopically to the thalamus, and thence to the sensory cortex. Ablation of the post-central gyrus leads to disturbances of tactile appreciation, and the ability to determine roughness. Stimulation leads to numbness and tingling referred to the contralateral half of the body. The role of the cerebral cortex in pain appreciation is not clear, although stimulation

(a)

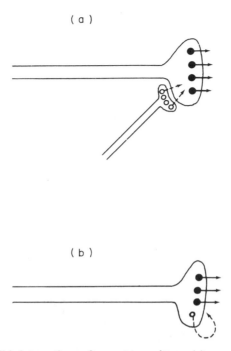

(b)

Figure 2.12. Possible interactions of neurotransmitters: (a) axo-axonal modulation; (b) autoregulation. ○→ monoamine, ○→ endorphin

almost never leads to pain. The monosynaptic connections between the thalamus and the frontal cortex are of interest, in view of the reported beneficial effects of leucotomy in some chronic pain patients (see Chapter 8). Using the technique of sequential degeneration it has been possible to demonstrate a pattern of interconnections of cortical sites related to the primary sensory areas, that shows a 'cascade' of projections which ultimately arrive at the limbic system (see Figure 2.13). While the visual and olfactory systems take a more direct path to the limbic system (Ref. 19, p.245), different sensory systems thus converge on to the same cortical areas in the superior temporal sulcus.

Information fed to the temporal lobes passes to the amygdala and hippocampus and thence, via the cingulate gyrus, fornix and stria terminalis to the septum, nucleus accumbens and hypothalamus. The latter, whose nuclei relate to such activities as hunger, thirst and reproductive behaviour has intimate reciprocal connections with the nucleus accumbens, the amygdala and the thalamus. The thalamus itself projects to the prefrontal cortex and other areas of cortex. The limbic system therefore is in a position to receive information about an individual's external environment from its neocortical inputs, and about the internal environment from its 'visceral' connections. It may emotionally colour sensory experiences, and be influenced by, or influence, the hypothalamus and prefrontal cortex. It has been suggested that

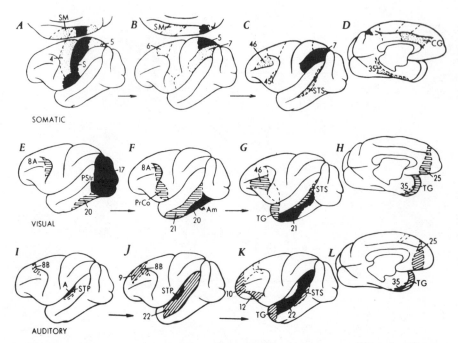

Figure 2.13. Sensory projections and the limbic system: a schematic diagram summarizing the outward progression of connexions from the primary somatic (A–D), visual (E–H) and auditory (I–L) areas of the cortex. Each new local step is shown in black and the further connexions of the new areas by light stippling or hatching. Notice that all sensory pathways converge in the depths of the superior temporal sulcus (STS). D, H and L are the medial aspects of the hemispheres shown in C, G and K respectively (Jones and Powell, 1970)

the frontal lobes synthesize emotional and somaesthetic information in order to guide behaviour (Ref. 19, p.273). Pleasure is experienced in humans following electrical stimulation of the nucleus accumbens, whereas unpleasant feelings are described after similar procedures on hippocampus and amygdala. Monosynaptic connections have been described between these areas and, for example, brainstem nuclei that control eye movements,[20] which may have relevance for the alteration of eye movements seen in certain disease states such as schizophrenia, and for the close association between the eyes and emotional states that occurs in everyday behaviour. The amygdala have been implicated particularly in the control of aggressive behaviour, which is also modulated by the hypothalamus, such that destruction of the ventromedial nucleus of the hypothalamus leads to a lowered threshold for aggression, which is remedied by destruction of the amygdala.

The hippocampus has a special function in relation to memory, bilateral destruction leading to amnesic states (see Chapter 6). The RAS is involved in arousal, and linked to the limbic system, the spinal cord and the cortex. Within its substance are neurones related to the control of respiration, cardiovascular homoeostasis, and sleep. The latter appears to be particularly under control of the serotoninergic raphe nucleus, and the catecholaminergic locus coeruleus. Increased serotonin activity leads to inhibition of behaviour, with sedation and diminished responsiveness.

Movements are clearly dependent on the peripheral motor apparatus and the descending supraspinal pathways, which themselves originate in the cortex. Stimulation of areas of the motor cortex produce discrete and not co-ordinated movements on the opposite side of the body, and information from the cerebellum, hypothalamus and thalamus seems involved in the initiation of movement (Ref. 11, p.196). The role of the basal ganglia in movement disorders is well established, although they appear primarily to be involved in collaboration between the cortex and the thalamus (Ref. 11, p.188). Weak stimulation or discrete lesions lead to abnormalities of cognitive performance rather than motor deficits, and it has been suggested that the corpus striatum is essential for sensory–motor co-ordination.[21]

Drugs which diminish catecholamine activity decrease spontaneous locomotion, and inhibit conditioned responses and exploratory behaviour. Self-stimulation experiments, in which animals are shown to reward themselves by stimulating electrodes placed in the diencephalon and limbic system, indicate that such behaviour is dependent on noradrenergic activity. Adrenergic and noradrenergic activity are also related to the control of blood pressure, body temperature, food and water intake, sexual behaviour, aggression, and, via releasing factors, hormonal output.

Dopamine influences patterns of locomotor activity particularly in animal models. The administration of dopamine agonists leads to stereotyped behaviour such as sniffing, licking, biting or gnawing, depending on the species involved. In addition increased locomotion, grooming and abnormal movements such as myoclonic jerks have been noted, and such models are used to test dopamine activity of drugs. Other systems that are used for this are based on stimulation of dopamine sensitive receptors by dopamine agonists, following selective destruction of dopamine pathways within the CNS. Thus if unilateral nigrostriatal pathway lesions are made, and a receptor agonist is given, rats move in circles away from the side of the lesion. Drugs that block dopamine activity prevent this rotation, and the circling activity can therefore be used for detecting dopamine antagonists. Such techniques, especially with direct intracerebral administration of dopamine, have provided evidence that the striatum, and the associated nucleus accumbens, both of which are richly innervated by dopaminergic neurones, are involved in the regulation of behaviour. In particular it has been shown in animals that the corpus striatum is involved in the production of stereotypy, while the nucleus accumbens–mesolimbic dopamine system is more related to locomotor activity.[22] This has led to suggestions that the mesolimbic dopamine system is related to motivational arousal, and the striatum to motor arousal, and that adequate functioning of these dopamine systems is essential for the integration of sensory inputs, memory, motivation, and motor expression.[23] The nucleus accumbens in particular seems to be a bridge bringing limbic influences to bear on motor function, and the close ontogenetic, phylogenetic and neurochemical similarities between it and the nigrostriatal system suggests a neurological basis for the observed relationship between emotional states and motor behaviour (see Chapter 10). The growing evidence that similar transmitter pathways are involved in motor disorders and some psychiatric illnesses (see Chapter 4) emphasizes the utmost importance of the basal ganglia, and their relationship to the limbic system, for neuropsychiatric theory.

CHAPTER 3

Psychopathology, its Assessment and Measurement

PSYCHOPATHOLOGY

Clinical assessment of patients in neuropsychiatry requires not only standard physical examination with particular attention to the nervous system, but also detection of psychiatric disturbance and disability by observation of behaviour, both verbal and non-verbal. Phenomenology is described as the attempt to give 'a concrete description of the psychic states which patients actually experience . . .' (Ref. 24, p.55). Such descriptions depend entirely upon what is present in the patient's consciousness, but assessment is undertaken assuming that these phenomena exist, and initially without any further speculation or interpretation of their meaning. It is customary in examining psychopathology to distinguish form from content. The latter may have meaning for the patient, or for the physician, but the form of the phenomena are of major interest for making diagnostic decisions.

DISTURBANCES OF PERCEPTION

Objects may be perceived as altered in intensity, quality or spatial form. Hyperaesthesia, especially for sounds, is not uncommon in neurotic patients, sometimes leading to bizarre interpretations of events. Hypoaesthesia is noted in depression when the tone of sensations deteriorate. Anaesthesia, especially hemianaesthesia, is common in some varieties of abnormal illness behaviour, being one of the positive diagnostic signs of hysteria (Ref. 25, p.246). In such conditions the hemianaesthesia affects the left side of the body more than the right, and very often involves the face, scalp, trunk and limbs. The changing shapes and colours of perceptions are sometimes commented upon in patients with psychotic illness, but are often associated with drug intoxications. Alterations in size such as micropsia and macropsia are noted in patients with ophthalmological disease, but also occur in lesions affecting the temporal lobes. In metamorphopsia objects are seen to change from one thing into another. Synaesthesia occurs when a perception in one mode is experienced in another, for example sounds may be described as painful, or colours described as sounds. These experiences are most often encountered in schizophrenia.

Derealization refers to a disturbance of feeling about the self in relation to the world. The latter is seen as flat or empty, two-dimensional, and things are reported as being 'different'. Some patients feel that objects are new and startling, and want to touch them in order to test their reality. In depersonalization the patient himself feels unreal, the capacity to empathize being diminished. These phenomena are usually distressing and associated with high levels of anxiety. They may occur *de novo*, or secondary to disorders such as depression, schizophrenia, or, more rarely, as aurae in complex partial seizures. Autoscopy refers to an extreme variant of this in which patients report that they can stand outside themselves and see themselves. This may be associated with parietal lobe disorders (Ref. 26, p.27). These phenomena need to be distinguished from nihilistic depressive delusions in which patients complain they have lost all feeling and deny their own existence.

The sense of time may be altered by either a speeding up or slowing down. The former is typical in manic states and in some intoxications, whereas the latter is more common in depression. Some schizophrenic patients suggest that time will 'stand still' or pass with extreme rapidity. In *déjà vu* states people feel that everything that they are seeing or experiencing has happened before. *Jamais vu* is the opposite state, when familiar things become unfamiliar. These may be experienced by normal people, but are also associated with anxiety states, and temporal lobe lesions especially of the right side.

The two commonest disorders of perception encountered clinically are illusions and hallucinations. An illusion is a misinterpretation of perceptions, as opposed to hallucinations which are perceptions in the absence of adequate peripheral stimuli. Illusions occur in normal people, especially during fatigue, inattentiveness, or in states of high expectation. So-called optical illusions may be readily manufactured in the right circumstances. In psychiatric states, illusions occur with acute organic brain syndromes, but also are reported in severe depression and schizophrenia. Pareidolia is the ability to produce an illusion from an ill-defined percept. For example, complex shapes emerge from a configuration in the clouds or from a pattern of sunlight on the wall.

Pseudohallucinations are hallucinatory experiences that occur in subjective space, are less clearly delineated, and lack objectivity when compared to true hallucinations. They are dependent upon the person creating them, and the images readily dissipate and have to be recreated. In true hallucinations the experiences are constant, occur in objective space, have concrete reality and are substantial. They are usually retained unaltered.[27] Hare suggested that the most important difference between pseudohallucinations and true hallucinations was the absence of insight which is noted in the latter.[28]

Hallucinations may occur in the setting of strong affective disturbances such as depression; in organic brain syndromes both acute and chronic; in schizophrenia; following damage to peripheral sense organs; and in the setting of sensory deprivation. Hypnogogic and hypnopompic hallucinations occur when patients are falling asleep or awakening, respectively. These may occasionally occur in normal people, but are also a feature of Gelineau's syndrome.

Hallucinations may occur in any sensory field, and if they occur in a setting of clear consciousness are highly suggestive of schizophrenia. In this condition hallucinations are usually auditory, although many patients experience them in more than one sensory modality. The voices reported are mainly of family, friends or God, and the main feature of schizophrenic hallucinations is that people argue or talk about the patient in the third person. Other hallucinations characteristic of schizophrenia are when a patient hears his own thoughts spoken aloud, or hears a commentary on his actions which is often critical.[29]

Visual hallucinations occur in schizophrenia but less frequently, and when they are present are often in association with other hallucinations. Visual hallucinations in isolation, especially when highly complex, are very suggestive of an organic brain syndrome. Visual hallucinations of small animals are noted in delirium, especially delirium tremens, when they are often associated with extreme anxiety. Formication, the sensation that animals are crawling under the skin or over the body, has been associated with cocaine psychosis. Visual and auditory hallucinations occur together in complex partial seizures, in schizophrenia, and in organic brain syndromes.

Hallucinations of smell may be a feature of depression in which the patient may report that his body odour is offensive, and, for example, he can smell his body rotting away. Smell hallucinations may also occur in schizophrenia, and in complex partial seizures of the 'uncinate' variety. In the latter the smell is usually very unpleasant but non-specific, and may be associated with gustatory hallucinations.

Somatic hallucinations occur in schizophrenia, particularly sensations of heat, cold or touch. These may be misinterpreted as sensory neurological symptoms. Often the patient interprets them as being brought about by an external agency, so-called passivity experiences. In coenaesthetic hallucinations the body or part of the body may feel distorted or changed, often in quite fantastic ways.[30]

In functional hallucinations a perception forms the basis of an hallucination. For example, a clock ticking may be reported as an hallucinatory voice.

DISORDERS OF THOUGHT AND SPEECH

The most characteristic thought disorder, which for centuries has been regarded as pathognomonic of madness, is the delusion. It may be defined as a false conviction, the content of which is not in keeping with the patient's cultural and social upbringing, which is held with unshakeable certainty. It implies '. . . a transformation in . . . total awareness of reality' (Ref. 24, p.95). Delusions proper, or autochthonous delusions, arise *de novo* and do not arise from preceding morbid experiences. They are psychologically irreducible.

Secondary delusions arise understandably from preceding mood states. In delusional perception abnormal significance is attached to a real perception without any logical cause; a delusional intuition is a sudden delusional idea; a delusional mood precedes a delusional perception, in which perceptions may seem to have some significance, initially non-specific. This is not a well-defined affect such as depression, and the delusional percept does not arise from it in the manner of secondary delusions.[31] In contrast to a delusion, an over-valued idea is a conviction, strongly influenced by affect, which is understandable in terms of the patient's personality and development.

Autochthonous delusions are nearly always diagnostic of schizophrenia. The delusional perception is said to be pathognomonic, provided that it occurs in the setting of clear consciousness. Secondary delusions are seen in schizophrenia, depression, paranoid states and in organic brain syndromes. The commonest delusions in schizophrenia are delusions of persecution, and most patients can identify their persecutors.[32] Others include morbid jealousy, grandiosity, guilt, love, ideas of ill-health, poverty and nihilistic delusions. These may be seen in a variety of psychiatric illnesses, especially schizophrenia and depression. In delusions of reference, objects and events are perceived as having some special reference for the patient. The content of delusions usually reflects the cultural and social upbringing of patients, and in schizophrenia primary delusional experiences become integrated into a more elaborate delusional system. When these secondary delusions are all based upon one underlying delusion the complex is referred to as systematized. The degree of systematization seems to be related to the integrity of the premorbid personality (Ref. 26, p.42).

'Formal thought disorder' refers to patterns of thinking which are seen in schizophrenia and organic brain syndromes. In the former, the presence of a good vocabulary is seemingly at odds with the patient's poor conceptual thinking. The essence of formal thought disorder is the disorganization and concretization of thought processes. Several authors have classified this according to their particular psychological approach. Schneider used such terms as 'fusing', 'drivelling', 'derailment' and 'omission'. In fusion, different thoughts are brought together such that the whole sounds senseless; derailment is a line of thought which suddenly slips into a new direction which is close to the original line; in omission the stream of thought is interrupted and part of the idea is missing; in drivelling there is one complex idea split into separate elements which are all muddled together leading to a confusion. Bleuler considered that the fundamental thought disorder was lack of association between ideas, which in turn led to autistic thinking. There were incidental associations formed between thoughts, thus leading to condensation, displacement, and inappropriate symbolism. Cameron used the term 'asyndetic thinking' to refer to clusters of vaguely related sequences of thought with poor focusing on a particular topic. He also pointed out how schizophrenic patients use personal idioms, interpenetration of thoughts, and over-inclusion in which there is loss of the boundaries of thoughts at hand (Ref. 33, pp.19–26).

Several authors have compared schizophrenic thought processes with those that occur in organic brain syndromes. Kleist commented on the similarities between the thought deterioration seen in schizophrenia and that in Huntington's chorea and Alzheimer's disease. He noted the paraphasic elements of schizophrenic speech and suggested it was similar to the speech of patients with sensory aphasia noted following left temporal lobe lesions.[34] Goldstein drew attention to the impairment of abstracting abilities with concrete attitudes in schizophrenic thought disorder. Schizophrenic patients were thus said to be unable to extract the essentials of a situation from its background, with impaired figure–ground relationships. Similar mechanisms were noted to occur in organic defect states, but in schizophrenia the world was enriched by personalized ideas, and was not so impoverished as in the former.[35] Critchley[36] examined the speech of aphasic and psychotic patients. He pointed out that in dementia there was essentially poverty of speech, no neologisms, but a 'gratuitous paralogism' and verbal mannerisms. This was often associated with restriction of mimicry, mime, gesture and gesticulation. In schizophrenia, on the other hand, there was no inaccessibility of vocabulary, and a qualitative rather than quantitative defect, with excessive use of pronouns, especially 'I' and 'my'.

Vorbeireden is talking past the point where there is evidence that the patient understands the nature of the question at hand. Classically it is seen in hysterical pseudodementia, but also occurs in schizophrenia. In perseveration the patient cannot alter the line of thought from a given direction. This is seen in schizophrenia and some forms of organic brain syndrome. In palilalia and logoclonia the last word and last syllable respectively of a sentence are repeated with increasing frequency.

When the speed of thinking is altered there may be flight of ideas in which thoughts come into the mind rapidly. This may lead to abnormal verbal associations such as clanging, rhyming, punning, alliteration and a general incoherence. Distractibility is common when external impressions lead to alteration of thought content, and immediate objects or events are included in the patient's talk. Accompanied often by pressure of speech, flight of ideas is seen in hypomania and mania, excited schizophrenia, and following some neurological lesions particularly in the floor of the third ventricle. Pressure of speech without flight of ideas is not uncommon in states of agitation, especially agitated depression.

Slowing of the train of thought is found in depression, and when accompanied by a diminution of bodily movements is referred to as psychomotor slowing.

Viscosity is used to describe 'sticky' thinking, which may be seen in patients with organic brain syndromes, especially epilepsy. In thought-blocking the line of thought is suddenly interrupted and may be replaced by new thoughts. This is characteristically seen in schizophrenia. Circumstantiality refers to a persistent tendency to wander slowly over irrelevant details of an event before reaching the final point. While it occurs in normal people, it is also seen following brain damage.

Patients may complain of abnormal feelings regarding possession of their thought processes. In obsessions, patients are unable to prevent thoughts coming into their minds, even though they realize they are senseless. Such thoughts are often incongruous for the individual, and cause anxiety and distress. In thought alienation the patient feels his thoughts are not his own and that they are under the control of others. There may be thought insertion, thought withdrawal, or thought broadcasting. In the latter, the patient knows that his thoughts are being shared with others.

These last three phenomena are characteristically described in schizophrenia and in a setting of clear consciousness comprise some of the 'first rank' symptoms of Schneider.

Aphasia is impairment of language caused by neurological disturbance. Mutism is complete loss of speech and is seen in a variety of psychiatric disorders, but very rarely following structural neurological illness. Akinetic mutism is caused by diencephalic lesions and the patient, although mute, remains aware of his environment with impaired consciousness. Neologisms are new words or old ones used in an unusual way so as to acquire new meaning. They are to be distinguished from paraphasias. In literal paraphasia there is substitution of one consonant sound for another, whereas in verbal paraphasia there is word replacement. Severe paraphasia leads to a speech pattern referred to as jargon aphasia which is to be distinguished from schizaphasia, the 'word salad' of severe schizophrenia. Paraphasias are seen in aphasic disorders, whereas neologisms are commoner in the schizophrenias.

DISORDERS OF MOTOR ACTIVITY

It is through motor expression that we primarily communicate our feelings to others, and it is not unexpected that in psychiatric illness there are always associated motor changes. Examination of motor performance in patients reveals much that may not be apparent from examination of the form or content of thought processes. Motor disorders generally can be divided into hypo- and hyper-kinetic categories. Parakinetic disturbances are those in which there is inept motor performance.

Hypokinesia includes a variety of phenomena, from the motor slowing of patients with retarded depression, through to catatonia in which the muscle tone is so high that passive movement leads to resistance. In flexibilitas cerea limbs can be maintained in various postures for hours on end. This is also referred to as catalepsy, and is encountered in schizophrenic patients, although it may be seen following encephalitis or as a side effect of major tranquillizer therapy. In negativism resistance to all instructions and actions occurs, and passive movements may be resisted by the same degree of force as is applied by the examiner (Gegenhalten). Stupor is a state of complete immobility with loss of reaction to all but strong external stimuli, in which patients are usually also mute. It may be seen in such illnesses as schizophrenia, depression and the organic brain syndromes, or occur as 'hysterical stupor'.

Hyperkinetic behaviour is typical in the manic phase of a bipolar affective illness and in excitement states of schizophrenia. Grimacing is facial distortion, and is often reported in schizophrenia. In Schnauzkrampf the lips are pouted. Mannerisms are unnatural exaggerations of purposeful and common motor acts; stereotypies are regularly repeated non-purposeful motor (and other) acts, which nevertheless are representative of normal actions. They are more fixed than mannerisms and have to be distinguished from dystonias in which sustained abnormal postures occur, often with slow or rapid, repetitive movements. Tics are rapid, purposeless, repetitive motor acts that may affect any muscle or group of muscles. In chorea there are continuous, abrupt, jerky movements, and in athetosis slow twisting, writhing movements. Many patients with tics and choreiform movements turn their purposeless acts into quasi-purposeful movements. A sudden jerk of the arm may lead the hand to the hair, which is then smoothed down.

In some patients, especially schizophrenic patients, movements are thought by the patient to be induced by outside agencies. These 'made' actions, (but also 'made' volitions, thoughts, and feelings) are referred to as passivity experiences. In the absence of an organic brain syndrome, such symptoms are pathognomonic of schizophrenia.

Automatic obedience to commands is seen in schizophrenia, chronic organic brain syndromes, and in a variety of unusual disorders such as latah. Echolalia and echopraxia occur in mental subnormality, dementia, delirium, schizophrenia, the Gilles de la Tourette syndrome, and disorders such as the 'Jumpers of Maine'.

CLINICAL ASSESSMENT OF COGNITIVE ABILITY

In addition to the assessment of psychopathology and of course collection of adequate biographical details, during an interview it is essential to determine if any of the clinical findings may be the result of structural organic brain disease. For this an extended mental state examination is required. In general the scheme for this first assesses the patient's level of consciousness, then language abilities, followed by memory functions, and finally examines for other signs of focal brain damage such as apraxia.[37] By using such a sequence, errors of interpretation will be minimized. Thus, if initial assessment suggests that the patient has gross disturbance of consciousness, then interpretation of abnormalities of language or memory will be different from the situation in which the patient is normally responsive and orientated.

Assessment of the level and content of consciousness

The level of arousal of a patient is usually assessed by observation of behaviour at interview and noting his ability to respond to general questioning. Lethargy, stupor, and coma are all easily recognized. In lethargy, the patient appears drowsy, his attention wanders, and he may easily drift into sleep if left unaroused. Coma, by definition, is unarousable unresponsiveness.[38] The patient's orientation for time, place and person is examined and he is asked how long he has been in the hospital. The level of attention is assessed by asking the patient to repeat digits. Successful repetition of six or seven means that attention can be maintained for short periods of time. Longer periods of successful attention (vigilance) are tested by reading the patient a series of letters (or numbers) and asking him to notify the examiner by tapping every time a certain one is called out. Failure to identify the correct item, or tapping to the wrong items indicate lapses in attention that should not occur in normal people. Other tests employed at this stage of the examination include Serial Sevens, a test in which the patient subtracts 7 from 100 and continues to take 7 away from the remaining number, and the repetition of numbers backwards.

Language abilities

The main attributes assessed under this category are speech, comprehension, repetition, naming, reading and writing. The quality and quantity of spontaneous speech are noted before more complex procedures are carried out. Attention is paid to the rate, rhythm, articulation, and speech errors such as paraphasias and neologisms that may occur. Any pressure of speech can be noted at this stage along with flight or poverty of ideas. Dysarthric and aphasic disturbances or thought disorder may be apparent. Comprehension is assessed by asking the patient to point to objects in the environment, or to perform other acts on command; repetition by asking the patient to repeat words and then phrases of increasing complexity. Naming objects by pointing to them is then undertaken. Uncommon items should be included in the list since many aphasic patients do well with common words but fail with ones they are less acquainted with. In addition, at this stage, naming of body parts, finger naming and colour naming can be tested.

Reading and writing are then assessed. For the former it is important to note whether the patient has comprehended what he has read, and for the latter that signing of the patient's name or writing the patient's name and address down is not adequate as these highly over-learned activities may not be sensitive to subtle forms of brain disease. It is preferred that the patient writes from dictation and then is asked to briefly write about some event spontaneously, for example, what he does for a living.

Memory abilities

Memory disturbances may be specific to organic brain disease as seen in dementia or various amnesic disorders, or secondary to disturbed attention and orientation. In addition, disturbed language abilities will interfere with memory processes. It is therefore important that before any defect in memory is interpreted, full assessment of the patient's performance on other aspects of mental testing described above has been carried out.

Immediate recall is usually assessed by asking the patient to repeat digits, the Babcock sentence, and a story such as the cowboy story. Babcock developed a number of sentences of gradually increasing length which are read aloud to a patient and then repeated by the patient until correct repetition occurs. The actual content of the sentence is irrelevant. The commonly used one for testing adult patients is: 'The one thing a nation needs in order to be rich and great is a large secure supply of wood'. The cowboy story is one of a number of stories that may be read to the patient which contains a series of facts that the patient is required to remember, and then repeat. The story is as follows: 'A cowboy went to San Francisco with his dog, which he left at a friend's house while he went to buy a new suit of clothes. Dressed in his brand new suit he came back to the dog, whistled to it, called it by name and patted it. But the dog would have nothing to do with him in his new coat and hat and gave a mournful howl. Coaxing was of no avail, so the cowboy went away and put on his old suit and the dog immediately showed its wild joy on seeing its master as it thought he should look.' If necessary, such a test may be quantified by noting how many separate items in the story are recalled.

General knowledge about recent events is then tested and this must be adjusted to the patient's cultural and intellectual background. The ability to learn new things is examined by asking the patient to remember four objects, re-testing occurring after 5 minutes and then later in the examination at around 30 minutes. Most patients recall all items at 5 minutes and at least three out of four at 30 minutes. Non-verbal learning can be assessed by asking patients to reproduce simple figures, again at various periods of time after presentation.

Remote memory testing requires asking patients about things that have happened earlier in their lives. Biographical details are often used, but obviously need to be checked with relatives or friends. Historical details may also be asked such as dates of wars, coronations etc.

Assessment of other disturbances of cognitive function

Testing constructional ability and thus examining for one variety of apraxia requires asking the patient to copy drawings, draw *de novo* some shape or figure, and to draw a clock-face with a certain time on it. Both two- and three-dimensional drawings should be attempted in the figure drawing. Match-stick construction is also carried out. The patient is given a small number of matches and asked to copy a square or star-shaped design with them. Examination of results from these tests may show perseveration of lines, closing in — where the construction is placed too close or even overlapping with the model given by the examiner, neglect of one-half of the construction, loss of spatial relations, failure of integration of individual parts, or rotation of the figure by more than 45°. Such errors are highly suggestive of organic brain disease (Ref. 39, p.104).

The patient's abilities to carry out purposeful movements to command are noted, such as the ability to put out his tongue, hold out his arms, or do a complex sequence of actions such as light a cigarette, or fold paper, put it into an envelope and seal the envelope. Failure on such tasks may indicate apraxic disturbances. At this point motor tests such as the fist–palm–side test may be completed, in which the patient is asked first to place his hand on the desk in the first position, then in the flat-palm position, and finally on its side, and to continue in this sequence until told to stop. Perseveration of movements may be noted, suggestive of frontal lobe pathology. An alternative strategy is to ask the patient to tap twice when the examiner taps once and vice versa. Again, this is difficult for patients with frontal lobe abnormalities.

Visuo-spatial difficulties are assessed by asking the patient with his eyes closed to indicate objects in the room around him; right/left orientation by asking the patient to demonstrate the right and left side of his body, and also of the examiner's body who is sitting opposite him; topographical orientation by noting the patient's ability to orientate himself to his environment, and to get around the hospital ward. Calculating ability is determined by using tests of simple addition, subtraction, and multiplication. Finally, proverb interpretation and tests of 'similarities' are carried out. In the latter the patient is asked to explain the 'sameness' between two different objects. Commonly used examples are apple–orange, desk–bookcase, eye–ear, poem–novel, dress–coat, praise–punishment. This test and the proverb interpretation test may lead to the detection of concrete thinking which is seen in organic brain disease and schizophrenia, or bizarre or fantastic interpretations as are seen in psychotic states. A brief summary of this scheme of bedside mental state testing is given in Table 3.1.

PSYCHOLOGICAL TESTING

The procedures and information outlined above relate to assessment of patients in the clinic or at the bedside. As has been noted, much useful diagnostic and clinical information can be obtained by these procedures. In neuropsychiatry signs and symptoms are never taken in isolation and are set beside information gained from full documentation of the family history, the illness history, and the personal history of the patient. Failure of full pscyhiatric history-taking is one of the commonest errors in clinical practice.

Following the gathering of all the data and the clinical examination, it is often necessary to refer the patient for certain specialized tests of psychological function. In essence these more complicated test procedures give some quantitative estimate of patients' performance which can be compared to standardized populations of non-patients, and as such may have diagnostic use in their own right. Some of the more commonly used tests will be described.

Table 3.1. Scheme for bedside mental state testing

Observe and assess orientation for time, place and person.
Assess attention and vigilance: digit repetition: Serial Sevens: digit reversal.
Test language abilities: rate, rhythm, syntax and semantics; errors in speech.
> Ask patient to point to objects in the environment.
> Ask patient to perform simple commands.
> Ask patient to name objects, body parts and colours.
> Ask patient to read, and test comprehension.
> Ask patient to write.

Test Memory ability:
> Repeat the Babcock sentence.
> Repeat a story.
> Remember four objects.
> Test general knowledge for recent events.
> Test knowledge for remote events.

Test for constructional apraxia:
> Drawings, stick figures etc.

Test for visuo-spatial difficulties:
> With eyes closed indicate geography of the ward.

Test for ideomotor and ideational apraxia:
> Perform more complex tasks on command: complete complex sequence of actions.

Test for perseveration: fist–palm–side test.
Test for right/left disorientation:
Test for calculation.
Test for proverb interpretation.
Test similarities.
Retest memory: recall earlier memory tests.

Intelligence

Although no satisfactory definition of intelligence has ever been coined, in clinical practice intelligence tests are widely used, and have been standardized over a number of years so that objective measures of a patient's performance may be obtained. In neuropsychological testing, such tests and variants of them have been used to detect deficits of higher cognitive function, and specifically to localize disease processes in one or other of the cerebral hemispheres. It should be noted that not all of the tests described have been adequately assessed for their reliability and validity. The former is an assessment of the test producing the same results in a similar situation on two different occasions, validity meaning that they measure what they actually set out to measure. Reliability is usually assessed by inter-rater measurements, and test–retest situations in which the same subjects are tested on two separate occasions and the two different scores correlated. Methods of testing validity include comparing results in two populations known to differ in the characteristics being measured, and by comparing the test scales under examination with other scales or clinical assessments that are theoretically known to be measuring the same phenomena.

Prior to the use of these tests 'standardization' is required. Standardizing procedures involve designating the precise way in which a test is to be given, whereas standardizing scores means translating a subject's raw score into one that is related to larger samples that have been tested, taking into account age, sex, and whatever other variables are considered to be important in interpreting the results.

Intelligence tests were introduced originally by the French psychologist Binet, and have been widely used and standardized over a number of years. The Stanford–Binet test is still used for testing children, and the scale gives an estimate of the child's mental age in relationship to his chronological age. The IQ (or Intelligence Quotient) expresses this relationship, since

$$IQ = 100 \ \frac{\text{mental age}}{\text{chronological age}} \ .$$

Later adjustments of this test led to the IQ being calculated directly from tables, thus allowing for a more accurate interpretation of results. In practice the Terman–Merrill or the Wechsler Intelligence Scale for Children (WISC) are more widely used for testing children.

For adults most assessments use the Wechsler Adult Intelligence Scale (WAIS). This is composed of eleven sub-tests, each of which examines a slightly different aspect of cognitive function and for which age and sex norms have been established. The sub-tests are divided into six verbal and five performance tests given in the following order: information, comprehension of certain statements, arithmetic, similarities, memory for digits, vocabulary testing, digit symbol substitution, picture completion, block design, picture arrangement, and object assembly. Most of these terms are self-explanatory. Digit symbol substitution refers to a patient's ability to substitute various shapes for a particular number according to a pre-arranged code. In block design coloured blocks are placed in accordance with patterns shown on cards, and in picture arrangement a set of pictures is ordered to form a meaningful story. The raw scores of these tests are converted into standardized sub-tests scores, and estimates of both verbal and performance IQ are given, as well as a full-scale IQ. As such the WAIS is widely used in research, and although profiles of sub-test scores have not been shown to be of diagnostic value, some sub-test patterns do suggest localization of particular neurological lesions. McFie presented a summary of results from over 200 adult patients, as shown in Figure 3.1. Vocabulary scores were lower in patients with left temporal lobe lesions; similarity scores were impaired in patients with left temporal and left parietal lesions; and digit span scores in left frontal, left temporal, and left parietal lesions. Right-sided lesions impaired performance abilities, in particular picture arrangement with right frontal and temporal lesions, and block design with right parietal lesions. It should be noted from this figure that digit symbol sub-test scores seem sensitive to lesions in many areas, and that picture completion seems relatively resistant to deterioration, and is said to correlate to some extent with the patient's premorbid general abilities in non-

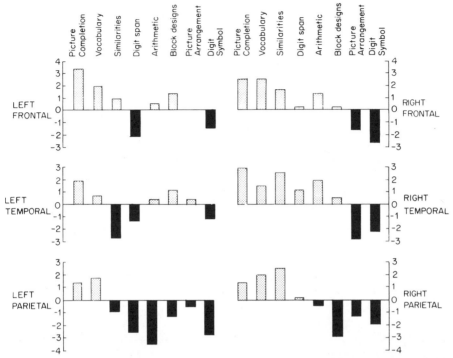

Figure 3.1. A summary of results of the Wechsler Adult Intelligence Scale (WAIS) obtained from over 200 adult patients, showing test correlations with various localized lesions (after McFie, 1975)

verbal tests (Refs. 40, 41, p.35).

Clinically, comparison of the age corrected IQ score with that which may be expected in relation to the patient's educational and occupational history is one method of assessing brain damage. Since verbal abilities seem less impaired than performance abilities in brain damaged patients, the verbal sub-test scores have been used as one measure of the premorbid IQ. An alternative method is to use the Wechsler Deterioration Index, which is based on the observation that with decline in abilities some tests 'hold' more than others. Vocabulary, information, object assembly, and picture completion thus show much less decline than the digit span, similarities, digit symbol substitution, and block design. The index is given by

$$\frac{\text{(sum of the 'hold' scores)} - \text{(sum of the non-'hold' scores)}}{\text{sum of the 'hold' scores}}.$$

Clinically there are many limitations to these methods. The result of WAIS testing is dependent on educational, cultural and social attainments of patients, and diverse results can thus sometimes arise in the absence of pathology (Ref. 42, p.138). For example 5% of normal subjects have significant verbal performance deficits. In addition the tests do not clearly differentiate groups of patients with organic brain syndromes from patients with psychiatric illnesses, since affective and psychotic disturbances sometimes markedly interfere with performance.

A major problem is determining if deterioration of abilities has occurred in comparison with premorbid levels of functioning. The Nelson Reading Test attempts to improve estimates of the latter. Based on observations that correlations exist between reading attainment in childhood and intelligence, a regression equation was established for use in adults to predict their IQ score from reading ability. In patients with dementia the reading ability score is taken to reflect the premorbid IQ, and this does not seem affected until dementia becomes severe.[43]

The Halstead Reitan neuropsychological battery has a number of sub-tests, the scores from which form the basis on the Halstead Impairment Index. This particular test was developed specifically to detect cerebral lesions and provides estimates of verbal and non-verbal abilities, concept formation, perception, language, and memory.[44]

The Raven Progressive Matrices is used as a quick assessment for non-verbal intelligence abilities. More and more difficult designs requiring completion are given to a patient, and since responses can be made verbally or non-verbally it is useful for patients with language deficits.[45]

Memory

Testing of memory requires specific procedures. One commonly used test is the Wechsler Memory Scale. This consists of seven tests, including personal and current information, orientation for time and place, counting, paragraph memory (in which recall of a paragraph read aloud is required), digit span, immediate visual memory, and paired associate word learning. The scores from these sub-tests are added together to obtain a total. Major disadvantages of this test are that it combines these separate scores, which may not be valid, and it is stronger in testing verbal, as opposed to visual, memory. More sophisticated techniques for assessing memory include separate evaluations of these two aspects of memory. The Walton and Black Modified Word Learning Test[46] scores the ability to learn the meaning of ten unfamiliar words taken from the Terman–Merrill Vocabulary Test. This test seems to discriminate between patients with organic brain syndromes and others, including those with psychiatric disabilities, although a proportion of the latter are still misclassified. A modification of this test for use in geriatric patients, in which words taken from the Mill Hill Vocabulary Scale and in which standardized definitions of unknown words are used, is referred to as the Synonym Learning Test.[40, 47] The Inglis Paired Associate Learning Test[48] is a good indicator of memory impairment which is independent of the general level of intellectual ability. The subject is asked to learn three pairs of words and is then presented with the first word of the pairs and asked to recall the second. The test is continued until the patient is able to give consecutive correct replies on three occasions.

The memory for designs test[49] involves reproduction of geometrical designs. They are briefly shown to patients who are then asked to reproduce them. The Rey–Osterreith Test uses one complex figure, which the patient is asked to draw after seeing it for 10 seconds. One way to score this relates to the number exposures a patient needs in order to make a good representational copy.

Warrington[50] has developed a battery of tests in which verbal and pictorial material are tested by forced choice recognition. Fifty items are presented, one every 3 seconds, and the patient is asked to respond 'yes' or 'no' depending on whether he 'likes' or 'dislikes' the item. The stimulus items are then paired with alternative distractor items, and on representation the subject is asked to pick out the previously shown items. Normal subjects show an excellent capacity to perform these tests and standardizations have now been carried out. While scores fall in any form of organic brain impairment, and lateralization is noted such that verbal performance falls with dominant lesions, and pictorial performance falls with non-dominant lesions, in Korsakoff's psychosis a dramatic decline in ability is described. These tests are far more sensitive than, for example, the Wechsler Memory Scale.

Frontal lobe

Patients with frontal lobe lesions show consistent deficits on certain procedures while performing perfectly well with many conventional tests.[51] In the Wisconsin Card Sorting Test patients are given a pack of 128 cards with symbols on them which differ in form, colour and number. Four stimulus cards are available for the patient with symbols on them, and the patient has to place each response card in front of one of the four stimulus cards. The tester will tell the patient if he is right or wrong, and he has to use that information to place the next card alongside the correct stimulus card. The sorting is carried out arbitrarily into colour, form and then number. Patients with dorso-lateral frontal lesions make more errors than others, especially perseverative errors. In addition, patients with frontal lesions perform badly on Maze Learning Tests, showing errors of 'breaking the rules' — for example, moving diagonally when such moves are disallowed.

ESTIMATING THOUGHT DISORDER

A number of tests have been designed to measure thought disorder in an attempt to distinguish schizophrenic patients from others. Perhaps the most widely used in research has been the Repertory Grid technique, although clinically it has found little value. The theory behind the experiments rests with the personal construct theory of Kelly. This theory suggests that people 'construct' their world actively such that their concepts allow prediction of what will happen. Events can thus be anticipated. In the Repertory Grid technique patients are asked to rank photographs of people using criteria such as 'hard-working', 'likeable', 'selfish' etc. Normal people show high correlations between similar constructs such that 'likeable' and 'good' for example would be ranked together. The higher these correlations the greater the 'intensity' of the relationships and thus the strength of the conceptual structure. A second set of photographs is then administered to patients and the procedure repeated. Thus 'consistency' of the constructs can be calculated by comparing the first grid to the second one. Low consistencies are seen as pathological, implying that a person's experience of the world is unstable. Schizophrenic patients shown both low 'intensity' and low 'consistency'.[52]

RATING SCALES IN PSYCHIATRY

In the same way that attempts have been made to quantify changes of cognitive abilities, a number of rating scales have been devised in order to assess more accurately moods and personalities of patients. The last 20 years has seen a rapid expansion in the use of such tests, which stems partially from the necessity to quantify clinical assessments for research, but also from the extensive use of computers that has enabled large amounts of data to be analysed with relative ease. A number of the more commonly used scales will be briefly described. They are divided into subjective and objective scales. In the former the patient is allowed to self-report his symptoms, whereas in the latter the scales are filled in by the tester. Some of these scales cover wide areas of psychopathology; others are used for specific mood assessment, for example anxiety or depression; still others for the assessment of stress, social environment, rehabilitation, ward behaviour etc. In research their main use is in comparing patients on different occasions particularly following treatments. The most useful tests are those that can be administered quickly, scored quantitatively, and used flexibly in a variety of situations. They are not recommended for diagnostic purposes.

Depression

The most widely used self-rating scale is the Beck scale.[53] For 21 items, each of which represents a depressive symptom, four or five statements of varying severity are available for the patient to choose from. Each of these statements carries a score, and a total score is compounded by adding the individual scores from different statements. It has been well validated both in psychiatric and general medical patients. The Zung scale[54] is a 20-item self-report scale which the patient rates on a four-point continuum.

The most widely used objective rating scale is the Hamilton scale. In one version there are 17 items rated on a 3–5 point scale ranging from symptoms absent to symptoms severe. The inter-observer reliability of this test is found to be high, and several studies have compared the validity of other scales against the Hamilton scale. Thus correlation with the Beck is at approximately 0.74 and with the Zung 0.79.[55, 56, 57]

Anxiety

The most important aspect of anxiety rating scales is that attempts have been made to distinguish 'trait' anxiety from 'state' anxiety. One of the earlier and most widely used scales was the Taylor Manifest Anxiety Scale in which 50 items, originally taken from the Minnesota Multiphasic Personality Inventory (MMPI), are answered as either 'true' or 'false'. The scores on this test give an estimate of 'trait' anxiety. Hamilton has also developed an anxiety scale assessing 12 symptoms and one behavioural measurement all rated on a five-point scale from 'absent' to 'grossly disabling'.[58] Spielberger[59] developed the State–Trait Anxiety Inventory. Items in this scale consist of 20 'state' questions asking how the person feels at that particular time, to which a four-grade response from 'not at all' to 'very much' is available. The 'trait' scale also has 20 items but enquires how the person generally feels, and the responses include 'almost never', 'often', 'always'. The State Scale may be used repeatedly during experiments to assess change, and the period of time varied to suit experimental conditions. Scores on this scale increase in response to stress, and decrease with relaxation. The Trait Anxiety Scale is highly correlated with other trait anxiety measures.

Multiple symptom scales and adjective check-lists

A number of scales have been used to assess wide areas of psychopathology. The Goldberg General Health Questionnaire[60] was constructed to detect psychiatric disturbance in the community both reliably and rapidly. The brief psychiatric rating scale[61] has 18 items rated on 7 point scales and is used as a rapid method for evaluating psychopathology, especially for in-patients.

Mood adjective check-lists provide adjectives which describe various moods, and subjects are asked to describe how they feel by ticking one of four alternatives available.[62] The choices are: 'not at all', 'a little', 'quite a bit', and 'extremely'. These are given scores of 0, 1, 2, and 3, respectively, and scores on adjectives which are related to different moods are then added together to get a total score. These tests can be adapted for trait or state measures. In the former, patients are asked how they feel generally, while in the latter they are asked how they feel now.

The Present State Examination has been developed by Wing and others over a number of years to standardize, as far as possible, the psychiatric interview.[63] The technique whereby patients are interviewed has been formalized and an agreed set of descriptions and definitions of symptoms are provided. The ninth edition rates the presence or absence of 140 symptoms and the results can be incorporated into a computer program, which sifts and combines information such that the patient is allocated to one descriptive class. These classes bear a close relationship to clinical diagnosis, and, while not intended to be diagnostic in their own right, provide a useful technique for standardizing diagnostic categories in psychiatric research.

Analogue scales

These scales, on account of their simplicity and ease of administration, have become widely used in psychiatric research in recent years. The symptom in question is represented by a line of standard length (e.g. 10cm), each end of this line representing the extreme degrees of severity. Symptoms are usually rated on a bipolar scale, for example one end of the line representing 'most elated', the other end 'most depressed'. The patient is asked to mark how he feels by a cross on the line at an appropriate point. These scales give accurate estimates of 'state' moods and may be used repeatedly over short or long periods of time. The results have been shown to correlate well with other scales.

Personal questionnaires

Shapiro and others[64] have described a technique for rating mood in individual patients which is based on questions that enable patients to repeatedly rate the intensity of their own symptoms, described in their own words, and calibrated in accordance with their own assessment of distress. In effect each patient constructs his own questionnaire. These scales are particularly appropriate for assessing short-term changes in intensive studies of individual cases, although their construction is complicated.

Personality questionnaires

A large number of tests have been developed for the assessment of personality although surprisingly few find use, even in research. Most are self-rating scales and vary in length and complexity. The most commonly used in Great Britain is the Eysenck Personality Inventory (EPI),[65] comprising 57 questions to which 'yes/no' answers are given. It takes only a few minutes to complete and provides an assessment of 'neuroticism' and 'extroversion'. The scale is based on Eysenck's theory that the traits of extroversion–introversion, and neuroticism, are continuously distributed in the population, and that anyone can be placed at a point on an orthogonal two-dimensional scale. The test incorporates a 'lie' scale to detect people who are inconsistent about their answers.

In America the Minnesota Multiphasic Personality Inventory is more widely used. It consists of 550 statements to which subjects answer 'true' or 'false'. It takes a considerable time to complete but does provide scores of a number of sub-tests, namely: hypochondriasis, depression, hysteria, psychopathy, masculinity–feminity, paranoia, psychaesthenia, schizophrenia and hypomania. Profiles can be drawn up for individual patients and examination of the profiles is used to predict psychopathology. Examples of such techniques are shown on page 151 where patients with chronic pain have been assessed with this scale. It is not intended for use in diagnosis of psychiatric illness, and the sub-categories mentioned above do not correlate well with psychiatric diagnostic categories.

Other scales sometimes used for the assessment of personality include the Leyton Obsessional Inventory for patients suffering from obsessional and compulsive disorders,[66] and the Foulds Hysteroid–Obsessoid Questionnaire.[67]

Projective tests

In these tests the subject is presented with an ill-defined situation such as an ink-blot shape on paper, a picture, or incomplete sentence and asked either to complete the situation or to state what the stimulus reminds him of. It is thought that the patient will project his own behavioural tendencies, needs, conflicts and desires into the answer, and that these may be assessed with the aim of throwing light on the personality of the patient. These tests have been widely used in North America but do not find great use in this country, the main disadvantage being their lack of quantifiability rather than the subjective interpretation of the results. The Rorschach test is the most widely used which consists of ten cards, each bearing an ink-blot, the shapes of which are symmetrical around the mid-line. Other projective measures include word association tests, in which the subject is given a series of words and asked to respond to each one with the word that immediately comes into his head, and the Thematic Apperception test, in which the subject is required to tell a story about a series of pictures which depict various ambiguous situations and relationships.

CHAPTER 4

An Introduction to Psychiatry

DIAGNOSIS IN PSYCHIATRY

Psychiatrists, like other physicians, are initially concerned to make a diagnosis. Without diagnosis, treatment of whatever sort cannot be initiated logically, unless it is so non-specific as to be of little value. In the last 30 years treatments in psychiatry, particularly with regard to psychotropic drugs, have become more specific in their action, and this has led to a renewed interest in diagnostic issues. It is often suggested that psychiatrists are particularly bad at making diagnoses and that little agreement exists between them on what constitutes an illness, if indeed they are dealing with illnesses at all. It is germane to note that at present neuropsychiatric diagnoses are based entirely on clinical assessment rather than on aetiological grounds, and that in practice the degree of diagnostic concordance reached between psychiatrists is no better or no worse than in other specialities. For example, the recent international studies on the diagnosis of schizophrenia indicate that when patients exhibit certain symptoms there is a 90% chance that they will receive a diagnosis of schizophrenia in countries as far apart as Taiwan and America. This compares to an accuracy of 79% for cardiac diagnoses based on heart sound recordings, or 74% agreement between radiologists diagnosing peptic ulcers from barium X-rays (Ref. 68, p.134). It is well-known that some 50% of appendices that are removed are normal pathologically.

Chapter 1 has indicated that certain diagnoses such as melancholia, dementia, or mania, have been clinically recognized for many years. These terms have been integrated into the diagnostic framework that is in use today. The study of abnormal personalities in contrast has a much more recent history, starting with Prichard who coined the term 'moral insanity'. It is suggested here that a patient's personality should be considered separately from any psychiatric illness that the patient may be suffering, a line of thought developed by Jaspers.

PERSONALITY DISORDERS

Personality means 'the particular way an individual expresses himself, in the way he moves, how he experiences and reacts to situations, how he loves, grows jealous, how he conducts his life in general . . . how he acts (Ref. 24, p.428). The classification of abnormal personality is a controversial issue, but in Europe follows the ideas of Schneider. Thus the abnormal personality is considered to deviate from the normal personality quantitatively as if 'normal traits' were statistically normally distributed within the population. Diagnosis is based largely on clinical judgement although some attempts have been made to quantify aspects of personality by the development of rating scales (See Chapter 3). An alternative system, used more extensively in America, assumes some qualitative difference between personality types. The following is based on descriptions taken from both the American and British literature.

Paranoid personality

This describes patients who, oversensitive and preoccupied with their own rights, often based in a degree of personal overvaluation, over-react to every-day events with feelings of suspicion, jealousy, or envy. They tend to blame others for their problems; have feelings that others are against them; and may hold beliefs so strongly that they develop an 'idée fixe' which absorbs considerable amounts of their energy. Their cognitive style may demonstrate denial, rationalization and projection.

Obsessional personality

These people are rigid and inflexible and have lives which seem well-ordered and disciplined. They tolerate upset of any routine poorly, and often find decision-making difficult. They may show rituals of touching, or checking, and have great insecurity. In contrast to paranoid patients they show isolation of the affect, with separation of the emotions from thought content. An alternative term used to describe such people is 'anankastic', and those with some anankastic traits in an otherwise apparently normal personality are often referred to as over-precise.

Cyclothymic personality

Such people have cyclical fluctuations in mood varying from depression to elation, or tend to have more persistent changes in mood, such that they have for example a long-standing depressed attitude to life.

Schizoid personality

Such personalities are shy, withdrawn and avoid close contact with others.

They are cold and aloof, and are said to indulge in autistic thinking with loss of the ability to clearly distinguish reality.

Hysterical personality

These personalities, 'far from accepting their given dispositions and life opportunities . . . crave to appear, both to themselves and others, as more than they are and to experience more than they are ever capable of . . . .' (Ref. 24, p.443). They have a shallow labile affect; emphasize emotional display with verbal exaggeration and imprecision that can lead to overt lying and pseudologia fantastica; are over-demanding and dependent in interpersonal relationships; are impulsive; and appear seductive but often have a fear of sexuality. When such traits are found in patients, but are within the bounds of normal variation, the latter are referred to as having demonstrative personalities (Ref. 69, p.70).

Antisocial personality

This term, which includes those who under the 1959 Mental Health Act were referred to as 'psychopathic', is confined to people who offend against society. They are said to include patients who 'show a lack of sympathetic feeling, and whose behaviour is not readily modifiable by experience including punishment (Ref. 70, p.17). They are immature, impulsive and lack judgement. They tolerate frustration poorly, and their behaviour brings them into repeated conflict with society and the law. Subdivision has been made into aggressive, inadequate, creative and sexual types.

Passive–aggressive personality

As implied, these people are both passive and aggressive. Instead of expressing their hostility openly they do so by obstructionism, procrastination and stubbornness which arouses hostility in others.

Explosive personality

Here such people demonstrate marked instability of mood and behave explosively in situations they do not like. Outbursts are very different from the patient's usual behaviour patterns and they may show remorse after the event. Unfortunately, such personalities have also been called 'epileptoid', although there is no evidence that there is any relationship of this pattern of behaviour to epilepsy. Antisocial acts are not a feature of this personality group.

Asthenic personality

This includes people who continuously have low energy with easy fatigability, oversensitivity to physical and emotional stress, and are often incapable of enjoying themselves. Such personalities are sometimes referred to as 'inadequate', and many of them are referred to as 'passive-dependent'.

Anxious personalities

Such patients have a long history of anxiety developing to all life's difficulties, actual or anticipated. Under stress they develop fear and panic. Anxiety is one of the mainsprings of our emotional activity, and excessive anxiety is seen influencing a wide variety of illnesses.

Borderline personality

The concept of the borderline personality has developed mainly from the writings of the psychoanalysts in America, particularly Kernberg.[71] Such personalities manifest anxiety; polysymptomatic neuroses which include bizarre conversion symptoms, dissociative states and hypochondriasis; polymorphous perverse sexuality; impulsive behaviour; and a tendency to addiction. They are said to be 'pre-psychotic' in their personality structure; to be prone to psychotic illness at times of stress; and psychodynamically to use primitive mechanisms such as 'splitting'.

Organic personality changes

These are discussed in Chapters 6 and 7.

There are many theories as to how personality organization is developed within the individual, but these will not be discussed here. However, it is important to note that amidst the various conflicting ideas certain facts emerge. Animal studies, and human genetic work, especially with twins, indicates more resemblance in personality between genetically related individuals than between unrelated ones. Shields noted that monozygous twins separated in early life, and thus raised in different environments, produced similar neuroticism scores on the EPI, and had similar mannerisms, habits and emotional styles.[72] Some neurotic traits such as enuresis were also concordant. Similar work with antisocial behaviour indicates higher concordance for monozygous as opposed to dizygous twins. Although some writers have suggested a specific relationship between somatic build and personality, such as Kretschmer's theory that pyknic people tend to be cyclothymic and leptosomatic people schizoid, and Sheldon's relationship of endomorphs, mesomorphs and ectomorphs to different types of personality, such views have not found a great deal of experimental support. However, there are some studies that suggest somatic links with behaviour patterns. In particular the electroencephalograph EEG has highlighted relationships between psychopathic behaviour and 'immaturity of the brain'. Antisocial personalities have more neurological and EEG abnormalities than the rest of the population. In particular they demonstrate bilateral temporal and central rhythmical theta activity of similar or greater amplitude than the alpha rhythm. Further, in some, posterior temporal 3 to 5 cycles per second activity is found. Sometimes this is unilateral, and may be associated with epileptiform discharges.[73, 74] In that these forms of abnormality are seen frequently in childhood, much less frequently in 'stable' adults, and occur more commonly in males than in females, it has been suggested that they represent immaturity of brain development. Williams[75] concluded that such changes were not due to structural brain damage, but were related to changes in the activity of the reticular activating system. More recently, abnormalities of the contingent negative variation, with erratic and inconsistent responses to successive stimuli, have been noted among prison inmates, lending further evidence to support neurophysiological differences between patients with different patterns of abnormal behaviour.[76]

Attempts to relate changes in genetic material to behaviour abnormalities have been unsuccessful except for the case of XYY patients. Such karyotypes demonstrate an increased incidence of EEG abnormalities, especially temporal slow activity; are overrepresented in prison populations; tend to be over-impulsive and prone to sudden violence and aggression, and have a lowered attention span.[77]

On the relationship between personality and psychiatric illness

The tendency of certain personality types to develop certain illnesses has received little attention in the literature. The relationship between personality and somatic symptoms is discussed in Chapter 5, and the changes in personality brought about by various neurological diseases are mentioned under the appropriate illnesses. With regard to psychiatric morbidity, there is some evidence that particular illnesses are found more commonly in certain premorbid personalities. Study of the relationship between obsessional neurosis and the obsessional personality has indicated that over 70% of the former have obsessional premorbid personalities, and a high incidence of parents and sibs with such personalities (Refs. 78, 79, p.151). Studies of depressive illness suggest a higher than expected incidence of premorbid obsessional traits.[80] Similar relationships have been suggested between the cyclothymic personality and manic-depressive illness; the schizoid personality and schizophrenia; and the paranoid personality and paranoid schizophrenia. The last of these associations has been a major area of controversy. Jaspers made the point that 'the investigation of the basic biological events and the meaningful development of the life history culminates in a differentiation of two kinds of individual life: *The unified development of the personality* . . . and the disruption of a life which is broken in two and falls apart because at a given time a *process* has intervened in the biological happenings and irreversibly and incurably altered the psychic life by interrupting the course of biological events' (Ref. 24, p.702). A similar view was taken by Schneider. Following this line of thought, clearly there is no necessary relationship between the premorbid personality and subsequent illness, and specifically a gradual transition from personality development to illness is excluded. Others, however, suggested that transitions occurred. Kretschmer defined 'Der sensitive Beziehungswahn,[81] or the 'sensitive delusion of reference', in which certain individuals, on account of their character, environment and experience, are prone to develop a paranoid illness. The psychoanalysts too would make the point that psychiatric illness always reflects abnormal personality development, early abnormalities becoming later fixation points for regression when it occurs.

PSYCHIATRIC ILLNESS

The broad groups of psychiatric disorders are shown in Table 4.1. The hysterical neuroses are discussed in Chapter 5, and the organic brain syndromes in Chapters 6 and 7. It is proposed here to deal with the other neuroses and the psychoses.

Table 4.1. Categories of psychiatric illness

Neuroses:	Obsessional
	Hysterical
	Depressive
	Anxiety
	Neurasthenic
Psychoses:	Manic-depressive psychosis
	Schizophrenia
	Paranoid states
	Schizoaffective illness
Organic brain syndromes:	Acute and chronic
Other disorders:	Autism and childhood disorders
	Gilles de la Tourette syndrome
	Sexual disorders
	Addiction states
	Subnormality
	Anorexia Nervosa and feeding disorders

Characteristically in the psychoses the patient loses insight into his condition whereas in the neuroses the patient retains insight. As variations of human existence, the latter are quantitatively rather than qualitatively different. 'Those psychic deviations which do not wholly involve the individual himself are called neuroses and those which seize upon the individual as a whole are called psychoses' (Ref. 24, p.575).

Anxiety neurosis

The principal feature of this condition is the presence of excessive anxiety. Somatic symptoms of anxiety are likely to occur in all bodily systems, and acknowledgement that many complaints with which the patients present may represent anxiety symptoms is important. Commonly these include palpitations; dyspnoea with a sense of choking; dry mouth; unpleasant abdominal sensations; nausea; loss of appetite, constipation or diarrhoea; sensory abnormalities; motor disturbances, especially increased muscle tone which leads to pain; tremor; frequency of micturition; difficulty in concentration; weakness, and memory difficulties. Often patients complain of a 'muzziness' in the head which is sometimes referred to as 'dizziness'. Patients describe sensations of tension, of being 'up-tight, which are unpleasant and often exacerbated by social situations. Some patients black out and have symptoms which are reminiscent of epilepsy.

When examined, patients with anxiety neuroses show physical signs including a fine peripheral tremor with fidgetiness, or more gross motor movements suggestive of agitation. There may be increased width of the palpebral fissure, with increased eye movements, flushing and sweating. The pulse, respiratory rate, and blood pressure are noted to be raised.

In neuropsychiatric practice, anxiety neurosis is probably the commonest neurosis encountered. This is because the manifestations of anxiety lead to motor and sensory neurological symptoms, and to abnormalities of higher cognitive function. Differential diagnoses can be difficult, but a clear understanding that somatic symptoms are a frequent accompaniment of anxiety should mean that anxiety neurosis is considered in a differential diagnosis of neuropsychiatric problems. The situation becomes clearer if the other manifestations of anxiety are present. The onset is often related to a traumatic event. There may be a preceding history of episodes of anxiety, or recurrent bouts of panic attacks with suggestions of long-standing dependency or immaturity within the personality. In addition there is often evidence of so-called neurotic traits of childhood. The latter include enuresis, nail-biting, finger-sucking, sleep-walking, night terrors, phobias especially of darkness, stuttering, encopresis and tics. As such these symptoms express a 'tenseness', and while in themselves they are not pathognomonic, their early presence is an indicator of the potential for later development of anxiety neurosis.[82]

Variants of the clinical picture include patients who develop severe anxiety states in mid-life in the absence of well-defined neurotic personality traits. This may occur after a trivial stress. *Phobic anxiety states*, in which fear of specific objects or situations develops, fall into at least two subdivisions: first, the monosymptomatic phobias which are commoner in childhood and respond well to behaviour therapy; second, disorders in which the anxiety is less well encapsulated. *Agoraphobia* is a variant of the latter type; the onset is often quite sudden, and patients express fear of leaving their home and going out into the street and public places. In such situations they develop anxiety symptoms and sometimes depersonalization and derealization. Agoraphobia is often associated with depressive features. The *phobic anxiety–depersonalization syndrome* is an anxiety state, accompanied by a depersonalization and derealization. Such patients present with feelings of detachment and unreality, sometimes so severe that patients feel like automata, and even detached from their own bodies. Depersonalization states may be a primary presenting feature with sudden onset, giving rise to a suspicion of epilepsy.

The aetiology of the anxiety neuroses is not well understood. Constitutional factors are important. Two schools of thought have prevailed over the actual mechanism of the production of anxiety symptoms. The James–Lange hypothesis suggested that the initial changes are primarily peripheral, and that following such changes people feel anxious. Cannon's hypothesis stated that the bodily changes and emotional experiences have a common origin within the brain. Recent understanding of the relationship of the limbic system to affective experience, and of the reticular activating system to arousal, has provided support for the latter ideas. In particular the amygdala, hypothalamus, hippocampus and accumbens nuclei have been shown to play a role in the mechanisms of anxiety. The facts that catecholamines seem involved in modulating arousal, and that precursors such as L-dopa can induce arousal, suggest the importance of the monoamines in the anxiety states. That peripheral mechanisms are somehow involved, however, cannot be doubted, since β-adrenergic blocking drugs which do not cross the blood–brain barrier can effectively control some anxiety symptoms.

Clinically, anxiety needs to be distinguished from depressive illness; thyrotoxicosis; epilepsy (in particular partial seizures with auras of panic); states of sympathetic overactivity, for example as seen in hypoglycaemia or phaeochromocytoma; and from a variety of other physical disorders that anxiety symptoms may mimic. Treatment involves superficial exploratory psychotherapy in an attempt to dissect out adverse situations, and patterns of patient behaviour that contribute to the patient's symptoms. Psychotropic drugs are often employed, ranging from β-adrenergic blocking drugs to minor and major tranquillizers. Monoamine oxidase inhibitors (MAOI) are often useful in the phobic anxiety–depersonalization syndrome. For many patients, especially those with monosymptomatic phobias, behaviour therapy is the treatment of choice. Such techniques employ methods of relaxation combined with exposure to feared situations, either slowly or rapidly, in vivo or in imagination.

Patients with anxiety neurosis not only have an increased risk of later development of chronic physical illness, but also have an increased mortality rate.[83]

Neurasthenic neurosis

The term neurasthenia was originally used by Beard to describe a heterogenous group of disorders characterized by irritability and 'nerve weakness'.

Although it is a diagnosis rarely used now, it is useful to describe certain patients commonly encountered in neuropsychiatric practice. Such patients complain of lack of energy and fatigue. They are incapable of completing their daily chores, find sustained concentration difficult, and complain of a variety of non-specific symptoms, often of a somatic nature, such as headache. In addition, neurasthenic symptoms are often described accompanying other psychiatric illnesses such as depression, or following physical illness particularly of a debilitating nature. In some patients the concern over their symptoms, especially their inability to concentrate, reaches hypochondriacal proportions.

Obsessional neurosis

In this condition, thoughts tend to force themselves into consciousness, or patients develop an urge to carry out an action which cannot be resisted. The latter is referred to as a compulsion. The patient struggles against these phenomena and if the actions are constrained anxiety results. The thought or thoughts which occur may be nonsensical, and may take the form of a phobia in which the patient fears something will happen although realizes this is entirely irrational. Contamination or infection phobias are typical. Sometimes ruminations occur and complicated patterns of thought may have to be completed before the patient feels at ease. Compulsions take a variety of forms which include touching, counting, checking, and looking. Many patients who develop such problems have premorbid anankastic personalities, the frank obsessional states occurring at times of stress. In others the obsessional illness develops slowly as a vicious circle, for example fear, leading to avoidance, leading to more fear; or abnormal thought, leading to anxiety, leading to a ritual, leading to more abnormal thought.

Patients with obsessional personality disorders appear to be prone to develop depressive illness, particularly during mid-life, and tolerate physical illness, especially central nervous system disease, poorly. In such patients the onset of the depressive illness may be heralded by the occurrence of frank obsessional symptoms. These symptoms may be encountered in the course of other psychiatric illnesses, and their presence in schizophrenia is said to be related to a good prognosis.[84]

The aetiology of the disorder is unknown, although the psychoanalytic explanation relates to anxiety arousal from unconscious conflict, which is counteracted by the thoughts and rituals. Minor forms of obsessive behaviour are frequently encountered in childhood, and society condones many rituals in adult behaviour. The finding of identical symptoms in patients with epidemic encephalitis, and the precipitation of them by L-dopa in patients with Parkinson's disease, may provide a further clue towards understanding their pathogenesis.[85]

Treatment options involve psychotherapy and behaviour therapy. The latter includes satiation training in which the patients are over-exposed to their obsessions, and restraint, in which they are prevented from carrying out their rituals, with management of the ensuing anxiety. Clomipramine (Anafranil) has been found useful in management, either alone or combined with behaviour therapy. For more severe illnesses, with long-standing crippling symptoms, psychosurgery may be appropriate.

Depression

Because of the controversy and confusion over the classification of depression, depressive neurosis and psychosis are included in this section. The term 'depression' has replaced melancholia in psychiatric literature. For some it represents a disease, others a symptom, others a reaction, and others a neurosis. Unfortunately, the term itself fails to distinguish everyday unhappiness from the severe states of depression that present clinically. Before discussing the symptoms, pathophysiology and treatment of depression, some of the problems of classification will be presented.

Depression or melancholia refers to 'a feeling of misery which is in excess of what is justified by the circumstances in which the individual is placed'.[86] As such it represents an illness rather than an understandable aspect of the patient's personality. Several ways of classification have been evolved and recently reviewed by Kendell.[87] While some authors, notably Lewis and Kendell, suggest that there is a continuum with only one type of depression, others dichotomize into such sub-categories as endogenous/reactive or psychotic/neurotic. The hallmark of endogenous depression is said to be clinical features indicative of hypothalamic disturbance, and lack of relationship to environmental events. It is also taken by some to be equivalent to psychotic depression, although strictly speaking, for a disorder to be called 'psychotic', psychosis should be present. Reactive or neurotic depression presents more difficulty. The term reactive is usually used to refer to depression that is caused by environmental stress, although more properly should refer to the quality of the depression, and its 'reaction' to environmental manipulation. A problem with the former, more widely used, definition is that many studies do not show clear-cut populations of patients with depression that conform to any dichotomy;[87] that studies of life events, which are an index of stress prior to the depression, do not demarcate a group that have a characteristic clinical picture in response to such events; and that life events occur as frequently before 'endogenous' as before 'reactive' depression.[88] In addition, the concept of reaction ignores why many people pass through similar life events and do not develop the same or similar symptoms. A major criticism of splitting up depression in this way is that it highlights the cartesian duality, and assumes two distinct types of depression — one in the body, and one in the mind. One way to overcome this problem is to recognize that stressful events may precipitate depression, but suggest that the features of depression are dependent on constitutional and personality factors, which are closely inter-related with the degree of stress required to precipitate the depression.

Two further classifications which have received attention and recognition

58

are those of the St Louis group, and that of Leonhard. The former divide depression into primary and secondary categories. Primary depression includes illness not preceded by other psychiatric illness, the secondary form being preceded by other psychiatric illness, or accompanied by physical illness. Leonhard introduced the terms bipolar and unipolar to describe clinical patterns of depression. Bipolar illness represents bouts of both mania and depression; unipolar illness recurrent mania or depression. Of all the classifications this last distinction has now gained widespread acceptance. It is suggested that for further discussion of depression, the classification used in Table 4.2 will be adopted. The term reactive will not be used except to express a clinical pattern of an established depression. The term affective disorder is sometimes used as a synonym for depression; however, it covers a variety of illnesses, the nature of which are 'emotional disturbances for which . . . one can have empathy' (Ref. 24, p.578).

Table 4.2. Classification of depression

Primary depressive illness	Unipolar
	Bipolar
	Masked
Atypical depressive illness	
Secondary depressive illness	To psychiatric disorder
	To physical disorder
	To drugs

Clinical features

The clinical signs and symptoms of depression have been well delineated by Lewis.[79] They are outlined in Table 4.3. Foremost there is a change of mood which affects the whole person and is reflected in changes of thoughts, movements and posture. In some patients the change of mood is denied or difficult to elicit, and the diagnosis rests on recognition of some of the other changes listed. Often depression presents in patients as somatic symptoms, especially neurological and gastrointestinal symptoms — so-called masked depression. Other patients have hypochondriacal preoccupation, their symptoms reflecting an underlying depression. Feelings of tension or anxiety are invariably present if asked for; in some this spills over to an observable motor unrest or frank agitation. Difficulties of thought and concentration are reported, which lead to poor performance, which itself increases patients' anxiety. If there is associated apathy and a degree of retardation, such a patient may present clinically as a pattern of dementia. Sometimes the retardation can be so severe that a state of depressive stupor develops. In severe depressions the sense of worthlessness and guilt becomes apparent and delusions may develop. Suicide is always a risk and preoccupation with suicidal ideas should be taken very seriously.

Table 4.3. Clinical features of depression

Change of mood: dysphoria; anxiety; irritability; hostility.
Changes of talk — form: increased in agitation; decreased often, mutism;
content: morbid, depressive.
Changes of action: retardation of over-activity; agitation; crying.
Changes of thinking: concentration difficulties; slowing of thoughts; difficulty in thinking; delusions; self reproach; guilt; suicidal thoughts; depersonalization and derealization; nihilistic delusions.
Changes of perception: hallucinations.
Loss of appetite, weight and libido.
Alteration of sleep pattern: especially early morning waking.
Diurnal variation: improvement towards evening.
Somatic symptoms: especially pain.
Restriction of activity: withdrawal.

Manic symptoms

As suggested in the classification, some patients who present with depression have a bipolar illness. They have manic symptoms either intermingled with depressive ones, or occurring at different times to the depressive ones, or precipitated by antidepressant therapy. Although occasionally patients have recurrent manic attacks, in most bipolar patients the depressive bouts are commoner than the manic episodes. Typical manic symptoms include a rapid flow in the stream of thought, often associated with a flight of ideas; an increased speed of thinking which may lead to rhyming, punning and word-play; increased motor activity; fleeting attention; grandiose ideas that may become delusional; and in severe forms a picture of delirium with confusion. Early symptoms of a developing manic phase include early waking with over-activity; increased talkativeness, and irritability, with an increased sense of well-being. The latter, typical of the manic state, is associated with euphoria, but sometimes the patient's mood is actually dysphoric and unpleasant, rather than euphoric. Mixed forms are occasionally seen of either depressed affect associated with a manic overactivity and dysphoria, or manic stupor. The term hypomania is used to refer to mild forms of the illness; chronic mania is a variant in which patients remain hypomanic for a number of years with little remission.

Atypical depressive illness

Amongst the atypical presentations of depression are included a group with marked phobic anxiety symptoms. Such patients are often young, appear anxious, and may have associated depersonalization or derealization. This has been referred to as 'atypical depression', and of importance in recognition of this sub-type is the often successful response to monoamine oxidase inhibitor (MAOI) drug therapy.[89]

Differential diagnosis

Although in many cases the diagnosis of depression is readily apparent from observing and listening to the patient, in some, especially in masked depressions with marked somatization, the diagnosis will only reveal itself after considerable searching of the patient's past history, family background, and symptomatology. It is of course important to establish whether the depression is primary or secondary and to consider the possible precipitants including drugs. Depression must be distinguished from schizophrenia, schizo-affective disorder and anxiety states. The admixture of anxiety with depression is well-known. It is very unusual to have a depression without some accompanying anxiety symptoms, although the reverse is not true — anxiety states exist in the absence of depression. The sudden development of anxiety symptoms in previously well-adjusted middle-aged patients is suggestive of a depressive illness. Depression may be the initial symptom of other central nervous system disease such as dementia, Parkinson's disease etc., necessitating physical examination of all patients. In the absence of other clearly defined episodes of similar illness, if psychotic symptoms are present, or if there is suspicion of personality change, EEG and further laboratory tests become essential. The presence of alterations of mood in the manic direction, especially after taking antidepressants, leads to the diagnosis of bipolar illness.

Pathogenesis of depression

Genetic studies indicate that the concordance rate for monozygotic twins is higher than for dizygotic twins. First-degree relatives of patients with depression have an increased incidence of the disorder, relatives of bipolar probands tending to have bipolar disorders, and those of unipolar probands, unipolar disorders. Linkage to the gene for colour-blindness and the locus of the Xg blood group have been suggested for bipolar illness. How such predispositions interact with environmental events and physical illness to induce depression is unknown. It is here suggested that the brain is the 'final common path' in the expression of the disorder, and various theories have been developed implicating brain dysfunction. Numerous abnormalities have been described in depressed patients, especially with regard to their hormonal states (see Table 4.4), and recently a number of theories based on neuro-biochemical hypotheses have been put forward.

The monoamine hypotheses will be briefly reviewed. Their central theme is that in depression there is altered bioavailability of certain neurotransmitters in the CNS. The concept gains support clinically from the many symptoms of depression, such as the sleep disturbances, loss of weight, etc., which suggest disturbed hypothalamic function, and the frequent association of depression with disorders of endocrine activity. Early observations indicated that depletion of monoamines by reserpine led to depression in 15–20% of patients, and that MAOI drugs were antidepressant. From these observations, the use

Table 4.4. Some physiological abnormalities noted in depressed patients

Mean plasma free and total cortisol increased.
Abnormal dexamethasone suppression of 17-hydroxycorticosteriods.
Increased residual body sodium.
Increased 17-hydroxycorticosteriod excretion and urine free cortisol.
Increased CSF cortisol.
Abnormal platelet MAO activity.

of precursors of the monoamines in treatment, and direct measurement of breakdown products of monoamines in depression was undertaken.

The serotonin hypothesis is supported by observations that L-tryptophan and 5-hydroxytryptophan possess antidepressant properties; reduced 5-HIAA levels occur in the midbrains of depressed suicide patients;[90] low levels of 5-HIAA are found in the CSF of depressed patients compared to controls, especially if the method of probenicid accumulation is used;[91] and plasma free-tryptophan is decreased in depression.[92] With regard to the CSF studies the abnormality persists after recovery: patients with low 5-HIAA are more likely to attempt suicide;[93] and both ventricular and lumbar CSF are abnormal in depression.[94] Changes in mania have not been consistent, showing alterations in either the same or the opposite direction as depression.

The catecholamine hypothesis is based on observations that urinary excretion of noradrenaline is diminished in depression and elevated in mania, as is the urinary output of VMA and MHPG, and CSF levels of MHPG are lower in depressed patients than controls.[95] However, there are inconsistencies in the data supporting this hypothesis, and observations that plasma catecholamines may correlate also with anxiety and psychosis[96] have led to suggestions that these biochemical changes reflect levels of motor activity. Observations on patients 'switching' from depression to mania, and vice versa, suggest that phase shifts in such parameters as temperature, sleeping and activity occur in association with the mood, although some biochemical changes may occur before the switch actually occurs.[97]

A variant of the catecholamine hypothesis is the dopamine hypothesis, which is based on observations that some depressed patients have low HVA in their CSF, and some respond clinically to dopamine agonists.

In order to make sense of these data, Van Praag has suggested there exists a group of patients with demonstrable serotonin deficiency that respond to antidepressants such as clomipramine (Anafranil), which is more selective in its action in the serotonin system, and that fail to respond to noradrenaline-potentiating antidepressants.[91] There may be a further group with noradrenaline or dopamine deficiency who respond differently and require alternative antidepressants. Thus patients with low HVA in their CSF respond to the dopamine agonists nomifensine and piribedil, and those with low MHPG excretion respond well to imipramine.[98, 99, 100] That even recovered patients have serotonin deficiency, however, suggests a vulnerability to the illness which may be amenable to correction with serotonin precursors.[100]

Although it is often argued otherwise, it is not unlikely that the aetiology of depressive illness involves some predisposition interacting with triggering factors. Predisposition may arise from a number of genetic and epigenetic factors. This would explain why people with certain histories, such as loss of a parent, especially a mother in early childhood, are more prone to later depression.[101] Triggering factors may include a variety of life events, especially further losses,[102, 103] hysterectomy,[104] drugs,[105] and physical illness, although they are not necessarily identical for all depressive illness.

Treatment

The main elements of the treatment of depression are some form of psychotherapy associated usually with psychotropic drugs. Full discussion of the latter is given in Chapter 11. Patients will require support, and where possible environmental manipulation to alleviate stress factors in their illness. Often this is impossible and more reliance has to be placed on psychotropic drugs, or where relevant a more protracted form of psychotherapeutic intervention. In more severe forms of the illness undue attention to the content of the depressed patient's thoughts is contraindicated, and drugs or electroconvulsive therapy (ECT) are the treatments of choice. Suicide must always be considered a danger and asked about. If the patient is thought to be a suicide risk then hospital admission should be considered. Rarely other techniques such as behaviour therapy and psychosurgery are used. For manic or hypomanic episodes some form of psychotropic medication is always necessary and delay in prescribing can have disastrous results. Occasionally ECT is indicated where florid symptoms fail to respond to medications.

Schizophrenia

As indicated in Chapter 1, the term schizophrenia was introduced by Bleuler and refers to a group of mental illnesses characterized by specific psychopathological symptoms and alteration of the personality. The exact symptoms, however, are a matter of debate, which partly reflects the historical origins referred to. Bleuler described both primary and secondary symptoms. The former included disturbance of association, and were thought to be due to the underlying disease process. The typical symptomatology described by Kraepelin, such as negativism, delusions, and hallucinations, were secondary symptoms. In addition, Bleuler distinguished 'basic' symptoms, including alteration of affect and volition, and autism, which were present at all times. Bleuler's ideas became influential in America, and the diagnosis of schizophrenia there is still based on his schema. European thought, however, has been faithful to the ideas of Kraepelin, and his subdivisions of dementia praecox into catatonic, hebephrenic, and paranoid types are still used. Although it is not the case that Kraepelin believed all schizophrenics deteriorated and failed to recover, generally it is held that the course is of gradual deterioration of the personality and later the intellect. Following Jaspers, Fish (Ref. 33, p.2) suggested that the only useful criterion of a schizophrenic symptom was that of lack of understandability. Schneider defined primary or first rank symptoms — 'ones which are always present'.[29]

Table 4.5. First rank symptoms of schizophrenia

Auditory hallucinations:	Audible thoughts (echo de la pensée)
	Voices commenting on actions
	Voices arguing in the third person

Thought withdrawal
Thought insertion and other interference with thought
Thought broadcasting
Delusional perception
'Made' experiences — in feeling, drive or volition
Experience of influences playing on the body

These are shown in Table 4.5. They represent varieties of thought and ego disturbance which if present, in the absence of an organic psychosis, confirm a diagnosis of schizophrenia. They do not, however, represent the gamut of symptoms in schizophrenia, and their absence does not make a diagnosis of schizophrenia untenable. Generally the symptoms of schizophrenia comprise disorders of thinking, perception, affect, volition and movement. Many types of thought disorder have been described (see Chapter 3), the main features being disconnection of thoughts with poor association of ideas. Otherwise unrelated thoughts are connected and often the listener is unable to follow the patient's trend of thought. There may be associated thought blocking, or pressure, with multiple confused ideas passing through the patient's mind. Thought disorder sometimes can be difficult to detect, and may only become apparent when the patient is specifically asked, for example, to interpret proverbs or repeat a story.

Hallucinations are usually auditory and occur in the setting of clear consciousness. Sometimes they consist of noises or inarticulate voices. The affective disturbance is typically described as 'flattened affect'. There is a loss of ability to feel the appropriate emotion for the circumstance, or alternatively some inappropriateness of affect with perhaps fluctuation over a short period of time. Transient states of ecstacy, panic or despair occur. The affective disturbances lead to difficulty in establishing rapport with the patient, giving the examiner a 'feel' of schizophrenia.

Patients may demonstrate negativism — a tendency to fail to do things asked or to even do the opposite. Their actions, thoughts, and will, may seem directed from outside, and these passivity feelings may be interpreted in a delusional manner. Motor symptoms are discussed in Chapter 10.

The diagnosis of schizophrenia, adopting Schneider's 'first rank' criteria, has the advantage that the signs required are objective, in the sense of being either present or absent, unlike, for example, 'loose association' or 'flattened affect' about which there could be disagreement. In that several countries of the world seem to use similar criteria to diagnose the disorder, some consistency is achieved. Using the PSE to quantify symptoms, similar groups of schizophrenic patients have been identified in several countries world-wide. In particular the presence of 'first-rank' symptoms leads to a diagnosis of schizophrenia in 90% of cases.

Hebephrenic schizophrenia refers to a disorder of emotion in association with loss of volition and thought disorder. In *paranoid schizophrenia* the emphasis is on delusions and hallucinations, and less on the destruction of the personality; of all the sub-groups this is the most homogenous and tends to occur in an older age group. With *catatonic schizophrenia* the emphasis is on the motor phenomena and negativism. Automatic behaviour and flexibilitas cerea may occur. *Simple schizophrenia* is used to indicate a slow progression of indifference and lack of drive, with gradual destruction of the personality, often in the absence initially of well-defined thought disorder.

Other variants of schizophrenia that are sometimes referred to include *schizophreniform psychosis* — a term used by Langfeldt to describe a syndrome resembling schizophrenia occurring as a result of 'psychogenic reaction' in a psychopathic personality. Others, however, have used this to refer to schizophrenia-like symptoms occurring with other illness such as epilepsy. *Cycloid psychosis*, introduced by Leonhard, refers to a 'psychotic episode which resolves completely and during which there are mood swings'. A variety of other features such as pan-anxiety, delusions and confusion or perplexity are also noted.[106] *Pseudoneurotic schizophrenia* was a term applied to a group of young patients with pan-anxiety, withdrawal from reality, and a tendency, especially under stress, to become psychotic. It is now referred to as borderline personality and as such is not a variant of schizophrenia. *Late paraphrenia* was used by Roth to define a senile paranoid psychosis in the absence of clear signs of dementia. Patients often have sensory deprivation, especially hearing or sight defects (Ref. 107, p.580). *Propfschizophrenia* is the occurrence of schizophrenic symptoms in people of low intelligence.

Diagnosis

In neuropsychiatric practice, diagnosis is often required in patients presenting with acute psychotic features, where the possibility of neurological structural illness is raised. Sometimes this is extermely difficult since the features of the illness as defined above are seen in a variety of organic brain disorders including epilepsy; following intoxications with drugs especially LSD, amphetamine and sometimes cannabis; vitamin deficiencies and endocrine disturbances; head injury; and a number of neurological illnesses such as tumours, Huntington's chorea, multiple sclerosis, and Wilson's disease.

Careful attention to family history, past history, and present psychopathology are important, and evidence of thought disorder, particularly one of the 'first-rank' symptoms, is highly suggestive of the diagnosis. The presence of rapport, with affective disturbance as a major accompaniment, is suggestive of an affective or schizoaffective illness. In order to rule out structural pathology or gross functional disturbance such as epilepsy, neurological examination is mandatory and EEG, radiology, serology and special tests for drug intoxications, vitamin deficiencies and endocrine disturbance will also be required.

Pathogenesis

There is no doubt now about the constitutional liability of some patients to develop schizophrenia. A number of studies indicate an increased incidence amongst first-degree relatives, and a greater concordance rate for monozygotic as opposed to dizygotic twins. Further, sub-types such as hebephrenic or catatonic types show genetic specificity. Recently studies have been carried out, using matched controls, on children born to schizophrenic mothers but removed from them in the first weeks of life, and of parents (biological and adoptive) of schizophrenic patients who were adopted. These demonstrated an excess of schizophrenia in the biological parents of schizophrenics as compared to controls, and increased psychopathology in children of schizophrenic mothers. There was also an increase in 'borderline' schizophrenia and psychopaths in the biological relatives of the schizophrenics, which has led to the suggestion of the inheritance of a 'schizophrenic spectrum' — the favoured mode of inheritance being polygenic.[108]

The fact that not all monozygotic twins of schizophrenics develop the illness has led to a search for environmental factors influencing the development of the disorder. Some theorists postulate, for example, abnormalities of family communication. The schizophrenogenic mother was described by Fromm-Reichmann; Bateson postulated the 'double-bind' in which parents say one thing but communicate an opposite by their actions; using the Rorschach method, Singer and Wynne have shown anomalous patterns of thought in the parents of schizophrenic patients; Lidz introduced the concepts of 'skew' and 'schism' to define distortions in family relationships leading to abnormalities in the emotional growth of patients. Unfortunately these studies have often been carried out uncontrolled, and replications in this country have not given such well-defined results.[109] More promising has been the attempt to predict the development of schizophrenia using childhood indicators. Developmental data including increased incidence of pregnancy complications, deficits of attention, poor motor co-ordination and psychophysiological variables suggest an early history of neurophysiological disturbance and may define at-risk children.

Neurobiochemical ideas have been numerous. Most emphasize changes within the limbic system of either neurotransmitter or receptor activity. The electroencephalographic abnormalities recorded in psychotic patients are discussed in Chapter 9. The association between schizophreniform illness and structural lesions in the limbic system, in particular tumours, epilepsy and

Table 4.6. Some biochemical abnormalities described in schizophrenia

Abnormal response to intradermal histamine
Increased serum aldolase and creatinine phosphokinase
Increased size of muscle motor end-plates
Increased trans-3-methyl-2-hexenoic acid in sweat
Reduced platelet MAO concentrations

encephalitis, is well-recorded.[110] Some of the abnormalities noted in schizophrenia are shown in Table 4.6. Two of the most promising biochemical hypotheses have been the transmethylation hypothesis and the dopamine hypothesis. The former, suggested by Smythies, is based on observations that the hallucinogen mescaline is an O-methylated derivative of dopamine. There may therefore be an endogenous neurotoxin that is a similar methylated substance. It is supported by reports that methionine — a methyl donor in transmethylation reactions — can induce acute psychosis in schizophrenic patients. Other methyl donors such as betaine and cysteine are reported to do the same. The methylated derivative of serotonin — dimethyltryptamine — has been reported to occur in the urine of schizophrenic patients, but to-date no clear differences between schizophrenics and controls are consistently reported.[111]

The dopamine hypothesis has received support largely from observations that drugs such as chlorpromazine, which are antipsychotic and not simply sedative, block dopamine receptors, and that amphetamine can produce a psychosis the symptoms of which are indistinguishable from those of schizophrenia. This and other evidence for the dopamine hypothesis is shown in Table 4.7.[112] As can be seen, the majority of evidence for this hypothesis is circumstantial, and to-date, there has been little direct evidence of abnormal dopamine function in schizophrenic patients. Recently abnormalities of CSF HVA have been defined in schizophrenia, increased accumulation following probenecid being noted. However, the correlation was with motor agitation and anxiety rather, than with any psychotic symptom *per se*.[113] Others have shown elevation of dopamine in the nucleus accumbens of post-mortem material from treated schizophrenic patients.[114] More significant, however, has been the suggestion that dopamine receptors, rather than dopamine turnover itself, may be more important to the disorder. Recent assessment of dopamine receptor function in post-mortem brains of both treated and untreated schizophrenic patients by the technique of labelled spiroperidol binding has shown increased binding, especially in the caudate, putamen and nucleus accumbens.[115] Some suggestion that the endorphins are involved in the disorder comes from observations of high β-endorphin levels in the CSF of schizophrenic patients, and of improvement of schizophrenic symptoms with the administration of des-tyr-gamma-endorphin, and β-endorphin.[116, 117]

The recent identification of cerebral atrophy on computerized axial tomography in chronic schizophrenic patients, associated with impairment of intellectual testing, suggests there exists at least one sub-group where there is

Table 4.7. Some evidence for the dopamine hypothesis

Amphetamine leads to a paranoid psychosis indistinguishable from schizophrenia.
L-dopa induces a similar psychotic picture in normal people and Parkinsonian patients.
Amphetamine and L-dopa exacerbate schizophrenic symptoms.
Drugs that block dopamine receptors are antipsychotic.
The antipsychotic action of such drugs is almost directly related to their potential to block dopamine receptors.
X-ray crystallography studies show the preferred conformation of chlorpromazine 'fits' the structure of dopamine.
Increased dopamine receptor activity is found in the nucleus accumbens and caudate nucleus of post-mortem brains.

associated structural brain pathology.[118] This is in keeping with the large range of neurological abnormalities noted in schizophrenia ranging from 'soft' clinical abnormalities to vestibular abnormalities, motor disorders and disturbances in ocular movements.[110] The latter include disturbed eye contact, altered blink rate, abnormal blink reflexes, abnormal lateral eye movements and irregular pursuit, which it has been suggested may reflect disturbed mesolimbic dopamine system activity.[119]

Treatment and prognosis

The use of major tranquillizers, and ECT, are discussed in Chapter 11. The emphasis in treatment of schizophrenia is on regular follow-up; hostel, day centre care, or hospital care where necessary; prevention of relapse with medication; and preferably avoidance of stress. Assessment of prognosis in the disorder is extremely difficult because of the lack of criteria in various studies, not only for the diagnosis, but also for 'cure' and improvement. It is generally accepted that certain clinical features, shown in Table 4.8, are predictive of a good prognosis, and that the diagnosis of schizophrenia does not necessarily herald an automatically gloomy future. In spite of the widespread use of neuroleptic medication, it is not clear that the long-term prognosis of the disorder is improving. Bleuler, in a 23 year longitudinal study of prognosis, suggested that although the numebr of mild chronic conditions has increased, and the number of severe cases decreased, the percentage of patients with a chronic illness progressing to a severe psychosis remained approximately the same.[120] Some 60% of all patients are said to be improved at follow-up, although a distinction has been made between 'atypical' schizophrenia, as defined by the Scandinavian authors (e.g. cycloid psychosis: schizophreniform psychosis) with a good prognosis, and 'process' schizophrenia with a much worse prognosis.[121]

The social circumstances of patients seem to be important in prognosis. Thus patients discharged to families that are hostile and critical are more likely to relapse. One index of this is referred to as 'Expressed Emotion' (EE).' Patients in an environment of high EE, having much contact with their close relatives and not on drugs, have a 92% chance of relapse, reducing to 55% on

Table 4.8. Indications of a good or a bad prognosis in schizophrenia

(a) *Good prognosis*

    Acute onset

    Well integrated pre-psychotic personality

    Onset associated with 'stress' — physical or psychological

    Admixture of affective symptoms

(b) *Bad prognosis*

    Age of onset under 20

    Schizoid premorbid personality

    Flat affect

    Insidious onset

    Positive family history

    Not married

maintenance drug therapy. This is much higher than the 15% relapse rate noted in patients from low EE homes not on medication.[122, 123] The increasing emphasis on community care, associated with the rapid resolution of acute symptoms in hospital by neuroleptic medication, has meant more rapid discharge back to the community. This has led to more strains within the family, and an increased number of re-admissions. Relatives find the patients' withdrawal, self-neglect, dependency, restlessness and socially embarrassing behaviour particularly difficult. They respond with anxiety, depression, guilt, anger, and often fail to receive the support and help necessary from the community. There is now increased acceptance for the idea that many patients should not be resettled with their families but require some form of intermediate accommodation, and, for a sub-group, long-term hospitalization still has an important part to play.[124]

Paranoid states

In these conditions there are delusional ideas, often elaborated and systematized, but no other features of a psychotic illness or evidence of personality deterioration. The delusions characteristically are persecutory or grandiose. However, they can present as complaints about the body image (dysmorphophobia), sensory symptoms or even pain problems. There is no agreement whether paranoia is a separate disease entity, or a variant of schizophrenia. Kraepelin separated it from Dementia Praecox, but others do not accept this distinction on the grounds that the relatives of such patients have an increased risk of schizophrenia, and that if the patients are followed up for long enough they will develop more characteristic schizophrenic symptoms. Paranoid psychoses are often seen secondary to other illnesses (see Table 4.9).

Schizoaffective illness

This term was originally used to describe a psychosis in which there was an

Table 4.9. Some causes of paranoid psychosis

Psychiatric illness: affective disorder, especially depression
Endocrine disease: thyroid and adrenal disorders
Intoxications: amphetamine and other stimulants, LSD, alcohol, barbiturates and cocaine
Neurological disease: epilepsy, Huntington's chorea, dementia, tumours, post-encephalitic Parkinsonism
Medications: ACTH, Pentazocine, L-dopa, anticholinergic drugs
Metabolic: uraemia, S.L.E., porphyria, vitamin deficiency (esp. B_{12})
Infections: syphilis, malaria, typhus
Other: post-operative, puerperal, Klinefelter's syndrome

admixture of affective and schizophrenic symptoms, the onset of which was associated with emotional stress.[125] Some view it as a sub-type of schizophrenia; others as a sub-type of bipolar affective illness, and still others as an independent entity. The prognosis of these patients seems to be more related to that of the affective disorders than to 'process schizophrenia', especially in schizomania. Family history and genetic data support the concept that some forms of schizoaffective illness form a separate group.[126]

CHAPTER 5

Liaison Psychiatry with Special Reference to Neurological Units

Over the last 40 years the expansion of psychiatric units in general hospitals has led to a recognition of the large number of psychiatric problems found in general medical patients. This has resulted not only in a need for psychiatrists to communicate their discipline to other physicians, but also to the learning of new skills in both the detection and management of psychiatric problems in these settings. In addition it has enabled physicians to highlight psychosocial aspects of somatic disease, and has led to a rapid explosion of knowledge regarding psychosomatic problems.

A number of authors have discussed the concept or process of 'liaison psychiatry'. Initially the psychiatric consultations were seen as 'patient orientated'. The psychiatrist on the medical or surgical ward emphasized diagnosis, treatment and disposition. This approach is still used by many, but is limited because the consultant deals primarily with the patient, responding only to explicit questions raised by a referring physician. A change of orientation came from Balint,[127] who emphasized that working with the referring physician was just as important as working with the patient. Schiff and Pilot[128] discussed the 'consultee-oriented' consultation in which the anxieties of the referring physician were recognized. The suggestion was that the request for psychiatric consultation reflected a breakdown of physician-patient relationships, or even discord amongst staff members resulting from different views about patients' management. In these situations the consultation involved dissection of the underlying reasons for the request in order to facilitate further patient management. Meyer and Mendelson[129] extended the concept further, pointing out that the consulting psychiatrist was essentially a participator in a 'small group' which they termed the operational group. This involved other physicians, nurses, hospital personnel and of course the patient. The request for psychiatric consultation was seen to reflect crisis within the group, the psychiatric emergency lying 'within the group itself and not with the patient'. They made the point that it was not the severity of the patient's psychopathology which necessarily led to referral but anxiety within the group looking after the patient.

Lipowski[130] has given the commonest reasons for the request of the psychiatric consultation as follows: 'diagnostic uncertainty; recognition of a gross psychiatric disorder; patients' deviant behaviour with regard to medical procedures and therapies, ward routine, etc., which disturbs smooth functioning of the medical team; crisis in the doctor–patient relationship; patients' admission of serious psychosocial difficulties'.

In practice, liaison psychiatric consultation requires assessment of the mental state and evaluation of the patient's problems in relation to knowledge regarding the patient's past and present medical history, and psychosocial status. It involves formulating an opinion, which then has to be communicated to the referring physician in language which is free of jargon, which discusses diagnosis, differential diagnosis, and treatment, in a logical fashion. Some assessment of the personality and the coping style of the patient should always be included in any assessment, since this is often closely interrelated with the patient's symptoms. Specific recommendations, regarding for example psychopharmacology or other treatments such as ECT, need to be made, side effects anticipated, and some explanation given as to why one particular treatment or drug is being selected in preference to another. Other recommendations, including the way in which nurses should manage the patient, or the way the patient's environment should be restructured to diminish psychopathology, should also be discussed.

PSYCHIATRIC PROBLEMS IN GENERAL MEDICAL AND NEUROLOGICAL PATIENTS

The prevalence of psychiatric morbidity in medical populations is variously given from 15% to 90% of patients interviewed. The variation in figures is dependent upon the techniques used for detection of psychiatric illness, the severity taken to indicate an illness, and finally upon the population studied. Following a review of the literature, Lipowski stated that some 30–60% of in-patients and 50–80% of out-patients suffered from 'psychic distress or psychiatric illness of sufficient severity to create a problem for the health professions'. Using objective rating scales, Knights and Folstein[131] indicated that 33% of patients admitted to general medical wards showed cognitive impairment, and 46% had psychiatric disorders. They noted that ward physicians failed to identify over one-third of these abnormalities. Kirk and Saunders[132] examined 2716 patients attending a neurological out-patient clinic and assessed them for primary psychiatric illness: 13.2% were so diagnosed, and of these 82% had neuroses or personality disorders, 1% schizophrenia, and 17% affective disorders. Of those with a psychiatric diagnosis, headache was the most frequently reported symptom, other common ones being dizziness, body pain and cognitive disturbance. Blackouts and facial pain were seen far more commonly in women, and multiple symptomatology was noted to be present in over 50%. Thirty-nine per cent of patients with facial pain had an affective disorder, and virtually all patients with back pain, black-outs and aggressive behaviour showed some neurosis or personality disorder. De Paulo and Folstein[133] studied 126 patients admitted to hospital for neurological disorders with rating scale assessments including the General Health Questionnaire, and noted that 30% had cognitive deficits and 50% had emotional disorders. In many patients the psychopathology went unrecognized by the resident neurologist. On re-testing prior to discharge, 50% of the patients with cognitive deficits and 67% of those with emotional disturbance remained abnormal. Of the patients with psychiatric disability detected by Kirk and Saunders, only 14% were referred to a psychiatrist, and similar rates of referral were reported by De Paulo and Folstein.

The actual psychiatric diagnosis of such patients varies from series to series, again dependent upon the referral population. Generally organic brain syndromes and depression are the commonest, followed by personality disorders and psychoneuroses. Schizophrenia or paranoid psychoses are reported with much less frequency. Lipowski and Kiriakos[134] have analysed 200 neurological and neurosurgical in-patient referrals to a psychiatric consultation service. Only 48% of their patients were discharged with a definite neurological diagnosis, and 38% had both a neurological and a psychiatric disorder. Depression was the commonest diagnosis, occurring in 30.5% of the sample; 20% had an organic brain syndrome in one form or another; 5.5% personality disorders; and 7% schizophrenia. The depression often presented with somatic symptoms, but in addition was noted to coexist with neurological disease.

The main reasons for referral fell into two major categories: these were diagnostic and/or therapeutic problems, and ward management problems. The first group related to questions about the relative contribution of neurological pathology to the production of symptoms, especially patients with fits of undiagnosed aetiology; pain without a clearly-defined somatic focus for the origin; the coexistence of multiple sclerosis and conversion symptoms; and the differentiation between organic and psychiatric disorders in producing such symptoms as depersonalization, fugues or tremors. Another area of consultation was the assessment of personality change and in particular the relevance of neurological disease to such change. In addition the differentiation between acute organic brain syndromes and psychiatric disorders such as schizophrenia and depression was a common problem. Ward management difficulties were related to handling patients with personality problems, in which conflicts with physicians or nurses or with others looking after them were occurring, or whose emotional behaviour was seen as extreme in relation to the neurological illness from which they were suffering.

THE PATIENT'S RESPONSE TO ILLNESS

As Schilder has pointed out, there is practically no symptom in any disease which is not finally modified by the attitude of the personality. Particularly in chronic disease, personality factors play an outstanding part (Ref. 135, p.194). Assessment of the personality and of the individual coping style of patients has therefore great relevance for understanding symptoms as they present. Any disease represents for the patient, injury, or threat of injury, and very often threat of loss of some ideal, body function, body image, role or job. In this respect neurological illness is particularly stressful and itself leads to psychiatric symptoms. The latter may manifest as a psychiatric illness such as depression or an anxiety state, but may also lead to lesser degrees of frustration, anger, withdrawal, denial, regression, and dependency. During illness the patient has to adjust to being in the hands of strangers and accepting a passive position, often being instructed to do things and obey commands in a way in which ordinarily he has not had to do.[136] Many patients are unable to make this adjustment and struggle against it, leading to a breakdown of doctor-patient or nurse-patient communications. As such these reactions are not specific to any particular disease but characterize the individual's usual way of responding to stress. A number of personality styles are defined, recognition of which is most helpful in clinical practice. The term 'style' refers to a form of behaviour that is identifiable in an individual by his or her actions, which in the medical context may be maladaptive for the patient. The more clearly defined relate to the personality disorders discussed in Chapter 4. Bibring[137] outlined seven categories of such behaviour and suggested appropriate management techniques when problems arose. These were: a dependent, over-demanding personality; the orderly, controlled personality; the dramatizing, emotionally involved, captivating personality; the long-suffering, self-sacrificing patient; the guarded, querulous, paranoid patient; the patient with feelings of supriority (narcissistic); and the patient who is uninvolved and aloof (schizoid). The suggestion is that each of these types react to the stress of illness and hospitalization with consequent anxiety which leads to an increased intensity of the basic characterological defences.

Lipowski[138] summarized the variables, in addition to personality structure, that influence any particular patient's response to disease. They included the meaning and importance for the patient of the affected part of the body or the actual lesion presenting and its relationship to the body image; beliefs about the causation of disease, including cultural and educational factors; the state of the patient's current interpersonal relationships; the extent of mutilation and loss of ability and the consequent socioeconomic disability for the patient; previous experience of disease; the patient's state of awareness and cognitive functioning; the degree of acceptance by the patient of the 'sick role'; and the doctor-patient relationship. With regard to the meaning of illness for individual patients, he pointed out that three major categories of meaning are recognized, namely loss, threat and gain. In neurological and neurosurgical practice a chief source of threat and consequent anxiety he suggested was the 'danger of impairment of highest integrative functions of the brain, and the impaired damage to the person'. The fact that in some patients illness paradoxically provides gain or relief for the patient must not be overlooked, and is implicit in certain varieties of abnormal illness behaviour discussed below.

While illness itself provides a potent source of stress for the patient, hospitalization likewise can lead to severe disturbances of behaviour. Wilson-Barnett,[139] in a number of studies investigating patients' emotional responses to hospital, has shown how certain patients who score high on the EPI Neuroticism Scale react strongly to even low levels of stress, which include the process of hospitalization itself or undergoing special tests such as barium X-ray examinations.

THE RELATIONSHIP BETWEEN PSYCHIATRIC AND SOMATIC ILLNESS

That there is a close link between psychiatric disorders and somatic illness is clear from a number of studies, some of which are discussed in this book. The relationship with regard to abnormal illness behaviour is discussed later in this chapter, and the problem of pain is discussed in Chapter 8. It is clear that neurological disorders, particularly those that affect the central nervous system, provoke a variety of psychiatric illnesses, some of which are specifically related to focal brain damage, but others of which closely resemble primary psychiatric illness. As indicated above, any physical disorder may aggravate predisposing personality disorders.

There are now a number of studies that indicate a relationship between a patient's life events and subsequent psychiatric and somatic illness.[103, 140] These studies have stressed how various life changes are followed by illness, and emphasize in particular so-called exit events, especially separations, including death of a child, spouse or close friend. A number of authors have commented on the close relationship between grief and bereavement and subsequent physical illness.[141, 142] Grief appears to be a definite syndrome with both psychiatric and somatic symptomatology, which may not occur immediately following loss but may be delayed. Somatic symptoms include feelings of exhaustion, digestive symptoms, loss of weight, rheumatism, rashes, headaches and panic attacks. However, not only is there an increased incidence of presentation to a doctor with somatic complaints following bereavement of a spouse, but also an increased subsequent mortality. Engel[143] in particular, has drawn attention to a psychological pattern that is associated with disease onset. He has termed this 'the giving-up/given-up complex'. The most characteristic feature is a sense of psychological impotence and a feeling that one is unable to cope with changes in the environment. The patient's coping mechanisms appear to have broken down, and in place of the smooth, almost effortless integration of behaviour normally seen, with confidence and mastery over events in the environment, there is a disruption in the patient's functioning and an alteration of self-perception. Patients express affects of helplessness and hopelessness, have a low self-image, and a loss of gratification from their life. He suggested that such a complex plays a significant role in modifying the ability to resist pathogenic factors, thus rendering patients liable to develop illness. Grief and bereavement were often associated with this state.

The possibility that emotional states are casually linked to somatic illness is an extremely old concept. A number of diseases have been defined as psychosomatic to express this relationship and several hypotheses have been put forward to explain the mechanisms including the symbol theories of the psychoanalysts; personality profile theories which suggest that specific personality profiles are aetiologically related to specific diseases; theories based on the physiological consequences of stress; ideas of the learning theorists; and some constitutional vulnerability theories.[144] Many of these concepts are firmly based in Cartesian dualism and most have failed to stand up to critical testing. Although a number of disorders are usually considered under the rubric of psychosomatic disorders, and these include asthma, migraine, peptic ulcer, colitis, hypertension and certain musculo-skeletal and cutaneous conditions, it is clear that in one sense all disorders have psychological and somatic components that can, and should be, taken into account. Recent advances in understanding brain-behaviour relationships and, in particular, observations that psychiatric disorders and 'stress' are associated with abnormal patterns of hormone release and changes in immunological responsiveness,[145] provide avenues for understanding psychosomatic mechanisms. The fact that disturbed function of an organ over time can lead to changes in structure is well known. The possibility that similar processes occur in the central nervous system cannot be discounted, and would explain many clinical observations on the relationships between psychiatric illness neurological disorders, some of which are outlined in other chapters of this book.

ABNORMAL ILLNESS BEHAVIOUR

In liaison psychiatry, abnormal illness behaviour and its variants provide some of the most interesting and yet puzzling phenomena encountered clinically. The term 'illness behaviour' was introduced by Mechanic to refer to 'the way in which given symptoms may be differently perceived, evaluated and acted upon or not acted upon by different kinds of people and in different social situations' (Ref. 146, pp.115–55). He pointed out how ethnic variations, cultural and developmental experiences determine a patient's reaction to threatening circumstances, and the great variety of response among different patients to the same illness condition. He says: 'Illness behaviour and the decision to seek medical advice frequently involve, from the patient's point of view, a rational attempt to make sense of his problem and cope with it within the limits of his intelligence and his social and cultural understandings, but this does not make it rational from a medical perspective'. Pilowsky, taking this concept further, defined 'abnormal illness behaviour' as 'the persistence of an inappropriate mode of perceiving, evaluating and acting in relation to one's state of health'.[147] This concept allows for further understanding of a number of overlapping clinical phenomena which are considered below including hysteria, hypochondriasis, Munchausen's syndrome, and factitious illness. As such, these names have provided conceptual difficulties for many physicians confronted with the clinical problems that patients present with, and have generated much sterile debate about their legitimacy as a diagnosis, their boundaries, and even their existence. As Pilowsky pointed out,[148] these diagnoses are usually initially made by physicians without psychiatric training on the basis of a perceived discrepancy between the degree of the objective somatic pathology noted, and the patient's reaction to it. He classified abnormal illness behaviour as shown in Table 5.1.[149] Of special interest for liaison psychiatry is the group he referred to as somatically focused abnormal illness behaviour. This presents either as 'illness affirming', in which the patient's says that he has some illness that the physician is unable to document, or as 'illness denying' when there is denial of illness that has been diagnosed or is apparent to another observer. In each of these categories the behaviour may be, in Pilowsky's categories, consciously or unconsciously motivated. Thus, consciously motivated, somatically focused abnormal illness behaviour covers malingering and the Munchausen syndrome. Unconsciously motivated illness

Table 5.1. A classification of abnormal illness behaviour (After Pilowsky[149])

Somatic focus
1. Illness affirming
   (a) Motivation conscious,
       e.g. Munchausen's syndrome, malingering.
   (b) Motivation unconscious,
       e.g. conversion phenomena, hypochondriasis (neurotic).
       Schizophrenia, monosymptomatic psychosis (psychotic).

2. Illness denying
   (a) Motivation conscious,
       e.g. to avoid insurance penalty or therapy.
   (b) Motivation unconscious,
       e.g. denial (neurotic or psychotic).
   (c) Neuropsychiatric,
       e.g. anosognosia.

Psychological focus
1. Illness affirming
   (a) Motivation conscious,
       e.g. Ganser states, malingering.
   (b) Motivation unconscious,
       e.g. amnesia, dissociative behaviour (neurotic).
       Delusions of amnesia (psychotic).

2. Illness denying
   (a) Motivation conscious,
       e.g. to avoid psychiatric consultation or hospitalization.
   (b) Motivation unconscious,
       e.g. denial in the presence of neurotic or psychotic illness
       with lack of insight.

behaviour of this category refers to hysteria, hypochondriasis, and conversion phenomena. Psychologically focused abnormal illness behaviour includes malingering, but in addition covers such syndromes as Ganser states, fugues and amnesias.

From this brief discussion it seems that the term abnormal illness behaviour has broad usage, yet fills satisfactorily the void left by those who suggest that, for example, hysteria or hypochondriasis do not exist (see below). Recognition of abnormal illness behaviour in the ward situation is most important since failure to make such a diagnosis will lead to unnecessary tests, which themselves may have both somatic and psychiatric morbidity, and possibly to inappropriate treatment with encouragement and reinforcement of the abnormal behaviour. The first step to recognition is the discrepancy noted between pathology elicited on examination, and the patient's presenting complaints. However, to finish investigation at such a stage and initiate discharge helps neither the patient nor the doctor. Full understanding of the patient's symptoms requires more elaborate assessment of personality, past illness behaviour history, present mental state, and the patient's current environmental and interpersonal stresses. As Pilowsky[147] pointed out this does not, and should not, require two separate examinations. Most relevant data can be obtained at a single interview if the appropriate technique is adopted. Often the initial examination of a patient, even when there is an early suggestion of abnormal illness behaviour, is entirely symptom and somatically focussed. This is followed by a number of investigations all of which turn out to be negative, at which stage the approach is suddenly 'switched' to a probing of the psychiatric status of the patient. This sudden turnabout may upset the patient, who then becomes indignant when asked to see a psychiatrist, since the implication must be that as 'nothing has been found' the symptoms are 'all in the mind' and thus imagined. It is far more logical and appropriate to make psychiatric and psychosocial enquiries at an early stage of any patient's investigation, pointing out to the patient, if necessary, that it is customary for patients to be asked a broad range of questions regarding themselves, their lives, and their illness so that all aspects of their problem can be adequately explored.

The mechanisms of the production of abnormal illness behaviour are poorly understood. However, as subsequent discussion on hysteria indicates, it is a widespread medical phenomenon, and to ignore it is to misunderstand the nature of symptom-formation in illness and to do patients misservice. Most studies that have been carried out indicate that abnormal illness behaviour is commoner in social classes 4 and 5, is commoner in large families, and is more frequently seen in the last-born of a family.[148] The influence of 'stress' is clear. Mechanic, in a study of 600 University students, (Ref. 146, p.129) showed that those with high 'perceived stress' used medical facilities far more than those within a low stress category. 'Distress' is therefore often more influential in ensuring that a patient will seek help from a doctor than the actual occurrence of a particular disease condition. Clinically the phenomenon of 'secondary gain', helpful diagnostically but by no means pathognomonic, is often elicited in these patients, and symptom-production is explained in terms of the stress reduction that occurs following attendant medical care.

Cultural differences in symptom production have been noted in a number of studies, the most often quoted being that of Zborowski.[150] He studied the ethnic differences in the expression of pain in patients presenting to a New York hospital. The Jewish and Italian patients responded to pain with emotional exaggeration, in contrast to the 'old Americans', and the Irish, who were more stoical and tended even to deny their pain. Italian patients primarily sought relief from pain whereas Jewish patients were concerned with the meaning and significance of their pain. His explanation of these differences lay in the different parental attitudes and responses towards health that the subjects received in childhood. The role of identification, symbolism, and past memories on symptom-formation has been stressed by authors such as Freud,[151] and Engel.[152] Freud,[151] and Pilowsky,[147] make the point that somatic sensations of some sort probably form the basis of every physical complaint. It may be physiological, such as a manifestation of anxiety which, while ignored by the majority, becomes the focus of preoccupation for patients with abnormal illness behaviour.

The relationship between abnormal illness behaviour and personality has been explored by Pilowsky.[148, 153] He specifically constructed a 53-item questionnaire called the 'Illness Behaviour Questionnaire' (IBQ), and noted that patients with abnormal illness behaviour were significantly different from other medical patients, showing illness conviction and symptom preoccupation, non-response to reassurance, and a need to deny a psychological component to their illness. From his investigations Pilowsky suggested that abnormal illness behaviour 'does not arise from the presence of physical disorder alone, nor is it characterized by an affective disorder but rather from a need to achieve a form of psychological equilibrium by adopting a particular sick role despite the belief of others that the role is inappropriate'.

Management of these problems is skilled and difficult. It is essential that patients are introduced early on in the course of their illness career to the idea that their symptoms may reflect psychiatric disability, and that once the suspicion of abnormal illness behaviour is high they are not instantly rejected as malingerers. It is not a physician's role to endow judgements about the rightness or wrongness of a patient's actions, but instead to understand their symptoms and to offer help that is needed. To quote Pilowsky again: 'The patient with abnormal illness behaviour is, in some ways, the ultimate test of our health care delivery system, for he responds and reacts to its every deficiency and shortcoming, and in so doing forces us repeatedly to re-examine our attitudes to every facet to illness from the pathological to the sociological, as they affect the patient, as they affect us, and as they affect the institutions in which we function.'

Hysteria

Of the various categories of abnormal illness behaviour, hysteria is the oldest referred to, and that which has provoked the most discussion. It appears to have been first mentioned in the Kahun papyrus of ancient Egypt in which various ailments were attributed to the displacement of the uterus. The Greeks continued the trend, and the word 'hystera' meaning uterus, was applied to the disorder. In the late middle ages Sydenham suggested it was the commonest chronic disorder encountered in his practice. The relationship to the female sex was reinforced by his suggestion that the equivalent disorder in men was 'hypochondriacal passion' — an ailment arising not from the uterus, but from the hypochondrium. The sexual theme was continued by others such as Charcot, who looked for ovarian pressure points in the disorder, and Freud with his concept of 'repression', primarily of sexual conflict, as a cause of the disorder. However, Willis is acknowledged as being one of the first to recognize that the brain, rather than the uterus, was involved; Sydenham, that there was a significant emotional component; and several authors, for example Landouzy and Charcot, that there was a relationship with 'organic' changes.[154, 155]

Chodoff and Lyons[156] drew attention to the semantic difficulties in the literature that hysteria presents, and clearly emphasized the separation between hysteria, a particular kind of psychosomatic symptomatology often referred to as conversion hysteria or conversion reaction, and the hysterical personality, a pattern of behaviour habitually exhibited by a certain individuals. In addition to these two separate meanings, other uses of the word include 'mass hysteria', in which there is an epidemic spread of symptoms in the absence of well-defined somatic pathology; and its use as a pejorative term which should be largely confined to the lay public. 'Anxiety hysteria' was used by Freud to describe a psychoneurotic disorder manifesting principally with phobias in which 'repression' was the principal defence mechanism. This use is now no longer employed. Finally, there is a growing literature on Briquet's hysteria, an apparently specific psychopathological entity named after the French physician, whose ideas later came to influence Charcot. Important issues to be discussed below include: (a) the relationship of the hysterical personality to hysteria; (b) the influence of neurological diseases in the presentation of hysteria; and (c) the relationship of sexuality to hysteria. Mass hysteria is not discussed here, and Briquet's syndrome is presented as a separate section.

The hysterical personality and hysteria

The essential features of the hysterical personality include egocentric attitudes, exhibitionism and dramatism, labile affects with excitability, emotional shallowness, flirtatiousness associated with sexual frigidity, dependency, and suggestibility. In its florid form this personality style is easily recognized, and experimentally, by use of standardized questionnaires, a number of authors have identified these trait patterns using factor analysis, and clearly distinguished them from, for example, obsessional personality traits.[157] Chodoff and Lyons, in a study of 17 patients with conversion phenomena, uncontaminated by known neurological disease, noted three with the hysterical personality, the others having a variety of personality disturbances, the main one being passive-aggressive.[156] Ljungberg, in a study of 381 patients, found 43% of the men and 47% of the women to have deviant personalities, 20.7% of the total having hysterical personalities.[158] Merskey and Trimble,[159] using a control group of patients with psychiatric illness, reported that the personality types of 89 patients with conversion symptoms included 17 with hysterical personalities, 17 with passive-immature-dependent personalities and 7 with obsessional personalities. In contrast, control psychiatric patients had a lower frequency of hysterical personalities, and a greater frequency of obsessional personalities. These data support the suggestion that there is an increased incidence of patients with the hysterical personality in those who present with conversion hysteria. However, it is also clear that the majority of patients do not conform to this particular style.

The relationship between neurological disease and hysteria

Gowers pointed out that hysterical symptoms frequently accompany diseases of the nervous system, and quoted Weir Mitchell who said: 'The symptoms of real disease are painted on an hysterical background.' Gowers reported that there was hardly a single disease of the nervous system that did not sometimes cause hysterical phenomena (Ref. 160, Vol. 2, p.988). Whitlock reported that 62.5% of patients with hysterical symptoms had significant coexistent or preceding histories of organic disorder, compared with 5% of the control group.[161] Merskey and Buhrich[162] reported that 61 of 89 patients with conversion symptoms also had organic disease, epilepsy being the commonest. Slater[163] assessed 85 patients diagnosed as 'hysteria'. Initially 19 had a combined diagnosis of hysteria and organic pathology. At follow-up he found that 12 others had died, four from suicide, and neurological illness developed in 22 which was not detected at the time of the initial assessment. Tissenbaum et al.[164] reviewed 395 patients with neurological disease and noted that 13.4% were diagnosed as 'functional' for up to 8 years before pathology was recognized. These data all indicate a close link between neurological disease and the presentation of hysteria.

The relationship of sexuality to hysteria

The early historical relationships have been noted. The modern era began with Freud's speculations on the mechanisms of hysterical phenomena. With Breuer[151] he suggested that undischarged affects could be 'converted' into somatic phenomena, and that symptoms were determined by 'repressed' experiences from an individual's past. The conflicts that led to repression were envisaged as sexual, and as the theory evolved were linked to infantile sexuality and Oedipal conflicts. The suggestion that repressed sexuality is linked with hysteria should mean that disturbed sexuality is a feature of patients with conversion symptoms. Few actual studies have been conducted on this relationship. Winokur and Leonard[165] examined a group of patients with Briquet's syndrome and commented on the deterioration of the sexual activity that occurred after marriage from a relatively normal premarital one when compared with control data provided by Kinsey. In particular they noted a decrease in the frequency of intercourse and orgasm, increased frigidity and increased extramarital coitus or divorce. However, there was not in this study an invariable association between hysteria, as they have defined it, and disturbed sexuality, although many of their patients had conversion symptoms amongst their complaints. Lazare and others, in investigations discussed above which measured personality traits by factor analysis, found that the factor loading for 'fear of sexuality' was low for the group of patients with the hysterical personality. Merskey and Trimble[159] assessed disturbances of sexuality in 89 patients with conversion symptoms, and found that compared with control psychiatric patients there was a signficantly higher incidence of abnormality in the conversion group, especially long-term frigidity. In addition they were able to relate sexual disturbance to personality type and indicated that the hysterical personality patients were more liable to be frigid than others.

Clinical findings

The frequency with which conversion symptoms occur in medical practice varies from 5 to 25%, depending on the population chosen. Some settings such as neurological clinics and wards attract a particularly high number of such patients. While it is often said that the prevalence of these complaints is declining, this is probably not the case, again particularly if special settings are taken into account. The prevalence of the diagnosis of 'hysteria' for the in-patients at the National Hospital, Queen Square, is given in Table 5.2 for three years selected from three decades. While a decline is seen to occur in the late 1950s, no further fall is seen for the 1960s or the 1970s. Other studies also note declines over the years although again it is mainly in the 1950s. The symptomatology of the patients from the National Hospital sample is shown in Table 5.3. In this setting it is seen that apart from a non-significant decline in the prevalence of motor disorders receiving a diagnosis of hysteria, the pattern has changed little over recent years. This is in contradiction to some other studies where a decline in the frequency of hysterical fits and 'mental conversion' has been noted.[166]

Engel has listed conversion symptoms as shown in Table 5.4.[152] They are divided into two broad groups: motor conversion symptoms, which include paralyses, spasms etc.; and mental dissociative phenomena, such as amnesias

82

Table 5.2. Incidence of the diagnosis of 'hysteria' at the National Hospital
for various years

	1951, 53, 55	1961, 63, 65	1971, 73, 75
No. of diagnoses	104	82	91
No. of admissions	6887	9608	9586
Percentage	1.55	0.85	0.95

$\chi^2 = 18.1, DF = 2, p < 0.001.$

Table 5.3. Symptom distribution of patients with 'hysteria' over three decades.

	1951, 53, 55	1961, 63, 65	1971, 73, 75
Total for all patients	171	144	159
Motor	51 (32.7%)	53 (36.8%)	40 (25.1%)
Tremors	2 (1.1%)	5 (3.4%)	7 (4.4%)
Convulsions	19 (11.1%)	19 (13.2%)	22 (13.8%)
Anaesthesias	10 (5.8%)	8 (5.5%)	11 (6.9%)
Visual	10 (5.8%)	12 (8.3%)	16 (10.0%)
Pain	43 (25.1%)	23 (16.0%)	36 (22.6%)
Amnesia, etc.	6 (3.5%)	8 (5.5%)	7 (4.4%)
Dizziness, etc.	16 (9.3%)	12 (8.3%)	15 (9.4%)
Other	9 (5.3%)	4 (2.8%)	5 (3.4%)

Note decline in frequency of motor symptoms in the 1970s.

and black-outs. Pain is the most frequently described symptom, although some authors would prefer not to include pain as a conversion disorder. Amongst neurological patients seizures are noted especially frequently, although all symptoms of neurological illness may present at one time or another. Where symptoms are unilateral they are more often seen on the left.

Diagnosis must rest not only on negative neurological criteria, but also upon positive psychiatric evidence, and where they can be demonstrated, positive neurological signs. The initial feature is the discrepancy between the observed pathology and the patient's complaints. The history may reveal other episodes suggestive of conversion phenomena, and a personality disorder with a propensity to seek medical help. Illness experiences in childhood need to be explored, especially illnesses that may have occurred in significant other persons in a patient's life. A number of patients may be found who have a long history of operations, investigations and complaints which, when carefully probed, all seem to indicate early episodes of abnormal illness behaviour. Psychopathology in the form of current affective illness may be quite clear and must always be looked for. However, often on account of the way the patient is presenting, it may easily be overlooked. Some authors write of 'la belle indifference' — a tendency to deny problems and to show unconcern regarding apparently serious symptoms. Although this is not regularly present, it may

Table 5.4. Conversion symptoms (from Engel[152])

Motor system
Generalized weakness (pseudomyasthenia gravis), fatigue
Paralysis or weakness of extremities
Muscle spasms, stiffness, contractures, pseudo-contractures, torticollis, camptocormia (bent back), writer's cramp
Abnormal movements, tics, tremors, localized seizures
Gait disturbances, astasia–abasia
Aphonia, dysphonia
Occular fixation, ptosis, blepharospasm, blinking

Sensory systems
Pain, aching, pressure, burning, fullness, hollowness, pruritus
Anaesthesia, hypaesthesia, dysaesthesia, hyperaesthesia
Sensations of dizziness, swaying, falling
Sensations of coldness, localized or generalized
Sensations of warmth, localized or generalized
Blindness, amblyopia, clouding of vision, tubular vision, scotomata, monocular diplopia, polyplopia
Deafness
Loss of taste, bitter taste, burning tongue

Level of consciousness
Fugue, amnesia
Stupor, coma
Convulsions, seizures
Syncope
Dizziness, lightheadedness, faintness, giddiness
Sleepiness, narcolepsy, somnambulism

Respiratory system
Cough, tickle, hoarseness
Dyspnoea, choking, suffocation, smothering, inability to breathe, hyperventilation
Sighing, yawning
Wheezing
Breath holding
Pain in chest, upper, or lower respiratory passages

Cardiovascular system
'Pain in the heart'
Palpitations
Dyspnoea, orthopnoea

Gastrointestinal system
Sensations of dryness, burning, 'acid' in mouth or throat
Anorexia
Bulimia
Thirst, polydipsia
Dysphagia, lump in the throat (globus)
Nongaseous abdominal distention, bloating
Pain, burning, fullness, and other abdominal sensations
Diarrhoea, frequent bowel movements, tenesmus, constipation
Anorectal sensations — fullness, burning, pruritus ani

Urinary system
Retention, incontinence, urgency, frequency, dysuria, pain

Genital system
Anaesthesia, paraesthesias, pain, pruritus, fullness, and other sensations
Dyspareunia, vaginismus
Pseudocyesis

lead to masking of psychiatric disturbance, and be easily missed by the inexperienced physician. So-called secondary gain may be clear at the outset, or only be discovered later in the course of the patient's illness. However, secondary gain is often based on value judgements by physicians rather than necessarily reflecting reality for the patient, and the danger of hinging a diagnosis of hysteria on evidence of secondary gain cannot be over-emphasized. Stress in itself is often a necessary, but not a sufficient, criterion for the emergence of conversion symptoms.

Of positive neurological criteria, the presence of hemianaesthesia or other clearly defined anaesthetic patches, not conforming to anaesthesias seen following neurological illness, is perhaps the most important. Often all modalities of sensation are affected, and in the hemianaesthesia the body and face of one side, most often the left, are affected up to the midline. Other neurological signs usually involve illogical findings in terms of established neurological illness, such as the absence of wasting and normal tone and reflexes in paralysed limbs; contraction of antagonistic muscles following passive movement or demonstration of movement in 'paralysed' muscles with special manoeuvres.[167, 168]

There are a number of studies on the morbidity, mortality and prognosis of patients with conversion symptoms. Slater's work has been referred to above, and the high incidence of the patients who are later diagnosed as having neurological or other organic illness is clear. Likewise he found a number of patients who go on to develop florid psychiatric illness. Of his 85 patients, four had committed suicide, two were schizophrenic, one was obsessional, and seven had recurrent depressions.[169] Slater's results, compared to the results of other follow-up studies, are shown in Table 5.5.[158, 163, 170-3] Although many show less overt morbidity than Slater's series, the figures do indicate that many patients diagnosed as hysteria or conversion phenomena do go on to develop more readily identifiable illness of both a psychiatric and non-psychiatric kind. Ljungberg[158] reported that after 1 year, 43% of men and 35% of women still had symptoms, and after 5 years the figures were 25% and 22% respectively. These latter figures were unchanged after 10–15 years' observation. He reported that the prognosis was better for patients with 'non-deviating personalities', and those who presented with astasia–abasia, paralysis, amnesia and aphonia. Patients in certain settings, e.g. military personnel at times of action, with acute onset illness have a much better prognosis than others.

The mechanisms of hysteria

As indicated, it is probably preferable to view hysteria as a variety of abnormal illness behaviour. A number of interrelated factors lead to the production of symptoms, the relative contribution of each one varying from case to case. The close interrelationship with organic illness is emphasized. This has led some authors, such as Slater, to suggest that 'hysteria is . . . a delusion but also a snare'.[169] Recognition of the interplay between the personality and somatic illness, and the probability that the location and pattern of symptoms presented are nearly always determined by somatic changes, avoids the problems raised by assuming that the diagnosis excludes organic changes. The most important aspect of the relationship between organic disease and conversion phenomena is that psychiatrists are fully aware of the detection and progression of neurological disease, and for the diagnosis of hysteria to be regarded as a disorder requiring follow-up and re-analysis from time to time,

Table 5.5. Follow-up studies on patients with hysteria[158, 163, 170-3]

Study	Age (in years)	No. No.	F.U. F.U.	Female (%)	F.U. (in years)	Disabled (%)	Psych. illness (%)	Organic illness (%)	Dead (%)
Carter (1949)	16-40	100	90	60	4-6	21	4	0	1 (1 suicide)
Ziegler (1954)	Mean 29	66	62	94	20-25	57	38	14	23 (1 suicide)
Ljungberg (1957)	Mean 43	401	381	61	7-23	38 (1 yr) 23 (5 yr) 20 (15 yr)	5	4	11 (6 suicides)
Guze (1963)	14-67	37	29	84	3-10	85	6	18	–
Slater and Glithero (1965)	Mean 38	99	85	53	7-11	85	13	58	12 (4 suicides)
Lewis (1975)	Mean 32	98	98	74	7-12	45	11	1	8 (1 suicide)

as opposed to being one which leads to immediate discharge of patients from physicians' care.

Schilder attempted to bring together the psychoanalytic interpretations of hysteria and the neurological findings, and developed the concept of 'organic repression' (Ref. 174, p.115). He emphasized phenomena which, at a structural level, repeated what was going on in other repressions at 'the so-called purely psychic level'. It is 'a similarity in the apparatuses which are in function or out of function, but very likely the agency which gets the apparatus out of function is different, and this agency works in a different way in the purely organic cases . . . .'. Psychoanalytic speculations regarding 'conversion' have not been verified experimentally, and while an increased frequency of sexual disturbance is noted in such patients, it is by no means universal. As Chodoff pointed out while referring to conversion symptoms: 'Miscarried sexuality probably does not play the major role in their pathogenesis, for our epoch at least'.[175] The term 'conversion' fails to contribute to the understanding of exactly what is being converted into what, and in many cases explanation of the symptoms can readily be obtained without reference to a Freudian libido theory. Some authors have attempted to explain conversion phenomena at the neurophysiological level. Charcot felt that the location of symptoms was in some way represented in abnormal neurophysiological activity within the brain. More recently, Ludwig[176] has put forward a neurobiological theory of conversion phenomena based on the suggestion of Whitlock that symptoms were related to a selective depression of the awareness of bodily function. Ludwig invoked the concept of corticofugal inhibition of afferent impulses, mediated by the reticular activating system. Walters took these ideas further stressing the role of the limbic system, with close connections to the parietal and fronto-temporal regions of the brain, as a possible mechanism for the altered perception and behaviour which occurs in relationship to past memories and feelings.[177]

In summary, conversion symptoms are more likely to occur in relationship to personality disturbances, not exclusively but often with the hysterical personality; sexual maladjustment; affective disturbances; and chronic brain lesions. Social circumstances and stress are often important precipitating factors, particularly in acute illness, some patients being much more vulnerable on account of personality factors to break down than others.

Treatments

Almost all treatments available for neuropsychiatric illness have at one time or another been used in the management of conversion phenomena. In the acute situation where the precipitating factors are clear, suggestion, hypnosis, or suggestion and abreaction under thiopentone have been advocated.[170] Behaviour therapy, using positive or negative feedback, desensitization and operant conditioning, brief psychotherapy, and occasionally psychoanalysis have proved useful. However, removal of the symptoms, especially if carried out in the absence of continuing support, can lead to the emergence of florid psychopathology and occasionally suicide.

Recurrent attention must be paid to the possibility of the development of recognizable neurological disease, and where suspected referral to an appropriate specialist made. Depression, psychosis and anxiety states or other psychiatric symptomatology should be treated as necessary. In long-term intractable cases, admission to a psychiatric ward in hospital in order to assess and explore the patient's behaviour more thoroughly can sometimes be rewarding. While removal from the patient's life situation in itself can be therapeutic, the acceptance by the patient that it is to a psychiatric ward rather than to any other ward that they need to be admitted is a major step necessary to any improvement.

Briquet's syndrome

A number of patients have been described, with clearly defined characteristics, which have been referred to by Guze and his colleagues as Briquet's syndrome.[178-80] The patients are all young females, polysymptomatic, and characteristically have a history of an excessive number of surgical operations and hospitalizations, numerous vague complaints, frigidity and often dyspareunia. This disorder has a genetic basis and is linked to sociopathic personality traits. While it has been suggested that Briquet's syndrome is a synonym for hypochondriacal neurosis, a variant of the hysterical personality disorder, or represents one end of a spectrum of hysterical disorders, the possibility that it exists as an independent entity is seriously maintained. It occurs in 1-2% of consecutive female patients attending for investigation, and in 10% of psychiatric in-patients. In that it is by definition an intractable disorder and extremely difficult to treat, recognition of such patients, particularly by general physicians, would seem to be of vital importance. Unnecessary surgical intervention, which clearly occurs, could be avoided, and the recommended management instituted, which includes reassurance, relaxation techniques, and low doses of non-habit-forming psychotropic drugs.

Hypochondriasis

For Sydenham, hypochondriasis was hysteria that occurred in males. It was not until the nineteenth century that the disorder came to be associated more specifically with a morbid preoccupation with health. As with the term 'hysteria', it has a pejorative lay meaning and medically there has been much discussion as to whether it exists as an independent entity. Its use is often unclear, describing symptoms, personality styles and behaviour.

Hypochondriacal symptoms preoccupy the patient's concern and sometimes completely dominate his or her life. Usually the complaints are multiple but monosymptomatic varieties occur, and merge with monosymptomatic delusional states and dysmorphophobia. Most commonly reported complaints involve the head, neck, abdomen and chest, and where the symptoms are unilateral they predominantly affect the left side. The most commonly associated psychiatric symptoms are depression and anxiety.

Kenyon[181] examined the records of 512 patients with a diagnosis of hypochondriasis and noted that pain was the most prominent problem, occurring in nearly 70%. This varied from specific symptoms such as headaches, to rather diffuse vague complaints. The bodily systems mainly involved were musculo-skeletal, gastrointestinal, and the central nervous system. However, a wide variety of other symptoms were noted, including cardio-respiratory, ophthalmological and otoneurological ones. The latter resulted in preoccupation with hearing, dizziness, vertigo, tinnitus and sinus trouble. Kenyon also listed concern over body appearance, and sexual hypochondriasis, amongst the spectrum of presenting problems.

Pilowsky[153] devised a questionnaire to measure hypochondriacal attitudes. On analysis he located three factors which corresponded to three dimensions of hypochondriasis described in the literature. These were bodily preoccupation, disease phobia, and conviction of the presence of disease with non-response to reassurance. In discussing the status of hypochondriasis, especially its relationship to hysteria and Briquet's syndrome, Merskey (Ref. 155, pp.131–3) tentatively offered the following classification:

(a) Delusional hypochondriasis: in which symptoms are part of a schizophrenic or affective disorder.
(b) Symptomatic hypochondriasis: which results from the development of a dementia. Delusional features may or may not be present.
(c) Hysterical hypochondriasis: this group may include Briquet's syndrome, and is marked by the occurrence of detectable motor conversion symptoms, some degree of satisfaction on the part of the patient, relative lack of disease phobia, and sometimes the classical labile histrionic features noted in the hysterical personality.
(d) Pure hypochondriasis.

The last group he suggested are those who do not have the conditions outlined in (a), (b) or (c), and do not have conversion symptoms or non-somatic complaints. They show the characteristics outlined by Pilowsky, and can clearly be shown to differ from patients with Briquet's syndrome. To quote Merskey: 'These patients show excessive concern with bodily function, a failure to respond to sympathetic management and reassurance by relinquishing their complaint, a marked fear of the occurrence of physical disease and a continuing or markedly recurring belief that they have got a disease. They show dependence on medical personnel and often are dissatisfied with them. A pattern of cultivated meticulous valetudinarianism may be prominent together with detailed ordering of the smallest items of daily life in terms of health and illness with cupboards overflowing with laxatives and home remedies, punctilious compliance with dietary fads, etc.'.

In stressing the existence of a pure form of hypochondriasis Merskey is in disagreement with Kenyon, who after a review of the literature and his own study felt that if it existed at all it was a rarity, and that the majority of cases should be considered as secondary to some psychiatric illness or personality disturbance.[181]

Although reported commoner in males, in social classes IV and V and amongst the young and elderly, the aetiology of hypochondriacal phenomena is not understood. Attempts to demonstrate well-defined premorbid personality styles have not been successful, and psychoanalytic speculations are even less well founded than those for hysteria.

Mild symptoms, such as sudden preoccupation with palpitations, often associated with minimal anxiety, may subside with examination and reassurance. In more severe forms minor or major tranquillizers may be required. However, hypochondriasis, especially in severe degrees, is often an associated symptom of more florid psychiatric disturbance or, especially in the elderly, early dementia, and in these cases treatment must be directed at the underlying problem. Delusions in particular need recognition since an unshakeable conviction of mistaken ideas, in the light of adequate reassurance and testing, is psychotic and as such requires antipsychotic treatments. In particular, monosymptomatic hypochondriacal delusional states have been reported to respond to pimozide (Orap). Rarely leucotomy has been necessary for severely disabled patients.

Munchausen's syndrome and related problems

A number of conditions are seen from time to time in practice in which excessive use of hospital facilities occurs, which for reasons to be discussed, are thought to differ from hysteria. These include Munchausen's syndrome, 'deliberate disability' and polysurgical addiction. Malingering, also included in this spectrum of disorders, is discussed in Chapter 7.

Munchausen's syndrome was first described by Asher.[182] He referred to it as a common syndrome and defined three types: the acute abdominal type; the haemorrhagic type; and the neurological type. The latter presented with paroxysmal headaches, loss of consciousness and fits. However, it is clear from the subsequent literature that a large variety of symptoms may be produced, which include psychiatric disability and feigned bereavement.[183]

Bursten[184] suggested three major features of the syndrome. First, the dramatic presentation of one or more medical complaints with a long history of hospitalization and operations; secondly, a pseudologia fantastica; and thirdly, the feature of wandering from hospital to hospital. It is this last feature that particularly distinguishes the disorder from some other varieties of abnormal illness behaviour.

The reasons for patients' behaviour in these cases is poorly understood. Some have suggested drug addiction; the need for board and lodgings; the desire to escape from the police; or even a grudge against doctors and hospitals which is satisfied by frustrating and deceiving. Other suggestions are that the patient's behaviour is related to masochism; a defence against psychotic disintegration; excessive dependency, or an hysterical defence mechanism, although none of these have been convincingly demonstrated. Patients with Munchausen's syndrome are said to be more aware of their manipulations than patients with hysteria, in this sense being similar to the malingerer. However, while 'aware' of what they do, patients are said to be 'unaware' of the actual reasons why they do such things. This differentiation with respect to both hysteria and malingering is shown in Table 5.6.

Table 5.6. The differentiation between hysteria, malingering and Munchausen's syndrome

	Hysteria	Munchausen's syndrome	Malingering
Motivation	Unknown*	Unknown	Known
Knowledge of act	Unknown	Known	Known

*Known or unknown refers to patient's knowledge.

What is clear is that exposure and confrontation leads to immediate indignation and usually self-discharge. Psychiatric consultation is nearly always rejected and difficult to achieve, although case reports indicate that nearly all patients have a severe personality disturbance, most appropriately called psychopathic. It is this personality disorder which distinguishes them from another group of patients described by Hawkins et al. [185] presenting with 'deliberate disability'. They described 19 cases, 16 of whom were female. The disability did not appear connected to immediate material gain or advantage, but all patients showed skilful simulation of illness, sometimes involving severe disfigurement, pain, or even threat to life. They noted a high proportion were nurses or related to nurses, and suggested that in the production of the patient's symptoms disturbed parent–child or sib relationships and emotional immaturity were more involved than secondary gain. In particular evidence of severe personality disorder in their group was lacking. At follow-up eight patients remained severely disabled. A high rate of medical and paramedical personnel, noted in their group, has also been commented on by other authors in relation to factitious hypoglycaemia and insulin abuse.[186] Identification with physicians and knowledge of medical techniques are probably important features leading to the clinical picture.[155]

CHAPTER 6

Organic Brain Syndromes: Acute and Chronic

Although a psychiatric presentation of organic brain disease is a common clinical occurrence, understanding the 'organic brain syndromes' is still at a rudimentary level. There is poor standardization of nomenclature, inadequate criteria for diagnosis, and a lack of knowledge of the mechanisms involved in the production of the clinical picture. The term 'organic brain syndrome' is used pragmatically to define psychiatric illness caused by coarse brain disease, or metabolic disturbances. It is not proposed that a clear demarcation exists between such illness and other forms of psychiatric illness, since it is becoming clear that, for example, schizophrenia has identifiable organic components, and some presentations of organic brain disorders are clinically indistinguishable from primary psychiatric illness. However, the importance of understanding and diagnosing organic brain syndromes is that the aetiology often resides in structural, as opposed to functional, brain changes, and that treatment is primarily aimed at the correction or halting of the disease process. In that an acute organic brain syndrome may precede severe brain damage or even death, its recognition is obviously important since prompt intervention may lead to significant change in prognosis.

The classification of the organic brain syndromes is shown in Table 6.1. Acute organic brain syndromes and the consequences of chronic focal disorders of the brain are discussed in this chapter, followed by a presentation of dementia, head injury, cerebrovascular accidents and multiple sclerosis in the next. Other neurological illnesses which may present with psychiatric illness are discussed in other chapters.

There is no clear-cut dichotomy between the acute and chronic organic brain syndromes. While the paradigm of the acute organic brain syndrome with global impairment is delirium, and dementia that of a chronic, often irreversible disorder, a spectrum of clinical pictures is encountered. The progression of a delirium into a dementia, the occurrence of delirium in

Table 6.1. Organic brain syndromes (after Lipowski[187])

Global impairment	Acute	(Delirium)
	Subacute	
	Chronic	(Dementia)
Selective impairment	Hallucinosis	
	Amnestic syndrome	
	Focal brain syndromes	

dementia, or the reversibility of a dementia, indicate that the terms 'acute' and 'chronic' have no necessary prognostic or aetiological implications.

DELIRIUM AND THE ACUTE ORGANIC BRAIN SYNDROME

Although an acute psychiatric illness consequent on physical illness was recognized for centuries, prior to the nineteenth century little attempt had been made to distinguish these phenomena from other forms of psychiatric morbidity. Any trauma it seems was likely to result in psychopathology, and the idea of a 'unitary psychosis' was accepted by many. In contrast to these views, Kraepelin suggested specific psychopathologies for various types of physical insults. It was however Bonhoeffer who first made a clear distinction between 'endogenous' psychoses, and the 'exogenous psychic reaction types'. Exogenous referred to insults arising outside the brain, and he described five resulting clinical pictures. Since his time the concept of the acute exogenous reaction type has been broadened, such that all severe physical disturbances, including intrinsic brain lesions, that lead to psychiatric disorders, are now encompassed by it.[188] Of the types he identified, delirium, twilight states, and hallucinoses are still used as clinical diagnoses. The term delirium refers to disturbance of consciousness with impairment of cognitive ability, consequent on disturbed cerebral metabolism.[187] It is synonymous with 'confusional state', although some authors distinguish between delirium — 'an obtunded state accompanied by incoherence' — and confusional state — 'incoherence accompanied by an obtunded state'[188] — suggesting that in the latter there is incoherent thinking without an immediately observable lowering of consciousness or the presence of accompanying illusions and hallucinations. Other authors have used the term 'delirium' for incoherence of cognitive processes plus increased motor restlessness and hallucinations.[189]

Lipowski[190] has suggested that the term delirium be defined by the following criteria:
(a) The individual is awake and usually capable of responding verbally.
(b) There is evidence of impairment of thinking, memory, perception and attention that fluctuates over time.
(c) There is an impaired ability to comprehend the environment and internal perceptions in accordance with the individual's past experience and knowledge.

(d) There is usually a concomitant change in the frequency of the EEG, which varies *pari passu* with the level of cognition.

The common factor in these states is an acute disturbance of consciousness, which is initially reversible, which presents as a global impairment of cognitive processes.

Using such definitions does not imply that patients with delirium are always over-active, hallucinated and deluded. Observation in general hospital wards reveals that many patients with delirium go undiagnosed, as their behaviour is not overtly disturbed, often being listless and apathetic. As defined, delirium is the most commonly occurring psychosis seen in general medical practice and estimates of its occurrence range from 5 to 10% of hospitalized patients at some time during their stay, with a much higher prevalence in the elderly. Lipowski quotes Bleuler *et al.* who estimated that some 30% of the 20–70-year-old population will sustain an episode of delirium within their lifetime.

The range of activity seen is very variable. In the early stages restlessness, irritability, fatiguability and sleep disturbances occur, while later many patients progress to develop florid psychiatric symptoms which may resemble depression, paranoid states, schizophrenia, or anxiety, and may mistakenly lead to the diagnosis of a primary psychiatric illness. Patients may show disturbed thinking with delusions of a paranoid nature, hallucinations which are predominantly visual, illusions, hyperactivity, apathy and stupor, aggressive outbursts and affective changes. Characteristically these symptoms of delirium fluctuate over a period of hours. So-called lucid intervals appear unpredictably, and last for minutes or hours. Usually the mental state of the patient deteriorates in late evening and night-time leading to the phenomenon of 'sundowning' (when the sun goes down the patient gets up).

Clinically, disorientation for time, place, and person is a most important diagnostic feature. Disorientation for time is usually the first symptom, followed by the others, and the degree of disorientation tends to fluctuate with the alteration of consciousness. Patients also show disturbed attention span with distractibility, impaired memory and a decreased capacity for abstract thinking, and occasionally confabulation. They perform badly on serial sevens, digit span, repeating digits backwards, and calculation tests, misjudging the passage of time. These tests may be used at the bedside to help make a diagnosis.

The electroencephalogram is most valuable in confirming a diagnosis. The basic frequencies are nearly always slowed, and the alteration of the α-rhythm frequency monitors the changes in disturbance of consciousness. This change may not always be apparent, however, if an initially fast α-rhythm falls into the normal range. Rare exceptions to this rule occur, notably with delirium tremens, when EEG fast activity is more frequently seen than slowing.[191] If there is any doubt about the aetiology of psychotic illness, especially if it is of acute onset and an acute organic brain syndrome is suspected, then an EEG investigation is mandatory. Where facilities exist, serial EEG recordings will enable the clinical progress of the patient to be monitored.

Table 6.2. Main differential diagnostic features of psychotic states: delirium compared with schizophrenia

	Acute organic brain syndrome	Schizophrenia
Hallucinations	Visual	Auditory
Clouding of consciousness	+	0
Fluctuation	+	0
Worse at night	+	0
EEG	Abnormal	Normal (?)

The main differential diagnostic features of delirium in comparison with schizophrenia are shown in Table 6.2. Another difficulty is differentiating a retarded delirium from a retarded depression. Again, correct mental status examination and an EEG will resolve the diagnosis.

Table 6.3. Aetiological factors in delirium

Infective	
Traumatic	especially head injury
Neoplastic	Primary, secondary or non-metastatic
CNS disorders	especially tumours, epilepsy, encephalitis, meningitis, etc.
Cardiac disease	
Cerebrovascular disease	e.g. hypertensive encepholpathy, C.V.A.
Respiratory disease	
Endocrine disease	
Renal disease	
Hepatic disease	
Metabolic	e.g. hypoglycaemia, porphyria, electrolyte disturbance, hypercalcaemia, alkalosis, acidosis.
Poisons	e.g. heavy metals and organic solvents, alcohol.
Drugs	especially polypharmacy: psychotropic drugs; alcohol, anticonvulsants and L-dopa
Others	steroids
	irradiation
	vitamin deficiency
	anaemia
	hypoxia
	heat

The medical causes of delirium are outlined in Table 6.3, and it can be seen that they cover a broad range of illnesses. However, as the final common pathway in the production of the disorder is disturbance of cerebral metabolism which affects those areas of the brain necessary for consciousness, delay in recognition may lead to permanent impairment of brain function and to the development of a chronic organic brain syndrome.

The final clinical picture and the progress of the disorder is dependent on a number of host and environmental factors in addition to the somatic illness. Lipowski[187] considered these in detail (see Table 6.4). Both younger and older

Table 6.4. Factors modifying the presentation of delirium (after Lipowski[187])

(a) Characteristics of the organic factors:	strength of noxious agent number of pathological factors global or selective involvement of cerebral structures rate of change of brain milieu duration of pathology static or progressive nature of pathology
(b) Characteristics of host:	age individual vulnerability to a given pathogenic factor personality factors sleep deprivation presence of chronic systemic disease presence of pre-existent brain damage current emotional state
(c) Characteristics of the environment:	sensory input — overload or underload social isolation unfamiliarity with surroundings quality of interpersonal relationships

patients are more prone to develop delirium, and in the latter group pre-existing mild chronic organic brain disease often lowers the threshold for its appearance. Multiple factors may be responsible, again particularly in the elderly age group. For example, a mild electrolytic imbalance, mild anaemia, and hypoxia combined with a mild pyrexia may be enough to precipitate the clinical illness. Although it is likely that everybody under sufficient physical stress will show some features of delirium, it appears that some people are more susceptible than others. There is no evidence of a hereditable diathesis, but both trait anxiety, and the cognitive style of field dependence may be predisposing factors, as may be addiction to alcohol and other drugs. Bleuler and others[192] studied 600 patients with brain tumours, and found 37% had some acute organic brain syndrome. The occurrence of the latter was not related to the site of localization of the tumour.

The clinical picture may be adversely affected by alteration of the patient's sensory input. Again it is the elderly who are the most sensitive to the disorganizing effect of restrictive or excessive sensory stimulation, and even moving the patient from home to the unfamiliar hospital environment may precipitate disintegration. Sensory deprivation may occur in hospital, when the patient is left alone in a monotonous environment, leading to a worsening of the mental state. Almost certainly the phenomenon of sundowning is catalysed by the turning off of the ward lights and restriction of communication with others that patients enjoy during the day-time. Similarly, the onset of delirium in certain situations, such as eye surgery or in respiratory tanks, is explained by this mechanism.

The clinical course of delirium is marked by fluctuation which, in the presence of the same physical illness, may well be primarily related to alteration of environmental factors. Symptoms of the disorder rarely last for more than 4 weeks, and while the overall tendency is to recover, in some patients the outcome is a chronic organic brain syndrome or even death. The latter may result from the physical illness that initially led to the delirium, or from the patient inadvertently harming himself while in a confused state.

The management of delirium

The major reason for making the diagnosis is to distinguish psychoses that require primary psychiatric intervention, from those requiring exploration of underlying somatic illnesses. When diagnosed, it is essential in management to treat the medical condition that is responsible. The origin may be multifactorial, and in some patients no clear single identifiable illness is implicated. In such cases attention to fluid and electrolyte balance, correction of any haematological abnormalities, and attention to adequate nutrition is important. Note must always be taken of any medication the patient is receiving since it may be the prime factor responsible for the delirium.

Since the majority of patients with delirium are general ward patients, there is often an immediate demand that they be transferred on account of the disruption they may be causing. However, this may not be helpful, especially if it leads to transfer to a psychiatric unit where general medical cover is not readily available, and a delay in the recognition and treatment of the somatic illness may occur.

General management must be aimed at keeping the patient as calm as possible. This should not be achieved by heavy sedation, which in itself may be harmful; but preferably initially by environmental manipulation and small doses of medications. Restraint, which leads to further restriction of sensory input and patient combativeness, should be avoided if possible. The patients should be nursed to provide adequate interpersonal contact for sufficient sensory stimulation and orientation, and close relatives may be helpful in providing familiarity to the surroundings and offering reassurance to a frightened patient. If necessary a special nurse should be provided round the clock to alleviate the anxiety of the routine nursing staff, and allow ordinary ward procedure to continue. Nursing should be carried out in a well-lit room, and at night the illumination should continue.

More irritable and aggressive patients need gentle handling, but again if managed correctly heavy sedation may be avoided. They should be approached in a calm, non-threatening manner and offered reassurance about where they are, and why they are there. They should be reminded about their temporary confusion, and if they are causing stress to others this fact pointed out. Any procedures that need to be carried out on them should be carefully explained beforehand. Physical restraint, if it becomes necessary, should be attempted only if there are enough people present to contain the patient. Where the situation demands it, patients can be compulsorily detained for up to 3 days in hospital by application of Section 30 of the 1959 Mental Health Act.

Medications for treatment include major tranquillizers, minor tranquillizers and sedatives. Generally the major tranquillizers are the drugs of first choice, although in states of alcoholic withdrawal or epilepsy they are contraindicated since they lower the seizure threshold, and may aggravate the situation by provoking a seizure. Chlorpromazine (Largactil), haloperidol (Haldol) or droperidol (Droleptan), are equally effective, although side effects such as hypotension occur less with the butyrophenones. These drugs may be given orally, intramuscularly, or intravenously, although oral doses are preferred if the patient will allow it. Rapid tranquillization may be attained with 5–20 mg i.m. or i.v. of haloperidol as often as every 30 minutes if it is essential.

Following the acute phase of the illness, oral maintenance therapy will be needed for several days, and should be continued until the patient is completely well.

Alternative medications used include chlordiazepoxide (Librium), diazepam (Valium), chlormethiazole (Heminevrin) and paraldehyde. The latter is effective, but generally not recommended on account of its pungent smell and liability to produce abscesses at injection sites. Chlordiazepoxide (Librium) and diazepam (Valium) are unpredictably absorbed when given intramuscularly, and intoxication can result if the patient's state is not carefully monitored. Rarely, in uncontrollable over-activity, ECT can be life-saving.

Prevention is always preferable to cure, and early recognition of delirium can prevent later catastrophes. Thus patients with early signs, such as anxiety, irritability, disturbance of sleep or complaints of mental confusion need to be detected, so that worsening of the clinical state can be avoided by intervention. At this stage small doses of chlorpromazine (Largactil) at night to regularize the sleep pattern may prevent deterioration into an acute psychotic illness, with all the difficulties of management that are then produced.

Hallucinoses

This refers to conditions of hallucinations in one or more modalities but usually auditory, in which there is absence of any evidence of other abnormal psychopathology, no clouding of consciousness, and no history of recurrent psychotic episodes suggestive of an alternative diagnosis. The hallucinations may be pseudo-hallucinations, and initially may be poorly formed, later becoming organized. It is most commonly encountered in alcohol withdrawal states, but may occur following intoxication with other drugs, such as LSD or cocaine, and occasionally associated with intracranial pathology. In a study of alcoholic hallucinoses, Victor and Hope[193] noted that the majority cleared within a week, and only 10% became chronic. In their series, half of the latter went on to develop a schizophreniform illness. In that these patients had no indication of premorbid schizoid personalities, and no family history of schizophrenia, it was suggested that the alcohol intake itself was implicated in the aetiology of the disorder.

CHRONIC ORGANIC BRAIN SYNDROMES

Chronic brain lesions lead to alteration of personality and behaviour, and two major categories are usually recognized. In focal brain damage certain areas of the brain are preferentially destroyed, and syndromes have been defined according to the area maximally lost. Patients with these syndromes show minimal, but selective impairment of cognitive function, and often have marked behaviour changes. In contrast, patients diagnosed as having dementia present with global brain damage. In this condition there is a deterioration of intellectual functioning across a wide spectrum, and personality change. Although the term has been applied to irreversible brain disease, it is now recognized that such a use is incorrect, and that reversible causes of dementia occur. In addition it was often applied only to severe brain damage, but it is now known that milder degrees of dementia exist in which the patient manages well until some untoward event such as bereavement, head injury, stress, or retirement leads to decomposition. Dementia may be preceded by, or combined with, an acute organic brain syndrome.

Focal brain syndromes

The symptoms of focal damage depend to some extent on the site of the lesion, but also upon the nature of the pathology, the rate of progression of the pathology, and the size of the lesion. The most common causes of damage are space-occupying lesions, especially tumours; trauma, especially penetrating head injuries; and cerebrovascular accidents. Rarer causes include encephalitis, demyelinating diseases, and brain abscesses. In some cases changes in personality and behaviour will occur suddenly, as for example following head injury. However, with slow-growing lesions change may be slow and subtle. Conventional neurological examination may be negative since the only manifestations of structural brain disease are often behavioural. In some patients changes occur over several weeks or even months following insult, and the patient's premorbid personality traits, and the subsequent development of secondary psychiatric illnesses such as depression, need to be taken into account when assessing the symptoms. Although the brain is not neatly divided into lobes, the focal syndromes are often defined as if this were the case. In defining frontal lobe, temporal lobe, occipital lobe, and parietal lobe syndromes it must be emphasized that in many patients admixtures of signs and symptoms are seen, and rarely are all the components of a particular syndrome seen in any one patient.

Frontal lobe syndromes

Since the early well-known case of Phineas Gage, the American who, in 1878 had his frontal lobes pierced by an iron bar, and whose personality and behaviour changed dramatically, observations of similar changes in patients with a variety of pathologies of the frontal lobes has led to the clinical recognition of the frontal lobe syndrome. Jacobsen's observations on primates in the 1930s[194], followed by careful testing of patients who received head injuries during the Second World War, or who received prefrontal lobotomy in the treatment of psychiatric illness, have led to the recognition of specific neuropsychological deficits associated with frontal lobe damage. Luria (Ref. 195, pp.187-225) distinguished between lesions of the lateral frontal cortex, most closely linked to the motor structures of the anterior part of the brain, which lead to disturbances of movement and action with perseveration and inertia, and lesions of the orbital and medial areas linked closely with the reticular formation and limbic system, which result in generalized disinhibition, and changes of an affective nature. The terms 'pseudo-depressed' and 'pseudo-psychopathic' have been used to describe these two types respectively.[196] Others, less certain about such sub-categories, emphasize that frontal lobe damage leads to personality disorders, alteration of motor activity, disturbances of cognitive function and 'paroxysmal disorders'.[197] There is euphoria, with lack of concern for the future. Some patients show inappropriate facetiousness with a tendency to pun (Witzelsücht). Disinhibition, erotic behaviour and outbursts of irritability and aggression may occur. The inertia is characterized by lack of initiative and spontaneous motor activity, but when exhorted to do things patients seem quite capable of carrying out every-day actions. The 'apathico-akinetico-abulic syndrome', seen with massive frontal lobe lesions, leads to a clinical picture in which patients lie passively unaroused, unable to complete tasks or even listen to commands. Such a presentation may resemble a severe depressive illness, and while these patients display lability of affect, especially transitions between euphoria and apparent depression, a depressive illness *per se* is not commonly encountered.

The cognitive disabilities encountered with frontal lobe lesions have been comprehensively studied, and tests specifically designed to detect abnormalities have been mentioned in Chapter 3. Patients show loss of abstracting ability with concreteness of thinking. Attention is disturbed, and memory difficulties of a special kind can be observed. Patients 'forget to remember',[197] have difficulty in judging recency, show lack of motor initiative, and are impaired in their ability to shift from one learning set to another. Stereotyped responses may occur with perseveration, and abnormalities of visual searching have been described. When patients look at a complex picture they fix their gaze at random, and answer questions about the picture with the first available guess rather than following logical deduction. Perseveration and inability to switch from one type of calculation to another leads to difficulty performing arithmetical calculations which require such operations. Serial sevens are performed incorrectly, as are carry-over subtractions. The paroxysmal disorders rarely occur, but consist of sudden periods of disorientation and confusion, sometimes associated with hallucinations.

The more the lesions extends posteriorly, the more neurological signs such as aphasia (especially with left-sided injury), paralyses, grasp reflexes and oculomotor abnormalities become apparent. Basal lesions may give rise to optic atrophy and anosmia.

Various mechanisms for the changes in behaviour and cognition following these lesions have been suggested. Luria emphasized the rich connections between the prefrontal areas, and the brainstem, thalamic structures and other cortical zones, such that the frontal lobes played a vital part in organizing and programming intellectual acts, and checking performance. With damage disintegration of intellectual activity as a whole occurred. Teuber,[198] following studies on patients with head injury obtained in war, suggested that the frontal lobes 'anticipate' sensory stimuli which result from behaviour, thus preparing the brain for events about to occur. The expected results are compared to actual experience and regulation of activity occurs. In contrast Goldstein[199] suggested that the lesions lead to impairment of 'abstract attitude'. Patients cope quite well with routine work, but are unable to handle new tasks and alter their mental set.

Temporal lobe syndromes

Because areas of the temporal cortex connect with speech pathways, one of the main deficits produced by temporal lesions is speech disturbance, in particular sensory aphasia. These are considered below in the section on aphasias. Of more relevance to neuropsychiatry are disturbances of the limbic system that are seen in patients with temporal lobe disease, which lead not only to overt personality change, but also to psychiatric illness and amnestic syndromes. Some relationships between chronic temporal lobe-limbic disease and behaviour are discussed in the chapter on epilepsy, where it is pointed out that an increased incidence of a variety of psychopathological symptoms is seen in patients with temporal lobe epilepsy, including personality disorders, aggressive behaviour disorders, and paranoid or schizophreniform psychotic states. Waxman and Geschwind[200] have described a syndrome of hyposexuality, religiosity and a tendency towards extensive and sometimes compulsive writing in patients with temporal lobe epilepsy, which reflects abnormal excitation and responsiveness of limbic system neurones.

Further examples of abnormalities are noted following head injury, with trauma to the temporal lobes,[201] and following surgery. Thus Kluver and Bucy[202] demonstrated striking behavioural changes in primates following bilateral anterior temporal lobe resection, including diminished aggressiveness, attention deficits, orality and hypersexuality. Similar cases have been described in patients. Malamud[204] has described how tumours of the limbic system, of a variety of differing pathologies, lead to a number of psychopathological syndromes, often indistinguishable from primary psychiatric illness. Such lesions may initially present without focalizing neurological signs, and early quadrantic homonymous hemianopias or visual inattention may be easily missed.

Williams[205] noted the importance of the temporal lobes for integration of sensations, both exteroceptive and interoceptive, and emotions, such that past and present were united to 'achieve the sense that 'I am' — subjective consciousness — and so to pattern consequent behaviour'.

Memory disturbances have now been clearly linked with temporal lobe/limbic abnormalities. Although there is some disagreement on terminology it is customary to divide memory into short- and long-term processes. This distinction derives primarily from experimental work which suggests two memory systems, differing with regard to speed of forgetting, mode of retrieval and capacity. Short-term memory refers to that of limited capacity showing rapid decay, as opposed to long-term memory with unlimited capacity for storage of well-rehearsed information. However, universal agreement does not exist on this dichotomy. The term 'primary memory' is sometimes used for that characterized by rapid forgetting, as opposed to 'secondary memory'. Other forms of memory classification include memory for skills and memory for events; or memory for words and concepts (semantic memory), and memory for personal experience (episodic memory).[206]

The process of memorizing involves perception and registration, retention and retrieval of information, all of which may be interfered with by disease processes. It is proposed by some that verbal information is initially processed by the short-term memory system, and unless rehearsal occurs the memory fades. Rehearsal ensures that it is encoded and then transferred to the long-term storage. The changes that occur in the central nervous system in order to allow consolidation are prone to disruption, the most noted occurrence of this taking place after head injury or bilateral ECT, where retrograde amnesia occurs covering several minutes or sometimes hours. The process of memory storage has not been clarified but suggestions include changes in neurochemistry, changes in neuronal pathways or changes in activity between neurones. Early theorists suggested that more permanent memory traces were related to patterns of electrical activity. Subsequent work, especially using ECT as a model, has discounted this. Others have postulated that some specific macro-molecules develop consequent to learning which represent alterations of neuronal DNA or RNA. Hyden[207] noted increased RNA associated with changes in the ratio of base composition in neurones from rat cortex following learning experiments. In addition he has identified specific proteins that increase in synthesis with learning. These, labelled s100 and 14.3.2, are noted first in the hippocampus, and appear later in the sensorimotor cortex.

Young (Ref. 208, pp.78–97), following numerous experiments with the octopus, suggested that memory is dependent on selection between alternative neuronal pathways, favoured pathways increasing and unfavoured ones decreasing in their effectiveness. Small interneurones help mould this process by producing inhibitory neurotransmitters.

Others emphasize the holistic nature of the memory process. For example Luria stated: 'Remembering can be regarded as a gradual process resting on a multi-dimensional system of connections incorporating elementary (sensory) and more complex (perceptual) and, finally, the most complex (cognitive) components (Ref. 209, p.4).

Clinically many disorders lead to disturbance of memory. In the 1880s Korsakoff[210] described a severe memory disturbance, especially for recent events, which sometimes resulted from alcoholism, associated with peripheral neuropathy. **Korsakoff's psychosis** is now used to refer to cases of memory disturbance, which usually appear as a sequel to Wernicke's encephalopathy, secondary to thiamine deficiency.[211] Lesions involving the mamillary body are thought responsible for the memory deficit, although some have implicated the medial dorsal nucleus of the thalamus. Victor *et al.*[212] studied 245 patients who had Korsakoff's psychosis, the majority of whom were alcoholic. In the acute phase many of them showed the classical signs of Wernicke's disease such as nystagmus, ophthalmoplegia, ataxia, neuropathy and clouding of consciousness. Of 104 patients followed up, only 21% made complete recovery, 54% having permanent severe memory disturbances Post-mortem brain examinations were carried out on 62 patients: 74% of these had lesions of the mamillary bodies, but the thalamic nuclei were also invariably involved, especially the medial dorsal group. Five patients had pathological changes in the mamillary bodies but no memory deficits. The memory disorder was characterized by Victor *et al.* as: (1) an inability to recall information acquired before the illness (retrograde amnesia) often of several years' duration; and (2) an inability to acquire new information (anterograde amnesia). Clinically the patients were able to repeat digits normally, and had relatively intact short-term memory. In addition they did not show major impairment of cognitive abilities in other fields. Although it has often been suggested that remote memories remain intact in these patients, in their series practically all patients also had impaired memory for events in the distant past. The retrograde amnesia tended to shrink with time, but the anterograde amnesia persisted, in some patients for many years without improvement.

Other symptoms of Korsakoff's psychosis include mood disturbances, especially apathy with an air of blandness and detachment, lack of initiative and insight, and lack of spontaneity. Confabulation may occur, but is not a universal feature, and generally the more insight the patient has into the amnesia, the less likely is there to be confabulation. Confabulation has variously been described as a defence mechanism; a factor related to patients' suggestibility; or a consequence of temporal disorientation. Mercer *et al.*,[213] after studying 11 patients with confabulation following a variety of organic brain syndromes, found it was not related to the severity of the memory deficit, or to the disorientation, but to the coincidence of four factors, which were: (1) the patient believing that a response was required; (2) an accurate memory of the answer lacking; (3) an overlearned and affectively significant response being available; and (4) an inability to monitor or self-correct the defective response.

While some authors have implicated a perceptual disorder as underlying the memory deficit in Korsakoff's syndrome, others have suggested apathy, a deranged sense of the flow of time, or coding and consolidation difficulties. What is clear is that by the use of specialized tests it can be shown that Korsakoff patients remember some information. Learning of motor skills, such as mirror drawing tasks or rotary pursuit skills, have been demonstrated. In addition, by presenting information partially, using fragmented pictures or words, Warrington and Weiskrantz[214] have shown that amnesic patients learn and have day-to-day retention. On the basis of these and other experiments they suggest that the main feature of the memory disorder in the amnesic syndrome is not the inability to take in material, or the failure of consolidation, but is an 'interference' from irrelevant memories during retrieval.

The anatomical basis for the memory disorder has been more clearly defined. Similar patterns of impairment have been described in other disorders, all of which have in common the destruction of the hippocampal-limbic system circuits. These include bilateral temporal lobectomy, occlusion of the posterior cerebral arteries with subsequent hippocampal infarction, anoxic damage, viral encephalitis usually attributed to herpes simplex which preferentially localizes in the temporal lobes, tumours of the third ventricle or tumours with bilateral temporal lobe involvement, subarachnoid haemorrhage, head trauma, and tuberculous meningitis. In order to assess whether the pattern of the amnesia is qualitatively the same in these various conditions, Cutting[215] examined groups of patients with Korsakoff's syndrome, alcoholism, dementia and temporal lobectomy on tests of verbal memory and picture recognition. While the alcoholic patients had a similar pattern of impairment to the right temporal lobectomy patients, the overall findings were not homogenous across the groups, suggesting that a 'uniform amnesic syndrome' may not exist. Others have found that in chronic alcoholics identical cognitive defects as seen in Korsakoff patients may be noted before the onset of Wernicke's encephalopathy,[216] and that the memory disturbance in Korsakoff's syndrome is different from that seen in post-encephalitic amnesic disorders.[217]

The hippocampus, via the fornix, projects to the mamillary bodies and although lesions, even bilateral lesions of the fornix in man, rarely produce Korsakoff-type memory defects, these sites and certain thalamic nuclei seem to be essential for the normal processing of memory.[218] Integrity of the Papez circuit probably subserves some elementary function related to the comparison of stimuli with traces of previous experience. However these systems do not operate in isolation, and clearly the ability to memorize and recall past events effectively is dependent upon attention, and in addition affective and perceptual mechanisms.

Other memory disorders are encountered in clinical practice. The capacity to recall recent events and to form new memories is impaired in a variety of organic brain syndromes such as dementia. These abnormalities are often non-specific, and associated with evidence of more generalized intellectual impairment. In such cases the pathology may be widespread although the early presentation of, for example, Alzheimer's disease may be with amnesic defects and localized pathology initially suspected. Material-specific deficits of memory occur in relation to cerebral damage at certain sites. Abnormalities of verbal learning are noted following left temporal lobectomy or damage, and impaired memory for visual stimuli following right temporal lobe lesions.

Short-term memory deficits with abnormally rapid forgetting have been described. Verbal short-term memory abnormalities are reported following lesions in the angular gyrus and supramarginal region of the left hemisphere, not accounted for by failure of perception, or by a motor speech abnormality or failure of long-term memory. The relationship of this defect to conduction aphasia has however yet to be clarified.[219]

Traumatic amnesia may result in a clinical picture similar to the Korsakoff's psychosis. **Transient global amnesia** is defined as a sudden global amnesia with some clouding of consciousness, which ends in recovery. The disorder is commoner in males of the 50–70 year old age group. Personal identity is retained, significant persons recognized, and motor skills unimpaired. It usually lasts for up to 24 hours, and when memory returns there is an amnesic gap for the period of the illness. Although single episodes usually occur, patients with multiple attacks have been reported. There is associated retrograde amnesia, which may extend many years previously, but which quickly shrinks although occasionally it may persist after recovery. Croft *et al.*[220] described 24 patients, nine of whom had two or more attacks. Physical exertion or exposure to cold or heat was sometimes noted associated with the onset. Patients complained of a defective memory, repeatedly asking questions and seeking information. On recovery the amnesia persisted only for the period of the attack itself.

The aetiology of this condition is unclear, although epileptic phenomena and cerebrovascular accidents have been implicated in a few cases, and in some patients it has been linked to migraine. The EEG is often abnormal during an attack.

The association between psychiatric illness and memory disorders has been relatively little explored. Memory is impaired in many forms of psychiatric disability, although often in a non-specific way. Depressed patients show abnormal short-term memory, but no involvement of long-term memory, the former improving as the depression clears.[221] Lishman[222] has shown not only that the emotional connotations of events are related to the ease of recall, such that normally pleasing material is recalled better than unpleasant material, but also that in depression the tendency to recall unpleasant material is enhanced. Treatments, in particular bilateral ECT and lithium therapy, may also interfere with memory processes.

Psychogenic amnesia is taken to refer to amnesia primarily determined by 'psychological' as opposed to neurogenic factors. However, in view of the close interrelation between organic and other factors in the production of abnormal illness behaviour (see Chapter 5), it is not surprising that psychogenic amnesia is often encountered in the setting of organic brain disease. Merskey gives the principal criteria of this form of amnesia as loss of personal identity associated with preservation of environmental information and complex learned skills (Ref. 155, p.76). Stengel emphasized the close association with depression, and suggested that fugue states, that is, wandering with amnesia, represent a form of suicidal equivalent.[223] During fugue states patients remain in good contact with their surroundings, and when they emerge from a fugue they either resume their identity with an amnesic gap, or they have a continuous loss of personal identity and amnesia for their whole life.[224] Kennedy and Neville[225] in a series of 61 patients with sudden loss of memory, noted an organic neurological cause in 16%, 'psychogenic' causes in 43%, and a dual aetiology in 41%. The features of the amnesia were the same in all groups, and a common finding was the patient's high level of suggestibility. Many recovered during a therapeutic interview or under hypnosis, most episodes lasting less than 48 hours.

Parietal lobe syndromes

Parietal lobe disturbances provide a rich field of neuropsychiatric signs and symptoms. The major ones include disturbed language functions, acalculia, disturbances of body image, visuo-spatial deficits, apraxias, neglect, right-left disorientation, prosopagnosia, anosognosia, and topographagnosia. Some of these presentations are seen preferentially after a lesion of one or other of the hemispheres, shown in Table 6.5. Often these deficits will be accompanied by neurological signs, such as sensory loss with impairment of the ability to recognize objects placed in the hand (astereognosis), poor localization of the placement of sensory stimuli, inattention and extinction, mild hemiparesis, etc., but on occasions, especially with right hemisphere lesions, the presentation is purely behavioural.

Table 6.5. Lateralization of parietal lobe symptomatology

Right side (non-dominant) lesions	Left side (dominant) lesions
Neglect of contralateral sensory field and anosognosia	Aphasia Agraphia Alexia
Disturbance of body image Dressing apraxia Visuo-spatial agnosia Topographagnosia	Right–left disorientation Finger agnosia

The aphasias

Aphasia refers to disturbance of established language ability secondary to disturbed brain function. It has to be distinguished from other language and speech impediments such as dysarthria, and the failure to develop language abilities during childhood.[226] A variety of different types of aphasia are defined. They are consequent on lesions of the dominant hemisphere which, for 95% of right-handed people, is the left hemisphere. In left-handed people the situation is more complicated, but some 50–70% have a dominant left hemisphere. The laterality of language functions is established in early life, but if young children sustain cerebral damage to the areas of the brain subserving speech mechanisms it is now known that transfer of these abilities to the opposite hemisphere occurs.[227] The possibility that in adults the potential for transfer still remains, and that some recovery of aphasia is due to this ability, remains speculation. Lesions that result in aphasia vary widely, although it occurs particularly frequently following cerebrovascular accidents involving the middle cerebral or internal carotid arteries. Aphasic symptoms are also seen following head injury, tumours, and degenerative lesions, but are rare in multiple sclerosis and Huntington's chorea.

While no universal classification exists, it is now customary to sub-divide the aphasias and to suggest that each one is related to some identifiable site of neurological lesion. It should be emphasized that some argue against this, preferring to suggest that language is a holistic process, and that while a single lesion may destroy articulation, language ability remains intact since language is the result of many different, extensively organized brain regions acting together. Others have implied that there is only one aphasia, the different clinical pictures that occur representing varieties of this basic syndrome. In clinical practice patients often present a mixed picture rather than with any clear-cut group of symptoms. Severe loss of all language ability is referred to as global aphasia. The clinical features of some of the aphasias is shown in Table 6.6.

Broca's aphasia (anterior aphasia; non-fluent aphasia; motor aphasia)

This type of aphasia, attributed to lesions of the posterior part of the dominant third frontal gyrus, is associated with a contralateral hemiparesis. There is non-fluent production of speech with restricted output, disturbed phonemic production, some dysarthria, and often loss of grammar abilities. Effort is required to produce verbal output. Repetition of speech is abnormal. While patients usually understand written and verbal instructions, complex instructions, for example asking the patient to point to several items in sequence, are often not followed. There is always an associated dysgraphia.

Wernicke's aphasia (posterior aphasia; fluent aphasia; sensory aphasia)

This form of aphasia is characterized by a failure of comprehension, and disturbed phonemic selection and sequencing. It results from lesions in the posterior part of the dominant superior temporal gyrus. Although speech output may sound normal, and is produced with little effort with correct grammar and intonation, it is frequently meaningless and on analysis will be found excessive in quantity with paraphasias and neologisms. Jargon aphasia may result. Reading and writing are also impaired in this condition.

Table 6.6. Varieties of aphasia

Function	Broca	Transcortical	Wernicke	Conduction	Anomic
Speech	*non fluent; agrammatical; produced with effort* decreased word frequency	fluent or non-fluent*	*fluent; grammatical; jargon with paraphasias; no effort*	fluent with paraphasias	fluent with paraphasias
Comprehension	normal	normal or abnormal*	*abnormal*	relatively normal	normal
Repetition§	abnormal	*normal*	abnormal	*abnormal*	normal
Naming ability	abnormal	abnormal	abnormal	abnormal	*abnormal*
Reading ability	impaired	impaired	impaired	abnormal	often abnormal
Writing ability	impaired	impaired	impaired	impaired	often abnormal
Hemiparesis	usually present	sometimes present	usually absent	usually absent	usually absent

*Depending on the site of the lesion.
§NOTE: In aphasia resulting from perisylvian lesions repetition is always abnormal.

Conduction aphasia

This form of aphasia is marked by an inability to repeat, although comprehension seems normal. Paraphasias occur in speech and the rhythm, although fluent, is broken, Repetition is disturbed by literal paraphasias. Although patients' reading abilities are abnormal, it is important that while they are unable to read aloud they often can read and comprehend silently. Many patients show some apraxia, and dysgraphia is usual. The location of the pathology in this disorder is unsettled, but it is thought to be due to a lesion in the dominant perisylvian region, probably affecting the arcuate fasciculus.

Anomic aphasia (nominal aphasia; amnesic aphasia)

Although 'anomia', which is the inability to name objects, occurs in most aphasic disturbances, it also occurs in non-aphasic conditions. It is seen in disorders which involve the nervous system diffusely, and may also present as hysterical anomia. In anomic aphasia there is primarily a disturbance of word-finding, and an inability to name objects. Comprehension is intact and speech fluent but circumlocutory, although paraphasias occur in naming objects. The lesion is thought to be in the region of the dominant angular gyrus, and other parietal lobe signs such as right–left disorientation may occur with it. However, the purest cases of anomic aphasia are seen following lesions in the basal portion of the dominant posterior temporal lobe.[203]

Transcortical aphasia

In this variety of aphasia, thought due to lesions that isolate language areas and thus involving frontal, parietal and temporal lobe border zones, there is difficulty in comprehension and lack of spontaneous speech, but normal repetition of words. Dependent upon the site of the lesion the terms 'transcortical motor aphasia' and 'transcortical sensory aphasia' have been used to describe the clinical pictures following anterior or posterior lesions respectively. Self-prompting, with motor actions to aid initiation of speech, is a feature of the former, and echolalia of the latter.

Pure word deafness

This rare disorder occurs in patients who have isolation of Wernicke's area from auditory inputs from the temporal lobe. Patients who are unable to comprehend spoken language are still able to understand written material and write.

Other syndromes of language impairment have been described. **Pure word dumbness** (aphemia) is a rare disorder due to acute brain damage, in which virtual mutism occurs in the presence of normal comprehension, reading and writing. In **alexia with agraphia**, patients cannot read or write, and lesions are found in the left angular gyrus. Patients may have associated anomic aphasia or apraxia. In **alexia without agraphia**, in contrast, patients are unable to read but write fluently. It occurs with left occipital lobe lesions, which also involve the splenium of the corpus callosum, and it is always associated with a right homonymous hemianopia. The disorder is of historical interest in that it was one of the earliest of the 'disconnection syndromes' to be described.[228] These, which result from disconnections between different cortical regions, result in a number of clinical pictures which have been identified and explained in terms of known neuroanatomical connections. In alexia without agraphia the left visual cortex is damaged, and although the right visual cortex can still receive visual information from the left visual field, it cannot so readily be transferred to the intact language areas, because of the partial corpus callosum lesion. Other disconnection syndromes described include pure word deafness, pure agraphia, and varieties of agnosias and apraxias.

The psychiatric disabilities encountered in patients with aphasia are multiple and frequently overlooked. Benson[229] suggested that the mental state following aphasia results from a sense of being 'locked in' and frustration. Unexpressed anger may lead to withdrawal and negativism with outbursts of hostility. Psychomotor retardation, apathy and blunting of affect may be noted. Independently from this, depression, often severe, may develop, although suicidal attempts and gestures are rare. Some patients, in contrast, demonstrate mild euphoria and a lack of concern over apparently severe language difficulties. The so-called 'catastrophic reaction' is seen when patients are presented with demands greater than they are able to cope with, and has to be distinguished from pseudo-bulbar palsy with uninhibited emotional expression to appropriate situations. Benson further suggested that the site of the lesion was related to the pattern of clinical presentation. Those who show concern, with frustration and depression, commonly have non-fluent aphasias and more anterior lesions, the unconcerned euphoric aphasias being more commonly fluent, with posterior lesions. Patients with aphasia sometimes show paranoid states, especially when severe comprehension deficits are present in association with dominant temporal lobe lesions. Pure word deafness is often associated with paranoid ideation and auditory hallucinations.[227]

It is not clear whether aphasic patients suffer from more general intellectual decline. Although some authors suggest that the impaired verbal and performance deficits noted with aphasia indicate a widespread disturbance of cognitive function, others note that patients often retain their non-verbal abilities, and suggest that any intellectual restriction is limited to language ability.

Treatment of aphasic disorders is complicated and difficult. Some patients, who remain seemingly unaware of their problems and have associated apathy, have a poor prognosis. Other indicators of a bad prognosis include old age, the presence of large or progressive lesions, and the presence of bilateral brain damage. Left-handedness favours a good prognosis, as does the absence of severe comprehension deficits. The mainstay of therapy has been speech therapy with individual or group sessions in which speech activities, reading and writing, are rehearsed with varying degrees of programming. In melodic intonation therapy, composed sentences and phrases with melodic patterns are given rhythmically to patients to learn and sing. The intoned pattern of the sentence is similar to the natural prosodic pattern of the spoken sentence, and the therapy eventually leads to the repetition of the sentence in normal speech.[230] Psychotherapy and social work exploration have an important part to play in the support of patients with aphasia, in particular helping them to cope with their problems, and rehabilitate in the presence of a severe sense of isolation. Antidepressants may be helpful for any emerging depressive illness, and unless there has recently been recurrent brain damage, aphasia itself is not a contraindication to ECT. Paranoid states are often difficult to treat, and may require hospitalization with major tranquillizer therapy.

The apraxias

Apraxia is the inability to carry out motor activity in the presence of intact motor and sensory systems, comprehension, attention and co-operation.[203] Ideomotor apraxia refers to the inability to perform actions to verbal command which can spontaneously be completed with ease. Imitation of the examiner is however often possible, and whole body commands are often performed well, while commands involving the limbs and the face are failed. Usually these disturbances are bilateral except when they occur in the left upper limb in association with aphasia and a right hemiplegia. Ideational apraxia refers to the inability to perform a sequence of actions correctly, although each component of the sequence can often be adequately performed by itself. Patients for example are unable to light a pipe using a box of matches. Constructional apraxia is a disturbance in the performance of tasks such as drawing or constructing objects in three-dimensional space, and dressing apraxia is an inability to put on clothes normally. Two varieties of the latter are defined. In the first, patients with unilateral neglect ignore one side of their body and therefore do not dress it; in the other, patients are unable to manipulate items of clothing successfully.

Although apraxia is usually associated with parietal lesions, the laterality of the lesions may be unilateral or bilateral. Ideomotor and ideational apraxia are usually associated with left hemisphere lesions, dressing apraxia with right lesions, and constructional apraxia with lesions of either hemisphere. Several different theories have been put forward to explain these disorders. Although some argue that the presence of associated unilateral neglect or aphasia makes interpretation difficult, or that some apraxias are really agnosias, the available evidence does not support these suggestions.[231] Geschwind uses the model of 'disconnection syndromes' to explain the deficits.[203] Lesions disrupt nerve connections between motor association cortex of one or other hemisphere and Wernicke's area, such that comprehension of a command occurs, but it cannot be translated to the brain areas responsible for the actual execution of the action.

The agnosias

Selected disturbances of recognition, in the absence of sensory disturbances or intellectual impairment, are described as agnosias. A variety of agnosias have been reported, for example for colour, sound, touch, pain, fingers, faces, and objects.[232] Astereognosia (tactile agnosia) is the loss of ability to recognize by touch, the nature of an object, and is usually associated with parietal lobe lesions. In visual object agnosia, patients have difficulty in naming objects visually presented, and cannot demonstrate or describe the use of the objects seen, although primary visual capacity appears intact. They can recognize objects by touch, but fail to match an object to a picture of it. In most cases bilateral involvement, especially of the occipital lobes, is reported. Visuo-spatial agnosia, common after right parietal lobe lesions, is virtually synonymous with constructional apraxia and patients are unable to carry out spatial tasks which require vision. In topographagnosia, also seen after right-sided lesions, patients are unable to follow routes on maps. Prosopagnosia is recognition difficulty for familiar faces only, and occurs following lesions, usually bilateral, in the parietal or parietal–occipital regions. In auditory agnosia, the ability to recognize sounds, musical pitch or noise of familiar objects such as a machine, is impaired. The patient may appear deaf, but on testing with pure tones hearing is intact. Although musical ability is related to right hemisphere function, auditory agnosia is usually associated with aphasia and bilateral lesions. Anosognosia is the failure to recognize disabilities, classically a patient not noticing a paralysis and behaving as if it were not present. It may represent more gross manifestations of the commoner unilateral neglect, noted particularly after non-dominant parietal lesions, especially acute lesions. Autotopagnosia is the inability to name on confrontation various bodily parts which either belong to the patient or to others.

The mechanism of the agnosias is obscure. Some authors suggest that visual agnosia as an entity does not exist, and that all cases can be explained in terms of intellectual or perceptual deficits. Others use the model of disconnection between two intact brain areas, or regard agnosias as perceptual disturbances independent of impaired sensory discrimination, dependent on the destruction of some central recognition process.[232-4]

Anosognosia has been interpreted as a distsurbance of the bodily scheme consequent upon non-dominant parietal lobe disease.[195] Others have suggested it implicates frontal lobe pathology, or some memory disorder in addition to the neurological loss. Weinstein and Kahn,[235] in a survey of 54 patients with explicit denial of disability, noted that denial occurred in patients who had tended to ignore and rationalize illness and inadequacies before disease developed. They felt the site of the lesion was relevant only in determining the type of disability denied. Lishman[42] suggested that it represents psychogenic elaboration of partially perceived defects.

The Gerstmann syndrome

This syndrome traditionally is described as a combination of finger agnosia (difficulty of identification and localization of fingers), right–left disorientation, acalculia and agraphia. To these Schilder[236] added constructional apraxia. A developmental Gerstmann's syndrome of childhood has also been described.[237] Although there was initial agreement that Gerstmann's syndrome was consequent on dominant parietal lobe pathology in the region of the angular gyrus, recently the whole basis of the syndrome has been called into question.[238] On statistical analysis of large numbers of patients, the components do not correlate well together as a separate entity, and occasional cases have been reported with focal lesions outside the dominant parietal lobe. Gerstmann's own hypothesis was that it was a disturbance of the 'body scheme'.

Occipital lobe disorders

The majority of symptoms produced by occipital lobe pathology are neurological, although resultant hallucinations may suggest florid psychiatric disturbance. The hallucinations, however, are not well formed, they are usually unilateral, and consist of, for example, stars, spots, or lines, which appear in defined areas of the visual field. Occasionally, formed hallucinations occur with occipital lesions,[239] and if associated with focal pathology, they imply more anteriorly placed lesions. A number of unusual symptoms may be reported following posterior lesions, including distortion of images, macropsia, micropsia, and palinopsia. *Anton's syndrome* is pathological denial of blindness, and is usually associated with bilateral visual loss.

Sub-cortical disorders

Lesions of structures such as the R.A.S. lead to alteration of states of consciousness and disturbances of attention. Some of these have been discussed under acute organic brain syndromes. *Akinetic mutism* (coma vigil) is the state when patients appear fully awake and alert, but respond poorly to the environment, and may do so only with strong sensory stimuli. It usually occurs following lesions of the R.A.S. and it has to be distinguished from the 'locked-in' syndrome, in which a fully conscious patient has complete paralysis of movement and expression, related to lower pontine or medullary lesions (Ref. 38, p.24).

Lesions of the thalamus interfere with attention and emotional control. Hypothalamic pathology may result in eating and drinking disturbances, often associated with fear, lowered threshold for aggression, loss of interest, and changes in personality. Patients with more severe lesions may become childish, show deterioration of their personal habits, and fatuous euphoria. Basal ganglia abnormalities alter alertness, cognition, and emotional behaviour

(Refs. 9, 240 pp. 130–40). Lesions in the diencephalon often produce fluctuating states of consciousness and sometimes frank delirium, and signs and symptoms of internal hydrocephalus such as headache, papilloedema and vomiting may also be seen. Attacks of sudden weakness may occur which, if combined with psychiatric symptoms, may be misinterpreted as hysterical.

Lesions of the cerebral commissures and inter-hemispheric differences

In recent years the concepts of 'dominance' of one hemisphere over the other have been questioned. While some asymmetry of function has been recognized for a long time, there has been growing speculation about the role of the minor hemisphere in cognitive and behaviour processes. Some of the above literature reveals marked differences between the left and right hemisphere as determined by neurological illness. Lesions of the corpus callosum and other inter-hemispheric connections, both in animals and in man, have led to an exploration of the individual role of each hemisphere when acting in isolation from the other. Clinically, corpus callosum lesions often produce non-specific changes in behaviour, but if associated with invasion of one or other of the hemispheres, then focal pathology relevant to that brain region will emerge. Disconnection syndromes also occur as mentioned above. Psychiatric symptoms are often seen early, and it has been suggested that such changes occur more frequently following tumours of the corpus callosum than with similar lesions elsewhere in the brain (Ref. 241, p.245). Symptoms include apathy, drowsiness and memory disturbances, but postural abnormalities resembling catatonia have also been reported (Ref. 42, p.27). Section of the corpus callosum *per se* does not seem to produce dramatic changes in either temperament or intellect, except for mild amnesic symptoms, and specialized techniques of examination are required to bring out hemispheric differences which enable information to be given only to one hemisphere. Studies on patients with these lesions confirm marked hemisphere asymmetry, in particular the lateralization to the left hemisphere of language production and 'conscious' experience, and some perceptual and spatial abilities to the right hemisphere. This work has led to renewed interest in the right hemisphere and its functions, in particular its association with emotional behaviour, the possibility that it may possess some linguistic functions, and be important in musical abilities and tactile processes. A summary of some of the differences between the hemispheres is shown in Table 6.7 (Ref. 19, p.352).

Localization of function within the brain

There are two general propositions. On the one hand it has been suggested that some 'function' (such as memory, speech, vision, etc.) is localized within the brain. This line of thought grew from early phrenology, and flourished with the observations of Broca and Wernicke on language disorders following cerebral lesions. Supporters of this concept have included Ferrier, Kleist, and

114

Table 6.7. Some attributes of the two hemispheres (after Popper and Eccles (Ref. 19, p.352)

Left (dominant) hemisphere	Right (non-dominant) hemisphere
Liaison to self-consciousness	No such liaison
Verbal	Mostly non-verbal
Ideational	Musical
Conceptual similarities	Pictorial and pattern sense
Analysis over time	Synthesis over time
Analysis of detail	Holistic
Arithmetical	Geometrical and spatial

more recently Geschwind. Their case is supported by the great success of neuropsychology in detecting specific patterns of cognitive impairment following brain lesions, and the prediction that certain post-mortem findings will occur following the presentation of various clinical syndromes. The alternative view, that the brain operates holistically, and is more than the sum of its separate parts, found early supporters in Hughlings Jackson and Marie, and followers included Freud, Lashley, Head, Goldstein, and Brain. Jackson pointed out that while it was possible to localize a lesion, this was not the same as localizing a function. It was noted that lesions such as tumours, while being localized in themselves, actually produced clinical effects at other brain areas due to pressure, displacement and circulation changes. The effects of lesions depended not only on the site and size of the lesion but also on the speed at which it progressed, and also on the actual personality that it affected. Acute temporary symptoms differed from residual symptoms. In addition, following injury and loss of a part of the brain, the symptoms produced represented the combined organization of the remaining intact brain, which in itself had become a new whole with its own reactions and behaviour.

One problem was that the early localizers at least assumed that areas of cortex actually represented the volitional events described, although few would probably hold such a view today. The greater understanding of the emotional consequences of neurological disease, the discovery of the neurotransmitters, the knowledge that some symptoms, particular psychiatric ones, defy localization, and the realization that behaviour is dependent upon the integrative action of multiple neuronal systems, with the recognition that regional factors and specific vulnerabilities play a role in determining the consequences of pathology, has led to a greater acceptance of a mid-ground position.[242, 243]

CHAPTER 7

Dementia, Head Injury, Cerebrovascular Accidents, and Multiple Sclerosis

DEMENTIA

The term 'dementia' originally referred to madness or mindlessness. Morel introduced dementia praecox to refer to such disorders that began in early life, and today dementia is usually used to refer to impaired ability consequent on organic brain disease. Although some authors use a restricted definition to include only a disorder with specific psychological and intellectual deficits, others broaden the criteria to include the behavioural consequences of disease, and emphasize social decline with failure to cope with an independent existence. Pearce and Miller suggest: 'Dementia is a symptom, arising from cerebral disease, often progressive, which is characterized by a decline of intellect and personality which reflect a disturbance of memory, orientation, the capacity for conceptual thought and often of affect' (Ref. 244, p.17). By definition, it is a chronic organic brain syndrome but it is not always irreversible.

It is estimated that 10% of the population over the age of 65 suffer from dementia, its incidence increasing with age. Whereas 2.3% of people in the 65–69-year-old age group have dementia, the figure rises to 5.5% for those between 75 and 79, and 22% for the over-80s.[245] In geriatric units, over one-third of patients show evidence of mental impairment, and chronic organic brain syndromes, especially of the senile and atherosclerotic variety, form a sizeable percentage of the diagnoses of long-stay mental hospital patients. However, fewer than one-fifth of patients with dementia are looked after in institutional settings, although surveys indicate that the severity of dementia in non-institutionalized patients is often as severe as in those in care.

Some authors refer to dementia under the age of 65 as 'presenile dementia', although the distinction between this and senile dementia is arbitrary. Nevertheless, there are now recognized a number of specific disorders that lead to dementia, and present in the 40–60 age range, which include Alzheimer's disease, Pick's disease, Huntington's chorea and Creutzfeldt–Jacob disease. While clinically the distinction between different causes for dementia is often difficult in life, some indicators of the underlying pathology may be gained from careful examination. Assessment of patients with possible dementia requires adequate history-taking, especially from close relatives or others who know the patient, in order to establish the onset and progression of the symptoms. A mental state examination assessing orientation, memory, and the content of the mental state, standardized psychometric testing with assessment of the patient's premorbid level of ability, and complete neurological investigation are also undertaken. Skull and chest x-ray, C.A.T. scanning, electroencephalography and, where necessary, examination of the CSF or more specialized radiographic techniques such as air encephalography, angiography, or isotope cisternography are used. Laboratory investigations performed should include electrolyte, B_{12} and folate estimations, serology, ESR, and thyroid, liver and renal function tests. It is important, if possible, to make an accurate diagnosis for the cause of dementia. Follow-up studies of patients with this diagnosis reveal a high incidence of errors, even after in-patient evaluation. Failure to investigate adequately is common, and frequent diagnostic mistakes include misdiagnosis of depression. In patients well investigated, possible causes for the dementia may be found in a high proportion, some 15% having conditions amenable to treatment.[246, 247]

SYMPTOMATOLOGY

Memory disorder is often a presenting problem in dementia. Patients usually report a difficulty in remembering new events, and as progression of the disorder occurs, the memory for past events also suffers. Experimentally, the capacity of the short-term memory store is found to be reduced, as is the retrieval or storage of long-term memory (Ref. 244, p.119). These features gradually become combined with other evidence of intellectual deficits reflecting concrete thinking and an impairment for abstract reasoning. Disorientation is noted, and performance on formal psychological testing declines, but language abilities remain relatively intact until late in the disease, when the capacity for reasoning and judgement is also lost. Thought disorder may emerge with delusions, which if combined with hallucinations lead to a florid psychotic presentation. Focal neuropsychiatric symptoms, which include apraxias, aphasias, and agnosias, may occur. In dementia due to such conditions as arteriosclerosis or neurosyphilis more widespread CNS damage occurs and other evidence of focal neurological lesions may appear. Motor symptoms, in particular Parkinsonism, may lead to poverty of the facial expression and postural disorders, and add to the slowness of movement and impaired ability to act. Premorbid personality traits are usually exacerbated, or focal deficits may give rise to a more clearly defined change in personality, such as disinhibition following frontal lobe lesions. As time progresses, apathy, personal neglect and vacuousness come to dominate the clinical picture.

Affective disturbances include early depression with an inability to cope, tearfulness and withdrawal. Delusions, sometimes bizarre, may colour the clinical picture. Hypochondriacal preoccupation may occur, with recurrent physical complaints and multiple presentations to doctors. Suicide attempts are not uncommon. Emotional lability may be noted, and later, if frontal lobe changes supervene, euphoria. Later still, apathy, shallowness, lability of affect, irritability and outbursts of aggressive behaviour may be seen. The so-called 'catastrophic reaction' occurs in some patients who, when faced with tasks that they find too challenging, react quite violently with anger, agitation or tearfulness.

ALZHEIMER'S DISEASE

This disorder is named after Alzheimer, who in 1906 described the pathological features associated with dementia in a 55-year-old female. It is one of the commonest varieties of presenile dementia. Although familial cases have been described with autosomal dominant inheritance, in the majority of cases multi factorial inheritance is suggested. The presentation is of dementia in the 50s or 60s, which is commoner in females. The disease progresses slowly over 5 to 10 years but typical early signs are amnesia with lack of spontaneity. As the disorder progresses the dementia becomes apparent and focal signs such as aphasia, alexia and apraxia may appear. Finally extrapyramidal signs, severe memory disturbances and advanced dementia result. Epilepsy is noted in a considerable number of cases, the majority presenting with major tonic-clonic seizures (Ref. 244, p.27; Ref. 42, p.542). Depressive and overtly psychiatric features may be seen early in the course of the illness, and psychotropic drugs readily precipitate an acute organic brain syndrome. The 'mirror sign' has been described in which the patient fails to recognize his own image in a mirror and talks to it as if a stranger were present.

The EEG is invariably abnormal in this disorder. Gordon and Sim[248] in a study of the EEG in 80 patients with presenile dementia noted approximately one-third of those with Pick's disease and Creutzfeldt–Jacob's disease had normal records, whereas all those with Alzheimer's disease were abnormal. Initially there was reduction of alpha-rhythm but later rhythmical theta and delta discharges or diffuse slowing was noted. In the Alzheimer patients there was a tendency for more severe degrees of abnormality to be correlated with more severe dementia.

The pathological changes are those of widespread generalized atrophy, and histologically there is loss of neurones, proliferation of astrocytes, and the presence of Alzheimer's plaques and neurofibrillary tangles. The plaques occur especially in the frontal, temporal, hippocampal and amygdala regions, and contain amyloid. The tangles, detected in silver-stained preparations are noted especially in the frontal and temporal cortex.

Recent neuropathological investigations have concentrated on neurochemical changes in the brains of patients with Alzheimer's disease.

Reduced amounts of choline acetyltransferase and glutamic acid decarboxylase have been found in the cortex, especially in the temporal lobe. This has led to the suggestion that some symptoms of the disorder, especially the memory deficit, may be linked to a neurotransmitter abnormality, particularly of acetylcholine.[249, 250] This is in keeping with observations that alterations of cholinergic mechanisms can disrupt memory in normal volunteers,[251] and has led to trials of cholinergic compounds in treatment. Since the brain does not synthesize choline, substances are used which increase brain choline, including dimethylaminoethanol (deanol), which, with the addition of one methyl group, is converted into choline, choline itself, and lecithin. Choline has not been shown conclusively to elevate brain acetylcholine except after massive doses, and with such doses a discomfiting fish-like odour occurs as a side effect. Lecithin has been shown to raise both brain choline and acetylcholine. However, to-date no clear improvements in the clinical state of patients with Alzheimer's disease have been consistently demonstrated with these substances.

PICK'S DISEASE

This was first described by Pick in 1892. He referred to a circumscribed atrophy of the frontal and temporal lobes in association with dementia. It is much less common than Alzheimer's disease, occurs more commonly in females, and familial recurrence has been reported. Some suggest that the inheritance is by an incompletely penetrant autosomal dominant gene (Ref. 244, p.32). At autopsy lobar atrophy of the frontal and temporal lobes is noted as the main feature, which is often associated with more generalized abnormalities. Microscopy shows neurone loss with gliosis. 'Balloon cells', which are swollen oval shaped cells, some of which have silver staining-inclusion bodies, are sometimes seen. Plaques and tangles are not a feature of the pathology of this disease.

In the earlier stages, the localization of the disorder may lead to clinical features that differentiate it from Alzheimer's disease.[252] Behavioural changes with aphasia are noted rather than memory disturbances, and psychotic manifestations are rare, as are epileptic convulsions. Basal ganglia involvement leads to the appearance of extrapyramidal signs. A curious 'hyperalgesia' has been reported in which mild pressure causes pain and deep pressure intense pain. The electroencephalogram is often normal or only mildly disturbed, even in later stages of the disorder. As with Alzheimer's disease, slow progression is noted over a number of years. The clinical distinctions between Pick's disease, Alzheimer's disease and a number of other forms of dementia are shown in Table 7.1

CREUTZFELDT-JACOB DISEASE

This disorder derives its name from the descriptions of Creutzfeldt in 1920 and of Jacob in 1921. They described a disease of the central nervous system with

Table 7.1. The differential diagnosis of dementia

	Alzheimer's	Pick's	Creutzfeld–Jacob	Arteriosclerotic	Hydrocephalic
Early signs	Memory	Behaviour change; aphasia incontinence	Neurological signs and symptoms	Acute focal deficit	Memory, psychomotor slowing; ataxia, incontinence
Focal deficits	+ +	+	+	+ +	– –
Orientation difficulties	Early	Late	–	+	–
Personality change	Late	Early	Early	Late	Early
Extrapyramidal signs	+	+	+	+	±
E.E.G.	Abnormal	Often normal	Always abnormal	Abnormal	Abnormal
Other features	'Mirror sign'	Hyperalgesia	Myoclonus	Pseudobulbar signs	

dementia, pyramidal and extrapyramidal manifestations.[253] In contrast to the two disorders outlined above, males are affected more commonly than females and progression is more rapid. Rarely, familial cases have been described. Initially, patients may present with vague symptoms including somatic complaints, mood changes, and personality changes, although quite soon pyramidal and extrapyramidal signs appear. Parietal lobe signs, muscle wasting, and later convulsions, especially myoclonic jerking, are reported. Delusions, hallucinations, and depressive symptoms also occur. In the final stages an advanced dementia is seen with decorticate or decerebrate postures, incontinence and unresponsiveness.

Pathologically, there is diffuse atrophy with widespread neuronal loss and gliosis. Demyelination of pyramidal and extrapyramidal tracts may be seen, but plaques and tangles are usually absent. The site of the pathological changes tends to match the clinical picture.

Nevin[254] described a rapidly progressive form of this disorder with an average duration of 14 weeks and death in 6 months. This tended to occur in older patients than classical Creutzfeldt–Jacob disease, and terminally myoclonic movements occurred associated with specific EEG abnormalities. On histopathological examination, an irregular 'status spongiosus' was reported.

Other forms described include the amaurotic variant of Heidenhain, the thalamic forms with dyskinesias, weakness and clumsiness, and amyotrophic forms with features of amyotrophic lateral sclerosis. Most investigators, however, prefer to regard the disease as a single nosological entity with a spectrum of presentations.

The EEG is always abnormal, with increased slow-wave activity and a diminution of the alpha-rhythm. The particular pattern of activity noted as the disease progresses, with bilateral slow spike-wave discharges which may accompany myoclonic jerks, is shown in Figure 7.1.

Of major interest has been the successful transmission of this disease from man to primates by a slow virus. The first degenerative disease of the human CNS shown to be due to a transmissable agent was *kuru*. This disease, found amongst the aborigines of New Guinea, was successfully passed to chimpanzees, and the pathological changes noted were similar to human disease. Creutzfeldt–Jacob disease has now likewise been transmitted to primates, and a number of other species.[255] Other disorders with similar pathologies in animals include scrapie, and transmissible mink encephalopathy. These are probably caused by a virus-like particle which fails to invoke the usual inflammatory responses in the brain or meninges. It has unusual resistance to radiation and a number of techniques that inactivate conventional viruses. This has led to speculation that these agents are infectious but lack nucleic acid, perhaps even being a self-replicating membrane fragment.

Recently there have been reports of transmission of Creutzfeldt–Jacob disease from man to man by corneal transplantation, and by neurosurgery via electrodes contaminated from an ill patient.[256] The possibility that other

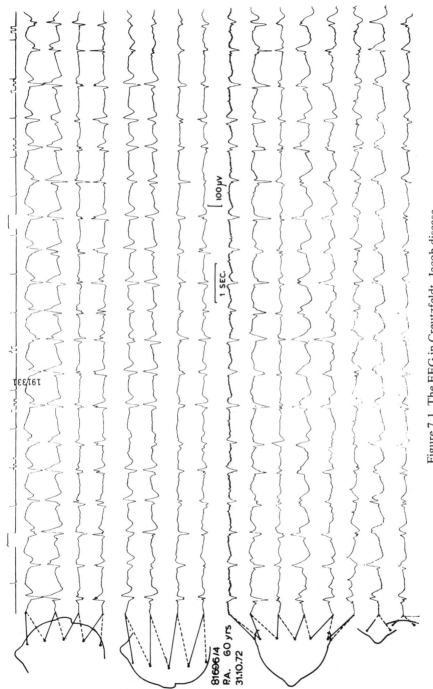

Figure 7.1. The EEG in Creutzfeldt–Jacob disease

central nervous system disorders, such as Alzheimer's disease or Parkinson's disease, may also be related to slow virus infections is seriously considered.[257]

ARTERIOSCLEROTIC DEMENTIA (MULTI-INFARCT DEMENTIA)

This form of dementia is related to recurrent cerebrovascular accidents. It is doubtful whether generalized atheroma of the cerebral vessels results in dementia without clearly defined episodes of infarction or haemorrhage occurring. Emboli arising from extracerebral sources, such as the extracranial arteries and the heart, are the most common cause of multiple cerebral infarctions. The sex incidence of the disorder is equal, and typically the patient gives a history of recurrent strokes, and may have been hypertensive in the past. Other evidence of arteriosclerosis may be found in the retinal or peripheral blood vessels, and there may be evidence in the history of an acute onset of cognitive disorder, with a history suggestive of a cerebrovascular accident. Alternatively, insidious changes in personality may occur which precede obvious intellectual impairment. On examination focal deficits are usually present. Pseudobulbar signs become part of the clinical picture, with emotional lability, bilateral hyperreflexia and extensor plantar responses; extrapyramidal features are often present, and epileptic seizures may occur.

Pathologically, multiple areas of softening and cavitation are seen, which are particularly common in the basal ganglia. The electroencephalogram usually shows severe changes, sometimes with focal features.

Cerebral blood flow studies[258, 259] show that in patients with dementia due to neuronal degeneration, the blood flow falls in relationship to the loss of brain tissue. In arteriosclerotic dementia fall in blood flow occurs early in the disease, is out of proportion to the degree of atrophy, and regions of abnormal perfusion are more widely distributed.

SENILE DEMENTIA

This term rather arbitrarily refers to dementia occurring after the age of 65 and is the most common form. While any of the varieties of dementia already described can present in patients over 65, the most common causes of senile dementia are arteriosclerotic dementia, and 'parenchymatous' senile dementia.

There are two main controversies. The first is the relationship between parenchymatous senile dementia and normal ageing. Since the brains of non-dementing elderly patients at post-mortem contain both senile plaques and neuro-fibrillary tangles, often associated with neuronal loss,[260] some argue that dementia is merely accelerated ageing. However, it has been shown that high plaque counts are a characteristic of the demented patients' brain, and a linear correlation exists between deterioration of intellectual abilities and the mean plaque count.[261] One suggestion is that when the neuropathological changes of ageing develop beyond a certain degree, qualitative cognitive differences appear and dementia results (Ref. 42, p.534). In support of this are the results of psychological testing that show the sub-tests that decline with age are different from those seen in dementia.[262] Genetic studies likewise favour differences. For example, the morbidity of first-degree relatives of patients with senile dementia is increased by a factor of 4.3, favouring a partially penetrant dominant inheritance, and monozygotic twins have a higher concordance rate for senile dementia than do dizygotic ones (Ref. 244, p.126).

The second is the relationship between Alzheimer's disease and senile dementia. Genetic differences between them, and the relative absence of extrapyramidal features, focal features and epileptic seizures in the presentation of parenchymatous senile dementia have led to the suggestion they are different disorders. Sourander and Sjogren[263] reported neuropathological differences, in particular noting the higher density of plaques and tangles in the temporal neocortex, amygdala and hippocampus from brains of patients with Alzheimer's disease. However, an alternative view was supported by Bowen et al.[264] following biochemical analyses of neurotransmitter enzyme activity in post-mortem brains. They demonstrated a reduction of choline acetyltransferase activity in Alzheimer's disease, not seen in normally ageing brains. No clear difference was noted between the Alzheimer group, and those presenting with senile dementia. In their studies they thus preferred to use the term Alzheimer's disease for this form of dementia irrespective of the patient's age.

Clinically, parenchymatous senile dementia has an insidious onset, usually with memory difficulties, affective symptoms, especially depression, and withdrawal. Focal signs such as aphasia or apraxia do occur, but are much less severe than in some other forms of dementia. Delusions, particularly paranoid, wandering, especially at night, and intermittent bouts of delirium are seen in response to changes in the environment, bereavement, or minor systemic illnesses.

HYDROCEPHALIC DEMENTIAS

The classification of hydrocephalic dementia is shown in Table 7.2 (Ref. 265, p.85). Non-obstructive varieties have been discussed above. Obstructive hydrocephalus is divided into communicating and non-communicating varieties. In the latter, obstruction to the flow of CSF may occur acutely or insidiously. A number of causes are recognized including tumours, colloid cysts of the third ventricle, ectatic basilar artery, and inflammatory changes in the outflow channels of the third ventricle. These pathologies interfere with the flow of the CSF between the ventricles to the subarachnoid space, and if the obstruction is partial the clinical picture may be that of dementia.

In communicating hydrocephalus there is no impediment to the flow of CSF from the ventricles, but either the fluid is unable to reach the convexity of the brain, or normal absorption through the arachnoid villi into the venous

Table 7.2. Hydrocephalic dementias (After Benson (Ref. 265, p.85))

Non-obstructive	Degenerative, e.g. Alzheimer's disease, Pick's disease, etc. Destructive, e.g. arteriosclerotic, traumatic.
Obstructive	Non-communicating — with ventricular obstruction. Communicating — normal pressure hydrocephalus.

channels adjacent to the sagittal sinus does not occur. Causes of such obstructions include subarachnoid haemorrhage and meningitis.

Adams et al.[266] described a number of patients in whom dementia occurred several years after head injury, subarachnoid haemorrhage or meningitis, and who in addition showed gait disturbances and incontinence associated with normal CSF pressure. Although it is now known that the CSF pressure in these cases if often raised, the term *normal pressure hydrocephalus* was used to describe this condition. The clinical picture is variable, and idiopathic varieties occur without clearly demarcated events such as haemorrhage or trauma. The dementia is often of recent onset and characterized less by impairment of memory, than by psychomotor slowing. Patients seem to lack spontaneity and initiative and are apathetic, a clinical picture that may be mistaken for depression.

The EEG is usually abnormal with diffuse slowing. On CAT scan the ventricles are large in the presence of normal or small cortical sulci. Air encephalography also shows large ventricles with little or no air passing over the cortex. The flow of CSF may be studied further by isotope cisternography. Radio-iodinated human serum albumin (RIHSA) is injected into the CSF and its pattern of distribution noted over the ensuing hours and days. Normally the isotope does not enter the ventricular system and is absorbed by about 48 hours. In normal pressure hydrocephalus there is immediate concentration in the ventricles, and little flow from the ventricles with time. Little or no isotope is seen in the cortical subarachnoid space especially in the sagittal region.

The possibility of treatment for this type of hydrocephalus has aroused considerable controversy. Shunting of the CSF, either to the atrium of the heart or to the peritoneal cavity, has been carried out, but not all cases respond, and the majority are left with residual deficit. Symon et al.[267] have shown by continuous monitoring of the intracranial pressure over a number of days that some patients show increased pressure during sleep, which often comes in waves of variable duration. These patients respond better to surgery than those not showing pressure waves.

SOME OTHER CAUSES OF DEMENTIA

A variety of other disorders may lead to a clinical presentation of dementia, some of which are readily amenable to therapy and are thus treatable. A list of these is shown in Table 7.3 (Ref. 244, p.43). Tumours, in particular meningiomas, must always be considered and if possible ruled out. Both folic acid and

Table 7.3. Treatable causes of Dementia (after Pearce and Miller (Ref. 244, p.43))

Trauma	Acute and delayed effects of head injury
Infections	Neurosyphilis Torulosis Cryptogenic abscess
Deficiency states	Vitamin B_{12} ? Vitamin B complex (B_1, B_6) Folic acid
Neoplasms	Hemisphere mass, primary or metastasic Carcinomatous meningitis
Intoxications	Barbiturates, Bromides Alcohol ? Amphetamines and hallucinogens ? Cannabis
Metabolic	Hypothyroidism Hypopituitarism Hypercalcaemia Cushing's syndrome Chronic renal failure Hepatic encephalopathy
Dynamic	Cardiac and extracranial vascular emboli

vitamin B_{12} deficiency can lead to neuropsychiatric changes and dementia. Macrocytosis is not always present and anaemia may be absent. Drugs, for example phenytoin in epileptic patients, may result in insidious deterioration of cognitive abilities, as can alcohol when taken excessively over a number of years.[268]

Hormone disturbances may lead to dementia, in particular hypothyroidism, which is usually accompanied by other clinical signs of myxoedema. Thyroid function tests will be abnormal, serum cholesterol raised and thyroid antibodies may be present in the serum.

Neurosyphilis, at one time a common cause of neuropsychiatric illness, may lead to dementia. General paralysis of the insane (GPI) presents as progressive deterioration and a variety of other symptoms including manic, depressive, and schizophrenic features. The disorder often starts insidiously, and memory soon becomes affected. Gross loss of judgement with florid delusions are well documented and without treatment the patient becomes profoundly demented and confined to bed. Death usually occurs from convulsions or infection. The disorder typically develops some 10–15 years following a primary infection, and is seen most frequently in the fourth to sixth decades of life. Pathologically, there is marked cerebral atrophy with meningeal thickening. Neuronal loss with astrocyte proliferation is noted, and iron pigment in the microglia and perivascular spaces is specific for the disease.[269] Treponema pallidum can be seen in the cortex of 50% of the cases using special techniques.

On examination, apart from the abnormal mental state, a number of physical signs may be noted including tremor of the lips, tongue and out-stretched hands. Speech disorder with hesitation and slurring occurs, and the characteristic Argyll–Robertson pupil is present in about 50% of advanced cases. Sudden episodes of unconsciousness occur, the patient on recovery having residual neurological deficits which gradually improve over a few days.

In the CSF there is elevation of total protein and lymphocyte count, a paretic Lange colloidal gold curve (first zone) and positive serology. The blood serology is positive in 95% of cases.

Although neurosyphilis is far less common than it used to be, cases are still reported especially from referral centres,[270] and screening of patients with a WR or VDRL and the TPHA tests is still mandatory. False positives are seen with a number of disorders and if the diagnosis is questioned, further tests, such as the treponema immobilization test (TPI) or fluorescent antibody testings (FTA), will be needed. Treatment is with antibiotics, usually large doses of penicillin. Steroids are often used in addition, to prevent the Herxheimer reaction, an acute febrile state with intensification of symptoms, which occurs usually within 24 hours of penicillin therapy. Mental symptoms may improve, but the Wassermann test in the CSF and blood may not become negative for a number of years. Relapses of the clinical manifestations are normally preceded by further CSF changes.

SUBCORTICAL DEMENTIA

Although dementia traditionally refers to cognitive changes consequent upon cortical damage, an alternative form of dementia may be seen in patients with a variety of neurological illnesses in which the major pathological changes occur in subcortical nuclear structures. Albert et al.[271] described the features of this syndrome as emotional or personality changes, memory disorder, a defective ability to manipulate acquired knowledge and slowness in the rate of information processing. They contrasted this pattern of dementia with cortical dementias, pointing out that in subcortical dementias, language abilities are well preserved and apraxias and agnosias are not seen. Such a clinical picture may be observed in progressive supranuclear palsy, Parkinson's disease, and Huntington's chorea. They supported this concept by quoting evidence that surgical lesions of the basal ganglia impair performance and problem-solving tasks, and that stimulation of subcortical structures leads to changes in cognitive performance. They also noted the similarity of the symptom complex of subcortical dementia to the behavioural syndrome seen in patients with frontal lobe damage. Pointing to the unique reciprocal connections between the frontal cortex and the limbic system with its subcortical components, they suggest a better name may be fronto-limbic dementia.

PSEUDODEMENTIA

The term pseudodementia covers a number of disorders including depressive pseudodementia, hysterical pseudodementia, and the Ganser syndrome. The clinical differentiation between dementia and depression can be extremely difficult, some of the major differences having been outlined by Post.[272] He noted that at any age both dementia and depression are characterized by impairment of psychological functioning, and that cognitive and psychomotor disruption can occur in severe depression. The early symptoms of both dementia and depression show overlap which can be difficult to disentangle, particularly in the elderly. Decreasing interest, increasing apathy, somatic complaints, memory disturbances, impaired concentration, disturbed sleep, slowing, and fleeting delusional ideas may be common to both. In making the distinction a clear history from informants is important. Earlier history of psychiatric illness, and gradual onset of depressive symptoms with classical depressive delusions, may then stand out in contrast to a more typical story of dementia with failing memory and mental ability over a period of time, with episodes of confusion and possibly failing physical health. The affective changes in dementia tend to be more labile and shallow, with fluctuations, and euphoria, anxiety, aggression, and other changes occur readily.

A more complicated situation occurs where dementia may coexist with depression. Post suggested that age changes in the brain facilitate the occurrence of depression, and thus depression is more frequent and severe in later life. Clinically, recognition of associated depression in dementia is important since it is treatable in its own right. ECT is not contraindicated although antidepressants are probably the initial treatment of choice. Close attention must be paid to the social circumstances of the patient, and attempts to overcome isolation, physical infirmities, and other stressful events undertaken.

The Ganser syndrome was described in 1897 and fully reviewed by Whitlock.[273] Ganser's patients presented with hallucinations, cognitive disorientation, hysterical stigmata, and vorbeireden. They were unable to answer even simple questions correctly, and although they understood the nature of questions, approximate answers were given. In that his cases were prisoners, Ganser considered malingering in the differential diagnosis but discounted it on account of the other signs and symptoms present.

Ganser syndromes have now been described in a number of disorders including depressive illness, epilepsy, schizophrenia, and chronic organic brain syndromes, mostly in patients not in prison. Whitlock suggested that vorbeireden alone was not sufficient to make a diagnosis, and that the syndrome implied an acute psychosis with clouding of consciousness and subsequent amnesia for the duration of the illness. In an analysis of the vorbeireden he commented that many patients' replies did not correspond to the concept of approximation, and it was their random and absurd nature which was striking. In some cases aphasia, or typical confabulation as seen in a Korsakoff syndrome, may have contributed to this particular symptom.

Hysterical pseudodementia has been equated by some authors with the Ganser syndrome, although others suggest that in hysterical pseudodementia patients show no disturbance of consciousness, and other features of abnormal illness behaviour may be noted in the history. It is more commonly seen in patients with low intelligence, and other hysterical conversion symptoms may be present. Lishman (Ref. 42, p.569) noted that in the Ganser syndrome the episodes of disturbance are typically brief with spontaneous termination, while in hysterical pseudodementia the disorder is often prolonged and relapsing. Successful malingering of mental illness is surprisingly difficult to achieve. Anderson *et al.*[274] asked a group of students to simulate mental illness, and compared their behaviour to patients with organic dementia and the Ganser syndrome. None of the normals were able to produce clinical pictures that resembled psychiatric disorders and syndromes, and even those that came close were only able to sustain it for a short period of time.

TREATMENT OF DEMENTIA

In the accounts of the individual disorders given above, some specific treatments have been commented on. In addition other therapies, especially drugs, have been advocated to improve cerebral blood flow, influence neuronal metabolism, and, it is hoped, ameliorate cognitive performance. Cyclandelate (Cyclospasmol) and isoxsuprine (Duvadilan) have both been reported to be of value in the treatment of arteriosclerotic cerebrovascular disease, although the pattern of improvement has been inconsistent, and in many studies the design has not allowed accurate assessment of the drug effects. Other drugs in this category include hydergine, pentifylline (Cosaldon) and naftidrofuryl (Praxiline). Amantadine (Symmetrel) has been shown to be of value in elderly patients suffering from psychomotor retardation, bringing about improvement in the general mental status, mood, and activity.[275] Where extrapyramidal signs are noted small doses of L-dopa may bring about improvements of intellect and motor function.[276] Psychotropic drugs are useful in alleviating some affective symptoms, in particular thioridazine (Melleril), and the benzodiazepines. For depressive symptoms antidepressants should be used, and where indicated ECT should not be withheld.

More general aspects of management include helping the patient to cope at home or work, and offering support to the family where breakdown is occurring. Where an elderly patient is living alone, help of the Social Services will be required to ensure that the patient is adequately cared for, and personal neglect is not occurring. Day care facilities should be used where necessary, and admission to hospital considered when it is clear that the patient can no longer look after himself in the hope of successful rehabilitation. Meticulous attention to health is important since it is easy to precipitate an acute organic brain syndrome in patients with dementia. In particular, vitamin deficiency, dehydration, and the subsequent development of a minor infective illness can lead to a disastrous situation which could otherwise have been avoided.

HEAD INJURY AND POST-TRAUMATIC NEUROSIS

It is estimated that in England and Wales some 150,000 patients are discharged annually from hospital having been admitted for head injury. Of these 7% are considered major head injuries. The commonest causes of injury include falls, road traffic accidents and assaults. Amongst adults road traffic accidents form more than half the admissions, and industrial accidents are responsible for 10%. As a cause of death, head injury accounts for under 1% of all deaths.[277] There is however considerable morbidity. This is dependent on a number of factors including the site and severity of the injury, the premorbid condition of the patient, and the presence or absence of the development of other complications such as epilepsy.

It is usual to assess the severity of the head injury by the duration of the post-traumatic amnesia. This is the time taken from the injury to the recovery of a continuous memory, and does not refer to the appearance of islets of memory which often occur before full memory powers are restored. In contrast, retrograde amnesia refers to the timing of the last clear memory prior to injury. It tends to be brief, up to a minute or so, and is nearly always shorter than the post-traumatic amnesia. Occasionally there is long retrograde amnesia, sometimes lasting months, but usually in these cases there has been severe brain injury, and the post-traumatic amnesia is equally long. Where retrograde amnesias are long they tend to show spontaneous shrinkage with time. Because of this peri-traumatic amnesia, details of the injury provided by the patient may be false. Such paramnesia is related to the development of an acute organic brain syndrome, and some patients show confabulation. Rarely a florid confabulatory syndrome may develop.[278]

Severe head injury usually refers to one in which there has been a post-traumatic amnesia of more than 24 hours. Another indicator of severity is the duration and depth of coma. This is often easier to gauge than the post-traumatic amnesia, and rating scales have been developed to quantify the impairment of consciousness in terms of verbal performance, motor responses, and eye opening.[279] Coma of more than 6 hours' duration represents severe injury.

Following severe head injury the mortality rate over 5 years is nearly 50%, younger patients surviving more than elderly patients but consequently resulting in greater social disability. Some 1500 patients annually are left with major disability from head injury, and either return to work at a level far below their former capacity or remain unemployable. Miller and Stern[280] examined 100 patients with head injury and post-traumatic amnesia of more than 24 hours. Approximately half had closed head injury, and overt neurological signs were present in 72. At follow-up of 92 patients over 3 to 40 years, they found that the average period of absence from work was 13 months.

A number of patients who previously had cranial nerve lesions recovered, and the outcome for spastic paresis was also favourable. Sixteen of the patients had psychiatric symptoms, ten showing some degree of dementia. Fahy *et al.*[281] followed up 32 survivors of severe head injury who had a craniotomy at the time of the injury, and thus objective evidence of brain damage was shown. Three had died of severe dementia, and residual neurological signs were found in the majority. Psychiatric disability was high, and both the psychiatric and neurological morbidity was positively correlated with the length of the post-traumatic amnesia.

The commonest neurological complications of head injury are intracranial haematoma, infection, and epilepsy. The latter is more likely to develop with a depressed fracture of the skull, with a post-traumatic amnesia of greater than 24 hours, and with the occurrence of a fit shortly after injury. If all three of these factors occur together then the chances of developing epilepsy are over 60%.[282] The epilepsy may be focal in origin but usually presents as a major tonic–clonic seizure.

The neurological sequelae of head injury depend to some degree on the site of the lesion, and focal signs and symptoms as outlined in Chapter 6 may be produced. However, many of the neuropsychiatric consequences of head injury cannot be predicted from such localization, and seem dependent upon several factors usually acting in combination (Ref. 42, p.207). Hillbom[283] conducted an extensive survey of 415 brain injured patients, 30% of whom had noteworthy psychiatric disturbance; 33 cases of psychosis were reported, the incidence being commoner in the more severely disabled and nine developed a chronic paranoid hallucinatory psychosis. Changes in personality were more frequent amongst the more severely injured patients, but in contrast, the neuroses, with the exception of the obsessional neuroses, were commoner in the less damaged. The psychiatric disturbances were commoner in patients who had left-sided injuries, 63% of the psychoses having such lateralization. Bilateral injuries were noted in relationship to the dementias and amnestic syndromes, frontal lesions were commonly associated with changes in character, and temporal lesions with the psychoses.

Lishman[201] studied the psychiatric morbidity in 670 patients with penetrating head injury in which detailed information was available as to the site and extent of brain damage. Both 'depth of penetration' and 'total brain destroyed' were significantly related to psychiatric disability. This finding was not due to accompanying intellectual deficits, although he confirmed that length of the post-traumatic amnesia correlated with the subsequent psychiatric disability. However, if the post-traumatic amnesia was less than 1 hour there was an inverse relationship with disability. In 345 patients the location of the brain damage was known. Left hemisphere lesions were associated with more psychiatric disability than right, and temporal lesions more so than frontal, parietal or occipital. In particular he noted the association between left temporal lobe damage and psychiatric morbidity. Lesions resulting in sensory-motor defects, visual field defects, aphasias and epilepsy were all significantly related to psychiatric illness.

In a further analysis of 144 patients he related various individual symptoms and syndromes to the site and size of the lesion. Intellectual and behaviour disorders had a close association with brain damage, especially to the left hemisphere. Affective disorders or somatic complaints had an association with right hemisphere damage. While depression, anxiety, irritability and difficulty in concentration had only a weak association with the site of lesions, apathy, euphoria, disinhibition, and the 'frontal lobe syndrome' were strongly associated with frontal lobe lesions.

Head injuries in childhood have also been examined with a view to assessing the psychiatric sequelae and the relationship to the brain injury.[284, 285] Depressed fractures are associated with a high degree of psychiatric disability, but in contrast to adult studies no relationship between the type of disorder and the site or size of the injury are shown. Children with psychiatric disturbances after head injury are more likely to have adverse social and family variables than controls, suggesting interactions between adverse environmental circumstances and brain injury leading to the consequent behaviour disturbance.

While brain damage itself seems to play a part in the production of neuro-psychiatric sequelae of head trauma, other factors must also be of importance. Lishman outlined these as shown in Table 7.4. From his own studies he calculated that the injury contributed to little more than one-fifteenth part of the total disability. He drew attention to the emotional impact of the injury which may precipitate psychiatric illness in the predisposed, and commented on the important place that the head holds in the body image and the consequent severe threat that injury to the head poses. The circumstances of the injury may have personal consequences for patients leading to unresolved conflict and guilt with consequent disability (Ref. 42, pp.207–11).

Table 7.4. Aetiological factors in psychiatric disturbance after head injury (after Lishman (Ref. 42, pp.207–11))

Mental constitution
Premorbid personality
Emotional impact of injury
Emotional repercussions of injury
Environmental factors
Compensation and litigation
Response to intellectual impairments
Development of epilepsy
Amount of brain damage incurred
Location of brain damage incurred

The development of neurotic symptoms following head injury is of particular interest. As noted above, this is more likely to occur following minor as opposed to major head injury, and is usually seen in association with closed rather than open head injury. Explanation purely in terms of localized brain damage is not tenable. Typically following an accident the patient develops symptoms referred to as 'the post-concussional syndrome'. Courville[286] examined 74 cases of patients who complained of symptoms following head injury. 94% had headaches, 71% dizziness, visual disturbances occurred in 53%, fatigue in 27% and tinnitus in 24%. A variety of nervous symptoms were reported which included anxiety, restlessness, irritability, sleeplessness, forgetfulness, confusion, poor concentration, and sensitivity to noise. In that there was some clustering of these symptoms, he felt that the post-concussional symptoms had a basis in organic neurological change, and could be distinguished from the symptoms of 'post-traumatic neurosis'. The main features of the latter were depression, exaggeration of pre-existing personality defects, the elaboration of symptoms both in statement and behaviour, the presence of hysterical components, and a multiplicity, changeability, and indefiniteness of the symptoms. More recently Lidvall et al.[287] surveyed consecutive patients suffering from concussion treated in a hospital emergency room over a 2 year period. The patients were followed up and examined neurologically and psychiatrically, and a group that developed post-concussional symptoms were compared with a group that did not. Using cluster analysis techniques, they were not able to conclude that the post-concussional syndrome was an entity. While headache and dizziness were dominant symptoms during the first week of injury, anxiety then appeared as 'the nucleus of the polymorphous late symptom picture'. However, they did report that a higher percentage of subjects with post-concussional symptoms had spontaneous and/or positional nystagmus on otoneurological testing, and that this was related to the later reporting of dizziness. Taylor and Bell[288] examined a group of patients with post-concussional symptoms and measured the mean cerebral circulation time. Significant differences were reported between patients and controls, the former showing an increase. Likewise Toglia[289] examined 309 patients whose main complaint was dizziness following whiplash injury. Specific attention was given to vestibular tests, including a search for latent and positional nystagmus. He reported lateral nystagmus in 29% of his patients, abnormal caloric tests in 57% and abnormal rotary tests in 51%. These studies suggest that subtle neuronal damage may occur following closed head injury and that some of the consequent symptoms may reflect such damage, especially early post-traumatic complaints.

Further evidence that neurological injury can result from mild head injuries comes from animal experiments, and studies of psychological testing of patients with post-concussional symptoms. Denny-Brown and Russell[290] induced experimental concussion in cats and dogs and observed physiological responses. They showed that even minor head injuries could lead to alteration of brainstem activity. Groat and Simmons[291] observed loss of neurones in brainstem areas following trauma, and a relationship between the amount of cell loss in regions such as the reticular formation and lateral vestibular nuclei, and the severity of the concussion. They concluded that 'some cell loss will occur in all concussions, even extremely light ones, and in some subconcussions . . .'. There are in addition a few studies of human post-mortem cases that show areas of neuronal damage following quite trivial head injury.[292]

Gronwall and Wrightson[293] performed psychological tests on patients with minor head injuries using a paced auditory serial addition test, which gave an indication of the rate of information processing ability. They found that patients who had typical post-concussional symptoms, and an inability to carry on with their normal work, showed reduced ability to process required information. In addition as the post-concussional symptoms improved, their test scores increased.

The mechanism whereby subtle brain damage could occur in minor head injury was explored by Pudenz and Sheldon.[294] They replaced the calvarium of monkeys with a transparent material to directly observe movements of the brain. High-speed photography was employed while they delivered sub-concussive blows to the heads of the animals. They found that brain movement lagged behind movement of the skull, presumably on account of the inertia of the cerebral mass. This glide was noted to be greatest in the parietal and occipital lobes, where tearing of the surface veins was noted, and least in the frontal regions. They suggested that the latter was due to comparative restriction of the frontal lobes by the rigid anterior fossa, and that this led to strains within the cerebral tissue of that region resulting in laceration and subsequent cerebral damage. Although they were unable to directly visualize the temporal lobes, they suggested that the latter would have the same susceptibility to damage.

Although it may be that many head injuries are associated with subtle neurological damage, and that many patients develop immediate post-concussional symptoms which have a physiogenic basis, there is much controversy surrounding the persistence of symptoms, and the later development of post-traumatic neurosis. Many such cases are involved in litigation, and the posssibility that the compensation is in some way responsible for the persistence of symptoms is often suggested. During the two World Wars a large number of neurotic illnesses, not associated with head injuries, precipitated by the stress of battle were observed, and terms such as shell-shock, battle neurosis and combat exhaustion came into use. It was apparent that these neuroses were very similar to those encountered in peace-time. Brill and Beebe[295] collected information on 955 Services personnel who were treated for psychoneuroses during the Second World War; 34% had neurotic traits recorded prior to their service, and stress was seen as a major factor in precipitating breakdown. At follow-up of those still disabled there was a significant relationship between the pre-service personality and adjustment to the continuing disablement, two-thirds of those disabled having symptoms that they had prior to service. Symonds[296] provided data on air force personnel diagnosed as having neurosis; 78% were found to have anxiety states, 9% depressive states, and 13% hysteria, and two-thirds of the cases had a family or personal history of neurosis. He attempted to evaluate the relationship between the stress involved and the predisposition, and noted that those with a strong predisposition broke down under mild stress, whereas severe stress was required to produce a breakdown in groups with no predisposition. He also collected information on military personnel injured by accidents that were not exclusive to being in the Forces, and may have occurred in civilian life. Of those with evidence of predisposition, suspected either by a family member or personal history of psychiatric disturbances or alcoholism, invalidism was twice as high as in those without. In a group of 111 flying personnel especially selected as being of sound mental constitution, only 12% were invalided by head injury, as opposed to 48% of other flying personnel, in spite of the injuries received by the two groups being comparable in severity.[297] Lewis[298] compared the past records of patients admitted to hospital with post-traumatic symptoms with a group admitted with neurosis but no head injury, and found no differences, which led him to conclude: 'the striking thing is that the long-standing, relatively intractable, post-concussional syndrome is apt to occur in much the same person as develops a psychiatric syndrome in other circumstances without any brain injury at all.' Similar results were reported by Guttmann.[299] Dencker[300] followed up unselected cases of closed head injury amongst twins using the co-twins as controls in order to keep constitutional factors as much as possible alike in the two groups. The head-injured twin differed significantly from the partner, showing more changes in intellectual capacity and antisocial traits, the difference being greater for the monozygotic pairs. However, the injured proband did not differ significantly in respect to temper, fatigability, tension, anxiety symptoms, obsessional ideas, depression, paranoid traits or psychosomatic disorders. In twenty of the pairs the head-injured proband was said to have undergone a change of personality after injury. However, even before the injury at least 15 of these had more of the symptoms or traits that dominated the change in personality after injury than their co-twins. Slater[301] studied over 2000 soldiers admitted to a neurosis centre during World War II. He commented that 'the monotonous character of precipiating cause and clinical picture was mirrored by a monotonous uniformity of the underlying personality. There were few who did not show some degree of psychic asthenia, a feebleness of will and purpose, coupled with tendencies to worry, pessimism and moodiness or hysterical traits'. A family history of psychiatric illness or epilepsy was obtained in 56% of the sample, and childhood neurosis was shown in 59%; 23% had had a previous nervous breakdown and 40% an abnormal personality. He confirmed the suggestion of Symonds that the tendency towards breakdown should be regarded quantitatively, the degree of stress required to produce breakdown being inversely related to the degree of neurotic constitution.

These studies emphasized the role of constitutional factors in the aetiology of post-traumatic neurosis. Another consequence of the examination of these states in the war setting was emphasis on the idea that 'gain' of one sort or another was related to production of symptoms. Post-traumatic neuroses were not reported in prisoners of war, and it was suggested that this was because they had no gain in being sick.[302] The concept of gain was incorporated into psychoanalytical viewpoints of the problem, and included realization of suppressed desires for sympathy, attention, revenge, and even masochistic longings. Some saw the gain as essentially financial. The term 'compensation neurosis' was introduced by Rigler in 1879 who noted the increase in invalidism after railway accidents following the introduction of compensation laws.[303] In England a variety of acts were introduced in the last part of the 19th century allowing for compensation to be provided for workmen who were injured during the course of their employment. Under the 1906 Workmen's Compensation Act, anyone who entered into a contract of service or apprenticeship with an employer was covered, even if negligence on behalf of the workman himself could be seen to have played a part in the accident. In the first 6 years after 1906 the numbers of accidents in industry rose by 44%, and the amount of compensation paid by 63.5%. However, non-fatal accidents increased at a greater rate than fatal ones, supporting the belief that it was compensation that led to disability.[304]

Miller[305] examined 47 cases with psychoneurotic symptoms following head injury. He found that such complaints occurred much more commonly following industrial as opposed to road traffic accidents, especially if the employers were large industrial organisations or nationalized industries. Neurotic complications were twice as common in men as opposed to women, were more prevalent in patients from social class IV and V, and an inverse relationship existed between the presence of neurosis and the severity of the injury and duration of unconsciousness. He re-examined 50 patients 2 years after settlement of their claims and found that only two were still disabled by their symptoms, recovery having occurred in 45.

Although the suggestion from these studies was that patients produce symptoms for financial gain, if the conclusion is that these patients are malingering, the difficulty is to know how to make such a diagnosis. Hurst[306] suggested that there are only two conditions that lead to a diagnosis of malingering with certainty. The person may be detected in *'flagrante delicto'*, in other words caught in the act, when he thinks he is alone or even perhaps unthinking. The second is when somebody actually confesses to malingering. Although others lay down criteria, such as that a malingerer is aloof, suspicious, hostile, secretive, etc., these are difficult to employ clinically. In addition the borderland between varieties of abnormal illness behaviour, such as hysteria and the Munchausen syndrome, and malingering is extremely blurred. The traditional distinction that in hysteria the gain is unconscious whereas in malingering it is conscious is impossible to establish clinically. To complicate the issue further, some authors suggest that malingering is a variety of personality disorder, thus falling within the spectrum of psychiatric diagnosis and itself amenable to psychiatric treatment. Kamman,[307] who felt that post-traumatic neurosis was related to a 'failure in the victim's total possibilities for adaptation', and that the neurosis was seen as a reaction to the injury, acknowledged the role of compensation in the production of symptoms in some people. However, he used the term 'attitudinal pathoses' to refer to a constellation of attitudes firmly held by patients, leading to a persistent mental set with regard to the accident, meaning that the patient would pursue his seemingly just cause through to its bitter ends. Likewise Good[308] described the malingerer as a psychopath who had no feelings of guilt about his malingering, and although the conscious element of his exploits was acknowledged, these were determined by unrecognized masochistic and infantile dependent attitudes.

Few follow-up data are available, and information collected has usually come from biased samples. The study of Miller is mentioned above. In contrast Russell[309] followed up 72 cases in which there was no question of compensation. A high percentage of patients complained of symptoms, in particular of nervousness and headaches. Balla and Moraitis[310] followed up 82 patients who had neck and back injuries following industrial and traffic accidents. They found that settlement of compensation made little or no difference to the patient's symptoms, and that early settlement of claims did not lead to a lessening of morbidity. Merskey and Woodforde[311] reported 27 patients who had minor head injury, in whom financial compensation was not an issue, who continued to have symptoms for a number of years after the accident. Ten of these showed little or no improvement at follow-up, five patients became unemployed, and six took a lower occupational status.

It would seem that the symptoms of post-traumatic neurosis arise from the interplay of a number of different factors. Subtle organic neurological damage undoubtedly plays a role in some cases, and the relationship between this and other parameters such as premorbid personality is probably similar to that seen in abnormal illness behaviour discussed in Chapter 5. Slater, in the study quoted above, noted that patients with organic states presenting to the Neurosis Centre had fewer neurotic traits. The organic injury leads to neurotic disability in its own right, predisposing to neurosis with less constitutional liability than would otherwise be necessary. This interaction between organic change and neurotic symptoms was also noted by Stengel who said: 'Often a neurotic syndrome forms round a nucleus of symptoms due to structural damage, especially where the latter is slight. It is difficult and unprofitable to attempt to demarcate the neurotic superstructure from what is called its organic basis . . . .'.[312] The recent advances in neurochemistry, in particular the knowledge that psychiatric disturbances are accompanied by changes in neurotransmitter function, which may be provoked by head trauma or neurological illness, may lead to further understanding of this very difficult area, and unite polarized views that post-traumatic neurotic symptoms reside either in organic changes, or are a consequence of malingering.[303]

TREATMENT

The immediate management of head injuries, particularly of severe ones, is of concern primarily to neurologists and neurosurgeons and is not discussed here. As noted above, a number of the neurological long-term complications gradually improve, and generally cause fewer problems for rehabilitation than might be anticipated (Ref. 277, p.61). Impairment of cognitive abilities may show improvement with time, and Lishman (Ref. 42, p.225) suggests that a firm prognosis should not be attempted with regard to the recovery of dementia until at least 2 or 3 years have elapsed since injury. In rehabilitation prolonged bed rest has been replaced by gradual mobilization with active physiotherapy and a programme of progressive activity. Supportive psychotherapy and social work help will allow exploration of the patient's fears regarding brain damage, and allow explanation to be given for symptoms that arise. Reassessment of the patient's ability to work may be required and retraining, or the provision of some form of sheltered workshop, provided where necessary.

Of all the complications of head injury it is probably the mental sequelae that interfere most with the patient's return to normal social life, personality changes and affective disorder being much more difficult to manage than physical injuries.[313] Roberts[314] in a study on patients amnesic or unconscious for over a week, noted that decline in level of employment was more related to personality or intellectual abnormalities than to neurological disability. Most disabling were frontal lobe personality changes, associated with intense irritability or uncontrollable outbursts of rage. Where indicated, antidepressant medication, antipsychotic medication, or ECT should be employed. Often small doses of minor or major tranquillizers help control irritable and dysphoric mood changes, and major tranquillizers may improve disinhibition. A number of studies have emphasized the consequences of head injury for the family. Again it is the psychiatric disturbances that cause the most distress. Two-thirds of close relatives require some form of psychotropic drug treatment, and many feel the support they receive to be inadequate.[315] Bond[316] commented on the profound effect that the patients' memory and personality impairment has upon family cohesion. A major complicating factor in rehabilitation is the patient's own lack of insight regarding his own limitations. This leads not only to increasing distress for relatives, but also to the pursuit of unrealistic goals by the patient, leading to frustration and further psychiatric morbidity.

CEREBRO-VASCULAR DISEASE

Cerebro-vascular disease is a common cause of morbidity with a prevalence of around two cases per thousand per annum, rising steadily with advancing age. Traditionally cerebro-vascular accidents are divided into emboli, haemorrhages, and infarctions. In one variety, small emboli result in the presentation of transient cerebral ischaemia, in which brief episodes of disturbed function occur followed by full recovery. Infarction occurs more frequently than haemorrhage, and follows emboli or thrombosis. Diagnosis of aetiology is often dependent on the characteristics of the symptoms, especially the rate of progression, associated clinical features, such as hypertension or evidence for a site of origin of an embolus, and the past history. In many cases examination of CSF, and the use of specialized radiographic techniques will confirm the diagnosis, and provide information regarding the cause of the insult. Usually this is related to atherosclerosis, hypertension, or an embolus from the heart or adjacent major blood vessels. Management of these problems, especially in the acute situation, is the province of the neurologist or the neurosurgeon. Long-term management involves a number of different specialities, although neuro-psychiatric complications have been relatively little explored. Focal symptoms such as those outlined in Chapter 6 will occur following specific areas of brain damage, and all acute insults may lead to an acute organic brain syndrome. Multiple small strokes may result in arteriosclerotic dementia as discussed in Chapter 7. Personality changes following strokes are common and include apathy, irritability, lower threshold for aggression and withdrawal. Depression is a frequent accompaniment, its occurrence often being dependent on premorbid personality characteristics (Ref. 42, p.465). Folstein *et al.*[317] studied depression in 20 patients with cerebrovascular infarctions, ten who had a right, and ten a left hemisphere lesion, 30 days after their strokes. They assessed psychiatric symptoms with the PSE and other rating scales, and as controls used patients with orthopaedic problems. The stroke patients, in particular the right hemisphere group, had notably more depression than the orthopaedic group, when matched for physical disability. They suggested that an explanation for this degree of depression was not explicable in terms of 'psychological reaction', since there were differences compared with the controls, and injury to the right hemisphere was particularly implicated. As catecholamine depletion occurs following experimental cerebral infarction in animals, they felt that monoamine disturbances may be more relevant, and advocated antidepressant drugs in therapy.

Psychosis following cerebrovascular accidents is rare. Davison and Bagley,[318] in a comprehensive survey, noted only a few reports of paranoid–hallucinatory states, and commented that cerebrovascular lesions were not over-represented in post-mortem brains from schizophrenic patients. They did suggest, however, that late onset schizophrenia may be significantly related to cerebrovascular disease.

Some authors have commented on personality structures of patients with strokes, suggesting that certain personalities are more prone than others. Ecker[319] noted long-standing personality difficulties in 20 patients, and emotional stress immediately prior to the stroke in most cases. In a more extensive study Adler *et al.*[320] also commented on certain personality features which were commonly noted before a stroke, which they referred to as 'pressured'. Such patients often had chronic problems with the control of anger, and 'an object-relating style' characterized by the assumption of personal responsibilities for gratification of needs. They documented a number of cases in whom a stroke had occurred when the patient was acting with strong emotional feelings, especially anger, hopelessness and shame. They were particularly impressed by the uniformity of the personality characteristics of their patients, and noted that similar findings had been reported for coronary disease and hypertension.

The psychiatric aspects of subarachnoid haemorrhage have received more attention. In this condition blood from one of the intracranial vessels leaks into the subarachnoid space. More than half of the patients affected have ruptured aneurysms, and a smaller number have primary intracerebral haemorrhage, or angiomas. Aneurysms usually occur at branches of vessels, the commonest sites being the anterior cerebral–anterior communicating artery complex, the division of the middle cerebral artery, and the origin of the posterior communicating artery from the internal carotid.[321] Mortality in this condition is high, and of the 25% of patients with aneurysmal subarachnoid haemorrhage that survive for 5 years, some 30% remain partly or totally disabled. Penrose[322] studied life events 3 months preceding subarachnoid haemorrhage in 44 patients. Those that had no demonstrable aneurysm had significantly more emotional disturbance in this period than those with an aneurysm or controls. Storey[323] investigated 261 patients with subarachnoid haemorrhage, 30 of whom had no demonstrable aneurysm; 11 of the latter gave a history of affective disturbance before the stroke, an incidence far greater than in the 231 patients with an aneurysm. In a further study of the histories of 102 patients with, and 101 patients without, aneurysms who had proven subarachnoid haemorrhage, significantly more of the aneurysm cases described physical activity at the time of stroke, and more of the no-aneurysm group had received previous psychiatric treatment. They felt that these figures suggested that subarachnoid haemorrhage could be precipitated by powerful emotional turmoil, especially in patients with normal angiograms and no aneurysms.

In further studies, Storey[324] followed up patients 6 months to 6 years after their illness, and noted a high incidence of psychiatric morbidity: 41% were considered to have personality impairment, severe in 4%, although a small number of cases actually showed some improvement in their personality. An increased chance of impairment was associated with increasing residual neurological disability, and it was significantly more common in patients with demonstrated aneurysms, especially middle cerebral artery aneurysms. Patients with anterior cerebral artery aneurysms had less intellectual impairment in the presence of personality deterioration than the others. Overall, the commonest changes in personality noted were irritability, increased anxiety, and apathy. Patients with middle cerebral artery aneurysms were most affected, and were reported to be dependent, emotionally labile, and fatuous. Those with anterior artery aneurysms often became uninhibited, less worried, and less irritable. Many patients showed a picture of ' "organic moodiness", a chronic shallow depressed mood often lifting quickly in response to some new stimulus, but rapidly falling back with apparent boredom, loss of interest and early fatigue'. The occurrence of depressive illness and anxiety were related to the premorbid personality characteristics of the patient. Storey commented on the similarities of these findings with those of Lishman in head injured patients.

Logue et al.[325] studied 79 patients with anterior cerebral or communicating artery aneurysms, 66 of whom were treated surgically. Memory deficits, especially for recent events, were more often noted, rather than overall impairment of intelligence. The predominant psychiatric changes were alterations of mood, an increased tendency to worry, affective flattening and lability, and irritability and outspokenness were found in nearly half. A number of patients were seen in whom elevation of mood and favourable personality changes had occurred which was attributed to a leucotomy effect.

Management of the chronic sequelae of cerebro-vascular accidents relies on control of any medical factors, such as hypertension, that may have caused the first episode, and tackling long-term rehabilitation. Great reliance is placed on physiotherapy, occupational therapy, social work help, and speech therapy. For a few, especially young patients, residential rehabilitation centres have been established. Special problems such as aphasia, which lead to even greater morbidity, have been discussed in Chapter 6. Psychotherapy of the supportive kind is essential to restore the patients' morale and motivation, and to help them come to terms with their limited ability. Hurwitz and Adams[326] discussed some of the 'mental barriers' to rehabilitation. They highlighted speech deficits, body image disturbances, apraxias, memory disturbances, lack of motivation, depression and dementia. They noted that the clinical features of some of these impediments varied from day to day, and that attention to these deficits is usually drawn to the doctor's notice by those looking after the patients, rather than the patients themselves. Their list of rehabilitation barriers and objectives are shown in Table 7.5.[327] Emergent psychiatric illness needs to be looked for and treated when apparent. Antidepressants that lead to minimal side-effects should be used, and small doses initially. The risk of precipitation of seizures is increased in these patients, and tricyclic antidepressants are best avoided. ECT is not contra-indicated providing the cerebro-vascular accident is not recent. Psychosis should be treated accordingly, although again the risk of precipitating seizures with major tranquillizers is increased.

Table 7.5. Some barriers and objective of rehabilitation (after Adams and Hurwitz[327])

Patients with no clouding of consciousness, without severe intellectual impairment, and with adequate hearing, vision, motor and sensory function, and coordination

Objectives	Mental barriers to recovery
Sit up	1. A defect in comprehension
	2. Neglect of the hemiparetic limbs
	3. Denial of disease
Stand up	4. Disturbance of body-image
	5. 'Space-blindness'
	6. Apraxia
	7. Motor perseveration
Walk	8. Memory loss of immediate events
	9. 'Mirror' and other synkinetic movements
Self-care	10. Loss of confidence
	11. True depression
	12. Too inattentive
	13. 'Don't want to do it'
Socially reliable	14. Catastrophic reactions

Generally the rate of improvement in rehabilitation is slow but may continue for several years after the initial stroke. Patients with right hemisphere lesions often make a worse recovery than those with left-sided deficits, probably related to subtle communicative deficits that occur following non-dominant hemisphere destruction. In particular, visuo-spatial deficits may be overlooked, and lead to the feeling that the patient is not trying, but also to an interference with the patient's own ability to successfully learn from rehabilitation procedures. Marquardsen,[328] in a long-term follow-up of 769 stroke patients, noted 407 immediate survivors, about half of whom became independent to the extent of looking after themselves without assistance. The rest were disabled to varying degrees, 12% being completely incapacitated.

MULTIPLE SCLEROSIS AND DISORDERS OF MYELINATION

The essential clinical criterion for a diagnosis of multiple sclerosis is the demonstration of multiple lesions in the CNS disseminated in time. In practice the lesions usually present as neurological problems, although initial presentation as psychiatric disability has been described.[329] The onset is typically between the ages of 20 and 40, and although in the majority the illness undergoes remissions, in 10–20% it is progressive. Particularly common presenting features are blurring of vision, diplopia, vertigo, limb paraesthesiae, weakness, impotence and bladder problems, although signs and symptoms are referrable to any part of the central nervous system. In some patients paroxysmal symptoms are noted, including transient weakness, pain, sensory symptoms, visual difficulties and bizarre movements.

Pathologically the lesions of multiple sclerosis are areas of demyelination which at post-mortem consist of scattered and discrete patches mainly in the white matter. Although diagnosis was traditionally made on clinical grounds alone, several laboratory tests have recently been introduced to enhance accuracy, especially the use of visual evoked potentials. A black/white pattern on a chequer board is alternated at a two per second frequency in front of the patient, and this produces a positive wave on occipital scalp electrodes. The wave peaks with a latency of approximately 100 ms in normals, but in patients with optic neuritis there is a delay, and asymmetry between the eyes.[330] This delay tends to remain even after resolution of an attack. In that many patients with multiple sclerosis have optic neuritis, the test is found positive in 70–90% of patients. Auditory evoked potentials and somatosensory evoked potentials have also been used in a similar way.

CSF changes in mutliple sclerosis include an elevation of protein, increased numbers of mononuclear cells, and an abnormal Lange curve. When the IgG gammaglobulin fraction is analysed, 70% have elevated values, with nearly always an oligoclonal pattern (2–4 abnormal gammaglobulin fractions detected by electrophoresis). EEG abnormalities in the form of slowing, focal or diffuse, are seen in the majority of cases in the acute stages of the illness.[331]

The psychiatric disability accompanying multiple sclerosis was commented on when the disease was first described by Charcot.[332] Cottrell and Wilson examined 100 unselected cases with symptoms lasting from a few months to more than 20 years' duration and reported 63 had euphoria, and 10 were depressed. They concluded that in every single case some change of mood was apparent, and emotional lability was one of the cardinal symptoms of the illness, more constant than any neurological sign. In addition they noted a sense of bodily well-being, which they called 'eutonia', to be an unexpected but nevertheless frequent accompaniment of the disease, which was not necessarily associated with euphoria. They attributed these symptoms to dysfunction of the thalamus and its connections. In contrast to these affective changes they found little evidence of intellectual deficits. Brain,[334] in a later review, pointed out that many early reports of mental changes should be discounted as they were made before neurosyphilis was a diagnosable entity, and added to Cottrell and Wilson's account of mental changes the 'predisposition to hysteria . . . long associated with this disease'.

There then followed a number of investigations in which authors suggested that certain personalities were predisposed to develop multiple sclerosis. This was assessed in detail by Pratt[335] in a controlled study of 100 patients. Using the techniques available for personality assessment at that time he concluded that no characteristic premorbid personality existed, and that in most cases emotional stress played no part in precipitating a relapse. However, in some patients severe emotional disturbances antedated their relapse or precipitated the onset of the disease. He confirmed the increased incidence of euphoria and emotional lability in the disorder, but in contrast to Cottrell and Wilson, noted a high incidence of intellectual impairment. He suggested this was associated with increased physical disability, and in some to disturbances of affect. Depression occurred slightly more commonly in the multiple sclerosis patients than in the controls.

Surridge[332] studied 108 patients and used patients with muscular dystrophy as controls. Two-thirds of his multiple sclerosis patients had intellectual deterioration, especially loss of memory for recent events and loss of conceptual thinking. Euphoria was found in 25%, and was not that of hypomania, but was associated with intellectual decline. It was accompanied by denial of disability and a cheerful complacency, often overshadowing an underlying depressive feeling. Depression was found in 25% of the multiple sclerosis patients and 13% of the controls, and did not appear to be associated with intellectual changes.

These studies all suggest that changes in the mental state are the rule in multiple sclerosis. In particular, lability, intellectual deficits, and affective disorders occur, and patients with euphoria are most likely to be the ones with severe illness and intellectual impairment. Other authors have indicated that the disease can initially present with dementia, sometimes rapidly progressive,[336] and it has been associated with a high risk for suicide.[337] While it is not more frequently associated with schizophreniform psychosis than would be expected by chance, the clustering of such presentations around the time of the appearance of neurological abnormalities suggests a link.[318] Occasionally presentation as psychiatric illness occurs several years before neurological signs develop.[338]

The aetiology of the disorder is unknown. The possibility that a transmissible agent is involved has been suggested by epidemiological data, serological evidence of raised measles virus titres in the serum of patients, and the presence in the blood of small identifiable agents. In addition an increased incidence of certain HLA antigens is noted in patients, suggesting the possibility that there exists a genetic deficit in immunoresponsiveness in the disorder determining susceptibility to environmental agents. To-date no particular agent has been identified,[339] and the mode of any interaction is unknown.

Present available treatments include unsaturated fatty acids, such as linoleic acid, immunosuppression, and for the acute phase ACTH. Although patients with the disease have low linoleate levels in their serum,[340] preparations designed to correct this have not consistently been shown to be effective in preventing relapse. ACTH, provided it is given within 8 weeks of the development of symptoms, shortens the relapse, although does not alter the eventual outcome.[339]

The mainstay of therapy is physiotherapy, drugs aimed at helping spasticity such as diazepam (Valium), or Baclofen (lioresal), and psychotherapy. The latter, which may be simple support, or more structured therapy, or even couple therapy with or without sexual counselling where necessary, is reported to help patients overcome their dependency problems, allow patients to express intense feelings, and improve their difficulty in interpersonal relationships.[341] The possibility that alleviation of distress by psychotherapy may alter immune mechanisms and thus alter the outcome of the illness has been raised.[342] Antidepressants and tranquillizers are useful adjuncts to therapy, and often alleviate stress in quite small doses.

OTHER DISORDERS OF MYELINATION

Although multiple sclerosis is the commonest disorder of myelination seen in practice, others occur and may be associated with psychiatric disability. In the dysmyelinating disorders there is abnormality of the development of myelin sheaths, as opposed to demyelinating disorders where developed myelin is destroyed. The dysmyelinations (for example Krabbe's disease) are rare disorders due to inborn errors of metabolism, and like the neuronal storage disorders in which abnormal substances accumulate in nerve cells, result in a variety of illnesses, usually in childhood, but which also can present in early or late adulthood. Generally the older the patient at presentation, the more likely it is that the main symptoms will be of a behaviour disorder. The enzyme defect in several of these diseases is now understood. *Schilder's disease*, an eponym covering several different neuropathological conditions, presents usually before the age of 10 with massive progressive demyelination, leading to early dementia and sometimes to a schizophreniform-like psychosis, especially of the hebephrenic or catatonic type. *Progressive multifocal leucoencephalopathy* is a rare complication of reticulo-endothelial neoplastic disorders, and may lead to progressive neurological deterioration associated with a dementia.

Metachromatic lecodystrophy can present diagnostic difficulties. This is now known to be due to an abnormal accumulation of cerebroside sulphate due to deficiency of the enzyme aryl-sulphatase A, and may present in an adult form as a schizophreniform illness. The development of similar psychoses in adolescence or early adulthood has also been found in association with disorders such as *subacute sclerosing pan-encephalitis, tuberose sclerosis,* and other neuronal storage disorders. In order to distinguish psychotic presentations of these diseases from other psychotic disorders in early life, the term *progressive disintegrative psychosis* had been suggested.[343] Such cases must be distinguished from *childhood autism,* where the abnormality of behaviour is noted in very early childhood, characterized by inability to relate to people and situations, associated with speech and language abnormalities; from *childhood schizophrenia* which usually starts over the age of 5, and is often associated with a family history of schizophrenia; and from *disintegrative psychosis of a non-progressive kind* in which there is normal development for a few years followed by loss of social skills and speech, with deterioration of interpersonal relationships, which can occur following overt brain damage, encephalitis, or in the absence of detectable organic disease. The hallmark of progressive disintegrative psychosis is advancement of psychopathology, often out of proportion to any environmental stress, to frank psychotic illness in which bizarre rituals, mannerisms, delusions and hallucinations may be seen. Recognition of this disorder is important, not only to establish the underlying neurodegenerative diagnosis, but also for management where undue emphasis on psychodynamic mechanisms may lead to parental guilt and ambivalence. Where such a diagnosis is considered, repeated neurological and EEG investigations are required.

Generally, detection of the dysmyelinating diseases, and other disorders such as the storage disorders requires, in addition to routine investigations, skull x-rays, EEG examinations, and specialized biochemical investigations for amino acids and abnormal metabolites in the urine and serum. Metachromatic leucodystsrophy is detected by aryl-sulphatase determination in the white blood cells and the urine, and is associated with slowing of peripheral nerve conduction and metachromatic material in freshly spun urine. Occasionally, rectal, peripheral nerve, or even brain biopsy are used to secure diagnosis.

CHAPTER 8

Chronic Pain

Many patients, with a variety of diseases and neurological lesions, have intractable pain, whose problems are dealt with by physicians and surgeons of a variety of specialities. Some however, on account of their behaviour, or because of a discrepancy between their apparent somatic lesion and their complaint of pain, are referred for psychiatric opinion. This section is therefore concerned with chronic pain, its understanding and management, as it presents to psychiatrists.

Merskey defined pain as 'an unpleasant experience which we primarily associate with tissue damage, or describe in terms of such damage or both' (Ref. 344, p.21). He placed emphasis on the experiencing of pain as an event, not dissimilar to the way in which we experience colour and pattern as a result of visual impulses from the retina, although it is clear that we can also experience similar phenomena in the absence of such impulses.

It is unfortunate that sometimes discussion of pain problems tend to result in debate about whether the pain is 'organic' or not. Patients may be led to adopt a defensive role regarding their problems, particularly if no overt pathology is detected after a number of investigations, and may feel that since their problem is not in their body, it must be 'in their mind', and hence imagined. This not only adds to patients' distress, but if their thoughts are reinforced by the doctor's own beliefs, it leads them to seek further consultations, with further tests, usually with the same results.

Assessment of the needs of chronic pain patients requires analysis not only of the somatic and neurological elements of their problem, but also of their psychiatric history, including their personality and coping style, previous pain experiences, and current mental state.

PATHOPHYSIOLOGY OF PAIN

The anatomy of the various nerve endings and fibre pathways thought to be implicated in the generation of pain are discussed in Chapter 2. Although it was thought that there were specific receptors for pain sensations, and that pain was carried by specific sensory nerve fibres, this 'specificity theory' is now questioned. In contrast, the 'pattern theory' of pain suggests that it is an alteration of the spatio-temporal balance of activity within the large and small nerve fibres that determine pain sensations. An extension of this theory is the 'gate theory' of Melzack and Wall.[345] Afferent impulses from the small fibres project to cells in the spinal cord, or the trigeminal nucleus, which can be facilitated or inhibited by afferent input from other peripheral fibres. Thus the end result of a peripheral stimulus is related to the number of nerve fibres active, the frequency of the impulses, and on the balance of activity between the large and small fibres. The 'gate mechanism' is located in the substantia gelatinosa of the dorsal horn of the spinal cord, and is capable of modulating activity in so-called central transmission cells (T-cells) of the dorsal horn, which are responsible for activating central pain mechanisms. The system envisaged by this theory therefore includes a central mechanism, activated by the large fibre system, and projecting to the gate mechanism, such that central influences are seen as directly modulating the pain experience (see Figure 8.1).

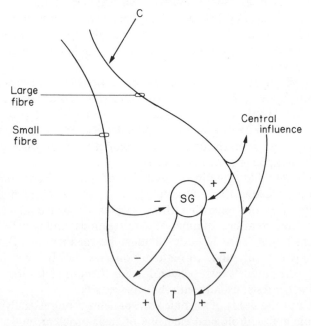

Figure 8.1. Schematic diagram of the nerve pathways envisaged as transmitting pain sensations according to the 'gate theory'. SG, Substantia gelatinosa; T, transmission cells; C, counterstimulation; + excitation and — inhibition

The theory accounts better than the specificity theory for many clinic observations, and has led to a search for new methods of treating pain problems, some of which, based on alteration of patterns of activity in the afferent neurones by low-voltage electric current stimulation, have had a certain amount of success. The theory has been criticized on account of the lack of experimental verification for it, and because it does not take into account certain neurophysiological observations regarding neurone impulses following experimental nerve fibre stimulation.

Since there are patients described that have had total spinal cord sections who can still experience pain from areas below the section,[346] central pain modulating mechanisms have been suggested which not only regulate the incoming experience of painful stimuli, but also respond to loss of stimulus input. The thalamus has been implicated because many fibres of the spinothalamic tracts terminate there, and pain is experienced either following lesions or stimulation of this structure. However, at this level individual sensory modalities are not separated, and stimulation results in diffuse pain. In the so-called *'thalamic syndrome'* there is poorly localized burning pain, which is exacerbated by touch. Pain of a similar diffuse kind has also been elicited following stimulation of the peri-aqueductal grey region of the midbrain, often associated with intense anxiety feelings. The role of the cerebral cortex in pain appreciation is briefly mentioned in Chapter 2.

The neurochemical mechanisms related to pain have been stimulated with the discovery of the endogenous opiate substances, the endorphins, since some of them possess powerful analgesic properties. Monoamines are also involved since it has been shown that parachlorophenylalanine, which inhibits serotonin metabolism, reduces the analgesic effect of morphine administration, while 5-hydroxytryptophan increases it.[347] In addition stimulation of the serotoninergic raphe nuclei also increases analgesia. It is of interest that many areas of the brain which are related to pain pathways, such as the substantia gelatinosa, the peri-aqueductal grey region and sites in the limbic system, contain both monoamines and endorphins in high concentration.

PAIN AND PSYCHIATRIC ILLNESS

Stengel[348] has indicated that pain is a common sign of psychiatric illness. In psychiatric clinics, pain, unrelated to overt somatic pathology, is found as a main presenting symptom in 45–60% of patients, and psychiatric illness is a major factor in determining the onset of the pain. In addition, pain presenting as a symptom in medical clinics is often associated with psychiatric illness, and as a symptom it may be equally as indicative of psychiatric, as of somatic, illness (Ref. 344, pp.31–45). It is seen in association with schizophrenia and organic brain syndromes, and may present as a symptom of depression, may lead to depression, or may be a substitute for depression. Pain occurred in 56% of Spear's patients with depression (Ref. 344, p.39), similar figures being given by others (Ref. 349, p.42). However, in psychiatric populations with pain generally there is a predominance of neurotic illness as opposed to depressive illness.[350] Pilowsky, in a group of patients with chronic pain,[351] found only 10% with depressive illness, and these were hypochondriacal with somatic preoccupation. That some patients may deny their depression, and concern themselves with their somatic problems is suggested by the results shown in Figure 8.2. This figure, showing a dip in the depression scores (D) compared with some other psychopathology scores on MMPI profiles in chronic pain patients, suggests that in some way 'conversion' of depression into somatic pain occurs. A similar related concept is that of masked depression, where pain is seen as a depressive equivalent.

THE PAIN EXPERIENCE

It is well-known that the intensity of physical pain differs from person to person dependent upon race, personality, previous experience and current affective state, and that an individual's pain varies from day to day. Some authors in discussing this problem distinguish between pain threshold, namely that level at which pain is actually felt, and pain tolerance, the level at which the subject requests termination of the pain. The former is thought to be more dependent on physiological factors, the latter on psychological ones.[344]

Pain is tolerated less well by females than by males; by Jews and Mediterranean peoples than by Northern European Caucasians; by the elderly compared with the young, and extroverts than by introverts. Studies using a variety of rating scales in chronic pain patients have shown differences between them and controls. Bond and Pearson[352] using the EPI, found that cancer patients with pain were more neurotic than those without pain, and that introverted pain patients were less likely to receive analgesics than extroverted ones. Others have noted, using the MMPI, high hypochondria and hysteria scores often associated with an abnormal, but less elevated, depression score. This so-called psychosomatic-V is said to reflect somatic preoccupation by patients, with a denial of emotional disturbance (Ref. 349, p.17) (see Figure 8.2). Whether such differences reflect a change of personality secondary to pain, or is a previous personality maladjustment, is not clear. Woodforde and Merskey[353] assessed 43 pain patients with the Middlesex Hospital Questionnaire and the EPI and found they resembled psychiatric out-patients, and those with pain and lesions were as neurotic as those who had pain and no lesions. Although they were unable to rule out certain selection factors, they suggested that the emotional changes noted in the first group were due to the continued presence of pain. Sternbach,[354] in studies of patients with low back pain, compared those with pain of less than 6 months' duration to a group with symptoms lasting more than 6 months. Using the MMPI, the psychosomatic-V triad was found in both groups of patients, but only the chronic patients had scores actually in the abnormal range (see Figure 8.2). They suggested there was an evolution of the abnormal personality profiles with chronicity, such that as the illness proceeded, patients became more concerned with their pain and more depressed. Similarly, patients who underwent surgery and obtained relief from their pain showed reduction in their hysteria and hypochondriasis scores, compared to those not relieved.[355] All these studies support the hypothesis that it is continued chronic pain that leads to the emotional changes. On the other hand Pilowsky's studies with the Illness Behaviour Questionnaire[356] have not shown changes in behaviour patterns that relate to length of illness in patients with symptoms varying from 6 weeks to 60 years. He argued that patients' attitudes towards illness are established at the outset and are not a consequence of it. Although the population of patients that Pilowsky examined was different from that of the other authors, in that only a few of his patients had any clearly-defined somatic pathology, reanalysis of his results on this 'organic' group still failed to detect any relationship between abnormal illness behaviour and chronicity. Pilowsky criticized Sternbach's data, pointing out that although surgery does lower estimates of psychopathology, the pain group as a whole still showed abnormal profiles, especially in the hysteria and depression scales.

This view, that some patients are pain-prone, receives support from the studies of Engel.[357] He assumed that from birth an individual builds up a library of pain experiences which are of importance not only for development, but also because they markedly influence later pain interpretation. Thus pain acquires for the individual meaning, as a warning of damage to the body, as a means of communication, especially leading to comfort by a loved person, as a means of punishment, as a means for expressing aggression and power, as an expression of sexual feeling, as a signal for 'badness' and guilt, and sometimes for the opposite, namely expiation of guilt. Pain is seen as a mechanism for the achievement of certain gratifications, and the attainment of psychic equilibrium. According to Engel, the 'pain-prone' patient shows some or all of the following features:

(1) a prominence of guilt with pain serving as the means of atonement;
(2) a background of predisposition of the use of pain for such purposes;
(3) a history of defeat and suffering, and an inability to tolerate success;
(4) unfulfilled aggression;
(5) development of pain as a replacement for loss;
(6) a sadomasochistic sexual development;
(7) the location of pain often determined by identification with a significant other — the pain being one either suffered by the patient when in conflict with another person, or a pain thought or actually known to be suffered by the other person;
(8) a variety of psychiatric illnesses.

Penman[358] provided further evidence in this direction from his observations on patients undergoing alcohol injection of the fifth sensory nerve for trigeminal neuralgia. Following operation he divided patients into five groups whose response varied from 'unreservedly glad' to 'patients in constant misery attributed by them to paraesthesiae'. About 20% of his total group developed neurotic symptoms or became constant sufferers. These dissatisfied patients had suffered pain from a few months to many years, and he felt that the loss of the pain had produced 'a gain on the physical roundabouts' but produced 'loss on the emotional and social swings . . .'. He believed that similar mechanisms could be seen in other pains, such as sciatica and peptic ulceration, in that given time the pain became not only the sufferer's chief occupation but also 'a refuge from some intolerable situation and hence an alternative to a neurosis . . .'.

Using the illness behaviour questionnaire Pilowsky examined 100 patients with chronic pain, and compared them to controls from other medical clinics, in order to establish more about their personality and modes of behaviour. The pain patients were found to show typical abnormal illness behaviour, in particular with conviction of the presence of disease, somatic preoccupation, and inability to accept reassurance from doctors. These results were the same irrespective of the presence of readily identifiable somatic disease. Generally they showed difficulty in expressing their feelings, especially anger, and a reluctance to acknowledge their life problems. Pilowsky suggested that for a substantial proportion of these patients 'the pain syndrome does seem interwoven with, and perhaps symptomatic of, a personality disorder or an essentially maladaptive response to psychological stress'.[359]

MECHANISMS OF CHRONIC PAIN

A conflict sometimes arises when attempts are made to understand pain as either being 'psychogenic' or 'organic'. As Szasz pointed out: '. . . the notions of "physical" and "mental" pain are meaningless . . . "the commonsense" view, which regards this matter as if there were two types of pain — one organic and another psychogenic . . . is misleading and is responsible for numerous pseudoproblems in the borderland between medicine and psychology'.[360] 'Psychogenic pain' has been defined as pain which arises independent of peripheral stimulation, or damage to the nervous system, and due to emotional factors; or else pain in which any peripheral change, such as muscle tension, is consequent on emotional factors (Ref. 344, p.19). It is sometimes distinguished from 'mental pain' which is more related to grief, and often expressed as a metaphor, such as 'pain in the heart'. However, attempts to identify differences in the pain experiences of pain patients with and without somatic lesions have not been successful — a fact that supported Merskey in his definition given above on page 145. There are sometimes distinctive qualities noted in the pain of patients with psychiatric illness, such as depression or schizophrenia when it may have a delusional quality, or may be in the form of an hallucination. Clinically, however, such cases are not common, and in such instances the pain either forms part of a more extensive delusional system, or is associated with evidence of a depressive illness. However, even in such cases it has to be explained why the pain should be felt in the location that it is, and not somewhere else. One possibility is that at some time peripheral tissue damage occurred which, with the onset of psychiatric illness, becomes the site of pain again. An alternative explanation for pain in some of these patients is through the mechanisms of symbolization and identification. Although most of the evidence for this is anecdotal, in individual patients these factors may be important determinants of the actual site of pain.[357] It is particularly for this reason that in pain patients it is essential to gather a 'pain history', especially noting illnesses in other persons significant to the patient. A common example is chest pain in somebody who has lost a close friend or relative with a heart attack, or headache in relationship with another's cerebral tumour. In these cases the association of a disordered emotional state, with a peripheral mechanism such as muscle spasm and in addition identification or symbolization may all combine to produce the clinical picture. Indeed 'muscle spasm' is often involved to explain pain of undetermined aetiology. It is known that anxiety can give rise to muscle contraction, and the latter can give rise to pain. It is easy to see how a vicious cycle is set in process as shown in Figure 8.3, and why such pains should readily respond to techniques that induce muscle relaxation. Whether or not similar or alternative mechanisms are responsible for the siting of pain which is an hysterical symptom is unclear. As the studies of Pilowsky have shown, abnormal illness behaviour is a feature of many chronic pain patients, and it is likely that in these situations there is an association between some, often subtle, somatic input and the patient's personality that leads to the pain problems.

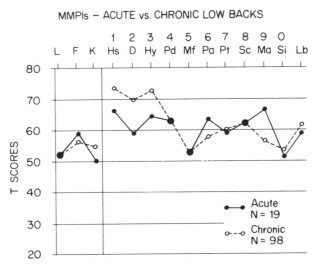

Figure 8.2. Comparison of profiles of 19 acute low back patients and 98 chronic low back patients. Scales 1, 2, 3, and 9 are significantly different for the two groups. (After Sternbach *et al.*, 1973, reproduced by permission of *Psychosomatics*)[349]

Other factors in the genesis of chronic pain, such as the role of secondary gain, or 'gratification' that such people achieve with their pain, may be apparent on close examination, but to assume a direct causal link may be dangerous, since satisfaction on the part of the examining doctor that the problem has been 'solved' may lead to ignorance of continuous progressive

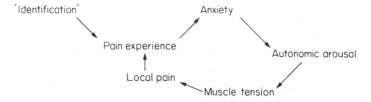

Figure 8.3. A suggested mechanism of pain production

somatic pathology. A good deal of anecdotal evidence collected together by Merskey and Spear stresses the relationship of guilt, hostility and resentment to pain. Prominent sado-masochistic and infantile dependent needs have also been suggested, the pain in some way solving psychic conflicts and providing atonement for guilt. It always has to be emphasized that pain is not the polar opposite to pleasure and that in some patients pain solves problems, and brings a psychic equilibrium that would otherwise be unattainable.

It is suggested that in attempting to understand the chronic pain patient, taking into account possible somatic inputs to the pain experience, personality factors, and associated affective illnesses will provide a more fruitful approach than attempting to decide whether pain is 'organic' or 'psychogenic'. An understanding of neurophysiological mechanisms, especially the neural substrates of the emotions, are important for understanding the close relationship between, for example, depression and pain, but also how emotional factors themselves alter pain tolerance and perception. The anatomical links between the reticular activating system, the thalamus, the limbic system, and the cells of the substantia gelatinosa, and the close relationship of these areas with both the monoamines and endorphins would seem important in forming these close links between the experience of pain and the emotional state.

SOME GENERAL COMMENTS ON TREATMENTS

The management of acute pain differs markedly from that of chronic pain. For the former good analgesic use is mandatory and, if problems of longer term abuse are avoided by careful prescribing, by definition treatment is successful and self-limiting. Chronic pain on the other hand requires a variety of techniques from divergent specialities. Recognition of this fact has more recently led to the setting up of pain clinics in a large number of centres.

(a) Analgesics

Generally it is advisable to start patients on non-narcotic analgesics, and progress to narcotic ones only if the clinical situation demands it. The latter are hardly ever justified in non-terminal chronic pain. The individual patient's response to all analgesics is variable and the danger of abuse is always present.

Table 8.1. Commonly used analgesics

(a) Non-narcotic

Acetylsalicylic acid	(Aspirin)
Paracetamol	(Panadol)
Acetylsalicylic acid + Paracetamol	(Benoral*)
Ketoprufen	(Alrheumat, Orudis)
Flurbiprofen	(Froben)
Phenylbutazone	(Butazolidin)
Indomethacin	(Indocid)
Ibuprofen	(Brufen)

(b) Narcotic 'partial' analgesics and narcotic analgesics

Pentazocine	(Fortral)
Buprenorphine	(Temgesic)
Dextropopoxyphene	(Depronal)
Dextropopoxyphene and Paracetamol	(Distalgesic)
Codeine phosphate	
Dihydrocodeine	(DF118)
Dipipanone	(Diconal)
Phenazocine	(Narphen)
Dextromoramide	(Palfium)
Pethidine	
Morphine	
Diamorphine	(Heroin)

*Each 10 ml contains 2.2 g of aspirin and 1.8 g of paracetamol.

There are a large number of analgesics that exist and are in clinical use, and some of these are given in Table 8.1. It is important to remember that while patients may not respond to medications on a p.r.n. basis, they may do well with regularly prescribed doses, with which satisfactory blood levels produce analgesia throughout the day. There is some evidence that therapeutic response is related to serum levels, and thus increasing the dose of non-narcotic drugs should be undertaken before changing to narcotic alternatives. Some patients lose the effect of the drugs after a while, and thus changing to an alternative preparation, and then re-starting the initial drug later, is a useful manoeuvre.

It is thought that aspirin and the non-narcotic analgesics act mainly at the periphery by blocking substances that activate pain chemo-receptors, such as the prostaglandins and various kinins, whereas narcotic analgesics act on the central mechanism presumably at sites of endorphin production.[361]

(b) Psychotropic drugs

These play a significant part in the management of chronic pain and are fully discussed in Chapter 11. Minor tranquillizers are useful in relieving any accompanying anxiety, and major tranquillizers possess some inherent analgesic activity. Both groups of drugs may make a useful adjunct to therapy, even when the somatic element of the pain is clearly a major one. Similarly antidepressants such as imipramine (Tofranil) have been shown to possess analgesic properties, although of course one of the main indications of this group of compounds is in the management of accompanying depression. Clomipramine (Anafranil), which appears to have selective action on 5-HT systems, is reported to be particularly useful in the management of chronic pain,[362] and this drug in combination with L-tryptophan to further increase serotonergic activity may be helpful clinically.

Combinations of phenothiazines and antidepressants may be valuable, and some authors add an antihistamine, such as promethazine (Phenergan), thus making up a psychotropic cocktail.[363] Dosage varies according to the patient, but clinical improvements sometimes only occur with larger doses.

Carbamazepine (Tegretol), although primarily used as an anticonvulsant, is the treatment of choice for some pain syndromes such as trigeminal neuralgia, and it seems to be a useful adjunct to therapy, sometimes in combination with antidepressants, in a variety of different types of pain including diabetic neuropathy, the thalamic syndrome, and phantom limb pain.

(c) Electrical stimulation and surgical treatment

Although electrical stimulation in one form or another has been used for many years to alleviate pain, the gate theory of Melzack and Wall renewed interest in such methods of treatment. Attempts have been made to stimulate the A-delta fibres of peripheral nerves transcutaneously, and dorsal column stimulation, with electrodes placed directly over the posterior columns, has also been used although with less success.

Surgical interventions have included nerve blocks, by neurolytic agents such as intrathecal phenol or alcohol, or direct surgical lesioning. The latter, which have included anterolateral cordotomy, percutaneous cordotomy, and posterior rhizotomy (section of the nerve root), are probably more suited to patients with chronic pain of malignant disease, or specific conditions such as lesioning of the trigeminal nerve in trigeminal neuralgia. Reported results from these procedures from selected cases indicate improvement rates of up to 64% with percutaneous operations,[364] to 60-75% for cordotomy and rhizotomy,[365] although most series record a high relapse rate. Other operations sometimes carried out include stereotactic thalamotomy, corticectomy, and frontal leucotomy. Thalamotomy has only a very limited place in pain management, being mainly successful following operations that damage the thalamo-frontal connections, thus influencing the emotional experiences of pain perception.[366] Leucotomy for pain was first undertaken by Freeman and Watts. The operation, while it did little to alter the patient's ability to feel pain, reduced the accompanying emotional aspects of the pain and following leucotomy 'the experience becomes less troublesome and less unpleasant' (Ref. 344, p.100). Generally, however, the indications for leucotomy are very limited, and the results disappointing.[367]

(d) Other treatments

In addition to the above, neuropsychiatrists have employed a variety of techniques for the management of chronic pain problems with varying degrees of success. E.C.T. is useful if the pain is associated with depressive illness, and there are reports of successful use in patients unresponsive to antidepressants.[368] Hypnosis and acupuncture have been used for many years Hypnosis probably alters the pain experience by alleviation of the affective components of pain, in particular fear and anxiety. Similar results may be obtained with biofeedback, either by alpha-training or, more effectively, by EMG biofeedback, in situations where anxiety leads to increased muscle tension, which in turn leads to further pain. Acupuncture may have non-specific effects, or in terms of the gate theory, alter impulse input into the spinal column, and perhaps even stimulate endorphin release centrally.

(e) Pain clinics

These clinics deal exclusively with the problems of chronic pain patients, and are multidisciplinary in their approach. They may include an anaesthetist, a neurosurgeon, a psychiatrist, a neurologist, a radiotherapist, a social worker, a physiotherapist and interested others. Each individual can bring his particular expertise to the patient's case, discussed in the immediate light of others working on the same problem. This approach has stimulated a great deal of interest in pain problems, and has allowed otherwise isolated disciplines to come into close contact, with beneficial results. Perhaps one great benefit of such a clinic is that it can act as a 'sanctuary' for both the patient's and physician's frustrations in dealing with chronic pain problems. If the patient can be maintained and supported by the clinic, it may put an end, for a while at least, to the relentless search for further consultations and treatments that characterize these patients.

The psychiatrist has several functions within a pain clinic.[369] First, to make a diagnosis, in particular a psychiatric diagnosis, if it is appropriate. In addition he should recognize patterns of behaviour which are maladaptive, and remind members of the pain team that certain relationships exist between psychic events and somatic processes that are of importance for the diagnosis and management of pain problems. The psychiatrist is also in a position to offer specific treatments for patients where necessary, including guidance and advice on the use of psychotropic drugs, psychotherapy, hypnosis, biofeedback and ECT. Where indicated, admission to a psychiatric ward can be arranged, often important for patients to come to some initial understanding that their problems are fundamentally psychiatric in nature. Finally, but most important, the presence of a psychiatrist in the pain clinic serves to emphasize the multi-dimensional aspects of chronic pain problems, and that the dichotomy between so-called organic and psychogenic pain is a false one.

SOME SPECIFIC NEUROPSYCHIATRIC PAIN SYNDROMES

Headache

It is essential in the first instance to make a decision as to the major aetiology of the patient's symptoms and, if they are caused by clearly-defined structural abnormalities, to decide on the most appropriate specialist referral. Often the pattern of a headache, and the ensuing neurological examination, will give clues to any structural pathology which may underlie the headache. The problem that often presents to psychiatrists, however, is of chronic or subacute recurrent headaches, which occur in the absence of overt neurological abnormalities, including migraine, tension headache, atypical facial pain, and pain secondary to other psychiatric disorders. In these various conditions the mechanism of the production of the headache is not well-known, although since muscle contraction can result in headache, it is the suggested mechanism for the production of tension headache. Such activity may occur below the level of awareness, but can be noted on the EMG, which, when quantified, is shown to be abnormal.[370] The intensification of headache from any somatic abnormality may occur by secondary muscular contraction, and in tense, anxious people this can rapidly lead to a vicious circle in which intense headache arises from some seemingly trivial noxious stimulation.

Migraine

This is defined as recurrent attacks of headache, of varying intensity, frequency and duration, which are often unilateral and associated with nausea and vomiting. They may be preceded by focal motor or sensory symptoms, or affective ones. A distinction has been made between 'classical' migraine, where the headache is preceded by such focal neurological phenomena, and 'common' migraine where these features are absent. As such, migraine is a common disorder that affects some 10% of the population. The onset is usually in adolescence or early adult life, its prevalence declining in elderly patients. The headaches typically are irregular in frequency, last for a few hours, and occasionally days, and then resolve for a period of time. Migraine headaches never occur daily. They may be associated with photophobia and other symptoms such as abdominal upsets, and present as dull, throbbing aches which become severe, and may involve the face and neck as well as the head. The attacks can occur at any time, and in some patients typically occur at holidays or weekends. For some hours before an attack patients may describe sensations of well-being or depression, and after their episodes may feel relaxed or even over-active. Some patients describe unusual body image disturbances associated with their migraine, including autoscopy and changes in proportion of various bodily parts.[371]

Variants of migraine include facial migraine, hemiplegic migraine, ophthalmoplegic migraine, and vertebrobasilar migraine. The latter may present with loss of consciousness and a variety of brainstem symptoms.

There seems little doubt that there is a genetic predisposition to migraine, some 50% of sufferers having an affected relative. Although it is often suggested that migraine patients are obsessional and striving, population studies using objective rating scales have found little evidence for this. However, sufferers, especially females, are more neurotic, showing more anxiety and depression, and higher levels of somatic complaints than others.[372]

The pathogenesis of this disorder is as yet poorly understood. It has been suggested that on account of vascular instability there is constriction of the cerebral arteries, which is associated with the prodromata, followed by a dilatation of the extracranial arteries which is associated with the headache. The cause for such change is unknown, although abnormalities of monoamine metabolism have been postulated. There is some evidence that an increase in plasma serotonin occurs, followed by a fall as the headache starts. Increased catecholamine levels have been reported 3 hours before certain types of migraine, and it is well-known that some foods, especially those containing tyramine, may precipitate attacks in some patients. Additional biochemical changes noted in attacks include water and sodium retention.[373]

The relationship of stress to migraine is very difficult to assess. There is no doubt that stress is often interlinked with tension headaches, and that migraine sufferers, at times of stress, may have an increase in frequency of migraine attacks, and develop tension headaches. The possible biochemical link of both affective disorders and migraine to, for example, the monoamines, may be important in this connection. It is interesting to note that noradrenergic fibres from the locus coeruleus have been shown to terminate on cerebral blood vessels.

Treatment in migraine is aimed at terminating an acute attack, or at prophylactic therapy for the prevention of further attacks. Some drugs used are listed in Table 8.2. For the acute episode, analgesics are given, often combined with an anti-emetic, and both major and minor tranquillizers can be useful. In severe episodes the patient should be placed in a darkened room, with peace and quiet to help bring about quick relief. The addition of metaclopramide (Maxalon) to any oral therapy is now recommended, since this increases gastric emptying, which has been shown to be delayed during a migraine attack.[374] This manoeuvre results in a greater serum level of the analgesics, and thus more rapid and sustained relief. Ergotamine is not essential in the management and should be avoided if possible.

Recent work on the effects of temperature biofeedback on migraine is promising, and some migraine patients may be trained to bring an end to their attacks by raising their peripheral temperature by a few degrees.

Prophylaxis usually involves some alteration of the patient's lifestyle, possibly psychotherapy, and attention to underlying affective disturbances if they are present. Any dietary factors that seem to be related to the attacks obviously should be eliminated. A variety of medications for use in such situations is shown in Table 8.2.

Table 8.2. Some drugs used in treatment of migraine

Acute attack		
	Analgesics	e.g. Acetylsalicylic acid
		Paracetamol
	Anti-emetics	e.g. Prochlorperazine (Stemetil)
	Tranquillizers	e.g. A benzodiazepine or phenothiazine
	Ergotamine tartrate	1–2 mg orally or sublingually to 6 mg,
		or 0.25–0.5 mg i.m. or s.c.
	Cafergot	Ergotamine and caffeine
	Migril	Ergotamine, caffeine and cyclizine
Prophylaxis		
	Tranquillizers	
	Antidepressants	
	5-HT antagonists	e.g. Pizotifen (Sanomigran)
		Methylsergide (Deseril)
		Dihydroergotamine (Dihydergot)
	Clonidine (Catapres)	
	Beta-blocking drugs	e.g. Propranolol (Inderal)
	Anticonvulsants	e.g. Phenytoin (Epanutin), Phenobarbitone,
		Carbamazepine (Tegretol)

Migrainous neuralgia

Migrainous neuralgia, or cluster headache, is a disorder which is probably related to migraine but with different characteristics. Bouts of headache occur over 2 to several weeks, followed by periods of relief. The onset is rapid, and the headaches last for a few minutes to hours, often occurring several times a day. They are severe, and unilateral, affecting the eye, frontal region, nostril and cheek and are usually associated with redness of the scalp and conjunctival injection. Lachrymation is common, and an ipsilateral Horner's syndrome develops in some 20% of patients. The headache itself is described by patients as deep, boring and intense. The syndrome is commoner in males and usually has an onset between the ages of 20 and 50. It has been suggested that patients with this disorder have a variety of personality disturbances including hysterical, obsessional and depressive personalities, often showing increased dependency needs.[375]

The pain is often so severe that patients get very apprehensive about their next attacks, and a depressive illness is often present. Treatments for this condition are similar to those for migraine, although lithium has also been used with limited success. The disorder should not be confused with *trigeminal neuralgia* in which transient, intense, stabbing pains occur in one or more of the divisions of the fifth nerve. Trigger mechanisms are often described by patients in trigeminal neuralgia, and it responds, in the majority of cases, to carbamazepine (Tegretol).

Tension headaches

The commonest form of headache is tension headache. These vary in duration and intensity, but when severe they occur throughout the day, and every day. They have no clear periodicity, are described as dull, constant, 'band-like', or tight, and are often bilateral, frontal, or occipital, associated with tender areas upon palpation. Patients may have associated nausea or photophobia, and characteristically these pains do not wake the patient at night, but may be present on waking. Patients suggest that they go to sleep with the pain, and wake up with it. Typically such pains are exacerbated by stress and noise, and relieved by relaxation and alcohol.

It is thought that these types of headache are in part the end-result of increased muscle tension, which is accompanied by vasoconstriction and accumulation of noicio-stimulant catabolites. On examination it is often possible to observe increased muscle tension in patients, particularly in the face, in the temporal and masseter muscles. Patients may look anxious, have increased peripheral movements or even tremor, and find it impossible to relax their neck or limbs. About one-quarter of patients who complain of tension headaches also have severe throbbing headaches, which are very similar to migraine, the symptom-complex being referred to as 'tension-vascular headache' (Ref. 373, p.78). Tension headaches usually have some relationship to be stressful life events, and may be reported, for example, after periods of excessive concentration. However, in a number of patients there is little evidence for this, and the question of the pain being a variety of abnormal illness behaviour arises. Psychiatric examination of patients with tension headaches reveals traits such as 'repressed hostility', dependency problems, and a variety of psychosexual conflicts.[376] MMPI evaluations indicate, in addition, increased scores on anxiety and depression,[377] the latter being especially common in younger patients, although the presence of any psychiatric symptoms seems unrelated to the length of time the patient has had the headache.[378]

Treatment of these headaches requires psychotherapy, often of a quite superficial kind, to explore their relationship to the patient's lifestyle and problems. Minor and major tranquillizers or antidepressants are used as necessary, and techniques such as biofeedback and hypnosis are helpful in certain cases.

There are a group of patients who present a clinical picture similar to tension headaches, in which depressive symptoms are more florid. Typically such patients have headaches with diurnal variation, and are associated with early morning waking, loss of appetite, loss of libido, and sometimes suicidal ideation. In such cases antidepressant therapy or even ECT is the most appropriate first line of treatment.

Other varieties include patients who, on account of excessive tension in their masseters, have face and head pains referred to as 'the facial pain dysfunction syndrome'.[379] These patients have been divided into 'nocturnal grinders' or 'diurnal clenchers'. They have pain and ache on moving the jaws, with pain radiating sometimes to the neck and the head. Tenderness is noted in the region of temporo-mandibular joint, and often the teeth are worn due to bruxism. Sometimes a bite-guard discourages the bruxism, and can bring relief.

160

Atypical facial pain

This term refers to face pains that do not conform to known patterns of neurogenic face pains, which, in the majority of patients, is accompanied by psychiatric disturbance. They are usually unilateral, but may be bilateral, are constant, deep and spread from the cheek area to involve the head, neck and occiput. In one series of 100 patients with such pain, 53 had defined psychiatric illness,[380] depression being the most common diagnosis. Such pains are often encountered in bereaved middle-aged females, who have dependency traits and notable loneliness. Although in some a clear history of trauma or dental operation is encountered prior to onset, it rarely responds for more than brief periods to further surgical or dental intervention, and attention to the psychiatric disabilities involved is more important. Monoamine-oxidase inhibitors may be especially useful in the treatment of this group of patients.

Sexual activity headache

Lance[381] has recently described a group of patients who have headache associated with sexual activity. Some of them had headaches similar to tension headaches which occurred during sexual excitement and others had throbbing vascular-type headaches during orgasm. Follow-up of patients did not reveal any structural lesions to explain these phenomena.

Backache

This common symptom, as with headaches, is sometimes associated with psychiatric pathology. Although examination to rule out structural lesions is obviously important, there are many patients who present continuing backache in the absence of clearly defined pathology. Wolkind and Forrest[382] examined 23 such patients using the Middlesex Hospital Questionnaire and noted that their scores were equivalent to those of a neurotic population. Many such patients have evidence of spasm and muscle tension in the appropriate muscles, and on examination tender points may be found. A major difficulty in assessing these patients arises if they have had one, or even more, neurosurgical operations, since in such cases a somatic input becomes clearly defined. Recognition of patterns of abnormal illness behaviour in patients with back pain is clearly very important to avoid the possibility of unnecessary surgical intervention.

Management of backache from the psychiatric point of view is similar to that of tension headache, especially if muscle spasm is readily apparent. Techniques are outlined above, but it is emphasized that EMG biofeedback may be particularly useful in cases with evident muscle spasm, and of course any coexistent depression will require appropriate treatment.

Phantom limb pain

Patients who have undergone amputation may have pain from a number of causes, one of which may be due to peripheral neuroma formation in the region of the stump. In contrast, phantom limb pain is felt in the projected image of the limb. It may occur spontaneously, or after movement of the stump, and is described as burning, continuous or intermittent, and seems related to the pain of causalgia. Only a small proportion of patients with phantom limb sensations actually have such a pain, and in these psychiatric morbidity is high.[383] There are patients described that have phantom limbs that share in altered sensation associated with other conditions. For example a shivering patient may experience goose-flesh in the phantom, or one with dermatitis may experience itching or irritation (Ref. 384, p.97).

The origin of the phantom itself is thought to reflect the persistence of mechanisms responsible for the cortical representation of the body image in the absence of the peripheral organ, and the 'image' is often experienced in the position of the limb immediately prior to the amputation. Phantom pains have also been described following amputation of the breasts, nose, tongue, anus and glans penis (Ref. 384, p.96). Treatment of a painful phantom limb is extremely difficult, notable relief only being achieved after either cerebro-vascular accident has occurred leading to a hemiplegia, or surgical ablation of the parietal cortex.

Congenital indifference to pain and pain asymbolia

In congenital analgesia patients perceive pain, but seem indifferent to it. This has a genetic basis, and is sometimes associated with mental retardation or chromosome abnormalities. It is to be distinguished from the behaviour of certain patients with mental retardation who self-mutilate, and seem at the time to show no clear indication of experiencing pain but are just as susceptible as others to pain inflicted from outside agencies. A second variety of indifference to pain is seen following degeneration of sensory nerves or dorsal root ganglia. Such patients have much morbidity from scarring and damage.[385]

Pain asymbolia refers to the condition in which patients fail to react normally to noxious stimuli, although they seem to experience pain. It is associated with parietal lobe lesions, and Schilder suggested that pain sensations failed to achieve meaning because they were not integrated into the patient's body image, and were therefore not acted upon (Ref. 386, pp.101–4).

CHAPTER 9

Neuropsychiatric Aspects of Epilepsy and Disorders of Sleep

EPILEPSY

Epilepsy is a disorder characterized by brief episodes of altered behaviour often associated with loss of consciousness. However, it represents an episodic or chronic disorder of neuronal function, which, when localized to one area of the brain, provides the neuropsychiatrist with a natural model for testing certain hypotheses about brain–behaviour relationships. In recent years the use of serum anticonvulsant drug monitoring the development of methods to record the electroencephalogram by telemeter, and introduction of newer anticonvulsant drugs, have led to changes in understanding and management of epileptic problems. In spite of this, 'epilepsy' itself still defies definition. The often quoted definition of Hughlings Jackson, of 'occasional, sudden, excessive, rapid and local discharges of grey matter' (Ref. 387, Vol. 1, p.100) lays emphasis primarily on fits and the acute paroxysms of the disorder, but fails to distinguish it from other possibly similar disorders such as migraine or acute panic attacks. Williams adopted a broader definition, saying: 'Epilepsy can be assumed when there are recurring discrete disorders of sensation or behaviour of any sort caused primarily by cerebral disturbance.'[388] This, as he suggested, 'takes the use of the word . . . to the doorstep of clinical psychiatry.'

CLASSIFICATION AND INCIDENCE

An abbreviated version of the classification suggested by the International League against Epilepsy is shown in Table 9.1.[389] Partial seizures are those of focal origin, which may remain focal or become generalized. Their symptomatology is described as simple or complex — the latter referring to interference with 'high level' cerebral activity, in which disturbance of consciousness occurs. Such patients present with a variety of experiences including hallucinations,

Table 9.1. Classification of the epilepsies

Partial seizures:	(a) Simple or Elementary	— Motor Sensory Autonomic Compound
	(b) Complex	— Impaired consciousness Cognitive symptoms Affective symptoms Psychosensory symptoms 'Psychomotor' symptoms Compound
	(c) Secondarily generalized	
Generalized seizures		Absences — simple — complex Myoclonic Infantile spasms Clonic seizures Tonic seizures Tonic–clonic seizures Atonic seizures Akinetic seizures
Unilateral seizures Unclassified seizures		

affective disturbances and thought disorder and usually have electroencephalographic or other evidence of temporal lobe abnormalities. Generalized seizures are due to bilateral disturbances, which are usually symmetrical. Two varieties that are commonly seen are simple absences, accompanied by 3 c/s spike and wave activity on the EEG — so-called 'petit mal epilepsy', and more disturbed and prolonged abnormalities associated with tonic–clonic muscular activity — referred to as grand mal seizures. Occasionally 'generalized' seizures fail to generalize and are unilateral, the abnormality apparently being confined to one hemisphere. A number of seizure types are encountered that fail to meet any of the given definitions, and are therefore referred to as 'unclassified'.

Although it is estimated that about 1 in 20 people may have convulsion in their life, the prevalence of epilepsy is far less, being around 0.5% for the general population.

CLINICAL DESCRIPTION

Classical tonic–clonic generalized seizures (grand mal) are almost unmistakable. The attack, which rarely lasts more than 2 minutes, has a sudden onset with loss of consciousness, tonic muscular contractions followed by clonic ones, after which the patient is unrousable for a period of time. Self-injury, incontinence and tongue-biting may occur, and there may follow a period of post-ictal confusion. If the attack has a focal origin, the patient may have an aura, which is a brief feeling or sensation that occurs immediately before the attack, representing the focal disturbance of electrical activity. It is to be distinguished from prodromata, which may serve to warn the patient about a forthcoming fit, and occur hours or even days before a fit. Prodromal symptoms are often changes of mood, although other symptoms such as headache or appetite change may occur. Other focal origins of the attack result in the spread of motor or sensory symptoms. The motor variants are called Jacksonian attacks. If the attack arises from the prefrontal areas, then the head and eyes are deviated away from the site of the attack — this is referred to as an 'adversive seizure'. Following an attack with focal origin a paralysis (Todd's paralysis) or sensory disturbance may be noted, and last several hours or longer. During an attack EEG changes occur with fast spike and wave activity in both hemispheres (see Figure 9.1a) and following the attack the record is marked by slow waves and lack of spiking activity. The focal origin of an attack may be detected by phase reversal of the spikes, sometimes only detected by special techniques (see Figure 9.1b).

Generalized seizures that present as absence attacks (petit mal epilepsy) impair consciousness for a few seconds only, and are virtually unaccompanied by motor signs. They occur primarily in children and in many cases cease before the age of 20, although about half the patients with petit mal epilepsy develop grand mal seizures. In a petit mal attack there is sudden arrest of attention, blinking and perhaps pallor with subsequent amnesia. The EEG in these states shows 3 c/s. spike wave activity (Figure 9.1c). A variant of this type of epilepsy, referred to as the 'petit mal triad' is an association of drop attacks and myoclonic jerks with the petit mal attack. However, it is not associated with classical 3 c/s. spike wave activity, and has a much worse prognosis.

There are a large number of simple partial epileptic phenomena which may or may not proceed to a generalized attack. In particular, focal temporal lobe attacks give rise to a whole gamut of psychic experiences (see Table 9.2). One variety, in which the patient experiences an unpleasant smell and taste which may be accompanied by chewing movements, and lip smacking, is referred to as an 'uncinate fit'.

Although patients may experience compound partial seizures, with a variety of experiences related to the focal origins of the attacks, in complex partial seizures there are disturbances of thought, perception, behaviour, affect, and consciousness. The term is preferred to temporal lobe epilepsy, as some manifestations of these seizures occur in attacks that originate outside the temporal lobes; and to psychomotor epilepsy — the term used to describe seizures with both psychic and motor phenomena. They may start at any age, are the commonest variety of epilepsy, and in the majority of cases the attacks are of temporal lobe origin. Any hallucinations are formed and complex, as opposed to those arising from primary sensory cortex which are simple. Characteristically the hallucination is constant with repeated attacks. Any recognized emotion may occur although the commonest affective experience is fear, sometimes intense, and often associated with a fear of death. Depression is uncommon but well-documented, and rage and anger as ictal events are very rare. Cursive epilepsy is the name given for running during attacks; gelastic epilepsy for laughing attacks.

Table 9.2. Some manifestations of simple and complex partial seizures of temporal origin

Motor:	Adversive attacks, lip smacking, aphasia, speech automation.
Sensory:	Visual, auditory or olfactory hallucinations; autoscopy; vertigo; unpleasant epigastric sensations rising to the throat; illusions; time distortions.
Affective:	Fear, panic, depression, euphoria.
Other:	*Déjà vu, jamais vu*, depersonalization, erotic experiences, forced thinking.

The term automatism was introduced by Hughlings Jackson for 'all kinds of doings after epileptic fits, from slight vagaries up to homicidal actions' (Ref. 387, Vol. 1, p.122). Characteristically, as he described them, behaviour is automatic and carried out unconsciously. Others have suggested the term should be restricted to apparently purposeful behaviour.[390] Automatisms have been divided into: (a) perseverative — in which the patient contrives to carry out actions initiated prior to the attack; or (b) *de novo* — in which a new behaviour is initiated.[391] During such episodes, which usually last less than 15 minutes, consciousness is altered and there is often, but not always, amnesia for the event. Patients may carry out complex quasi-purposeful behaviour, although violence is unusual unless the patient is interfered with during the automatism, when conflict can be provoked. Even then the behaviour is poorly directed and unlikely to be dangerous. Automatisms arise either as an accompaniment of the ictus, or in the post-ictal period, and neurophysiologically are associated with bilateral involvement of the amygdaloid-hippocampal region.[390] The majority of patients who perform automatisms have temporal lobe abnormalities.

Status epilepticus is a term used to denote recurrent epileptic seizures without return of consciousness between attacks. Persistent focal seizures are referred to as epilepsia partialis continua. An unusual variety of the latter is where complex partial seizures are continuous, which can lead to prolonged states of confusion with automatisms resembling psychosis. During such attacks continuous epileptiform activity from the temporal lobes will be detected.

Two other conditions of prolonged disturbance of consciousness related to seizure activity are to be noted. These are absence status, with typical

166

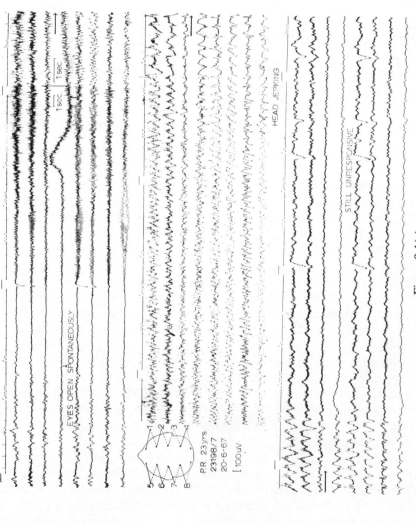

Figure 9.1(a)

167

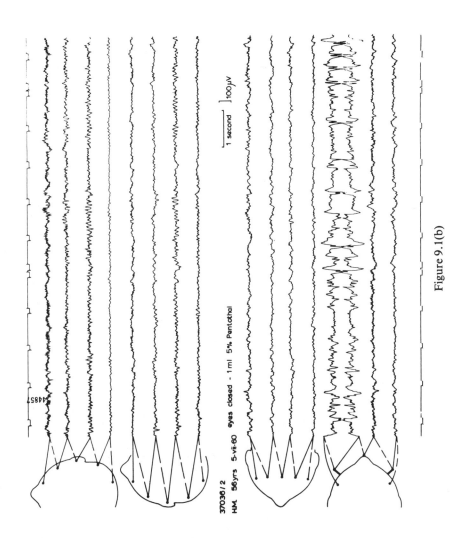

Figure 9.1(b)

168

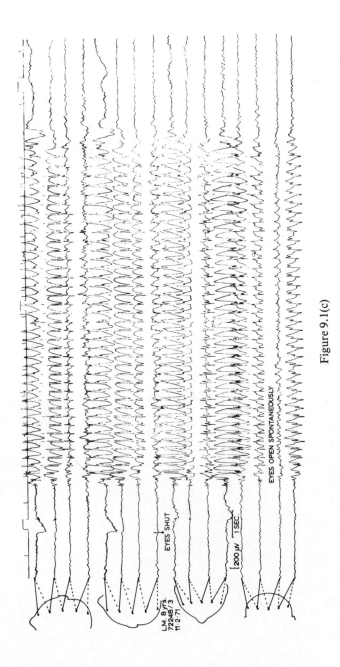

Figure 9.1(c)

Figure 9.1. (a) generalized tonic–clonic seizure — showing pre-ictal flattening and post-ictal slowing of the EEG; (b) partial seizure originating in the temporal lobe — detected by the use of sphenoidal electrodes; (c) generalized seizure — absence (petit mal epilepsy) spike-wave complexes on the EEG, and post-paroxysmal twilight states, in which the EEG will show diffuse theta and delta activity.

Myoclonic seizures

These present as brief, local or generalized, usually bilateral, myoclonic jerks. They may be a prodromal sign of an impending generalized seizure, or occur as part of other syndromes such as progressive myoclonic epilepsy of Unverricht-Lundborg, familial myoclonic epilepsy, cerebellar dyssynergia myoclonica, subacute sclerosing panencephalitis, and post-anoxic brain damage.

AETIOLOGY AND PATHOGENESIS

Why patients should have epileptic convulsions when they do is usually unknown. However, it is customary to divide epilepsy into idiopathic and symptomatic groupings. The assumption is that in the former there is some form of inherited or acquired mechanism which leads to a person having a low seizure threshold, whereas in the latter there is a more clearly identifiable cause which provokes the attacks, such as tumour or scar tissue. In practice such a distinction is often difficult, and since not all patients with tumours have epilepsy, presumably even in symptomatic epilepsy other factors than the presence of a local lesion are necessary to lead to a seizure.

Symptomatic causes of epilepsy are outlined in Table 9.3. There is variation in association with age. Causes of neonatal seizures include prenatal events (cerebral malformations, rubella embryopathy); damage during birth from hypoxia, and trauma; and post-natal events such as hypoglycaemia, hypocalcaemia and hypomagnesaemia, meningitis, inborn errors of metabolism, and drug withdrawal.[392] In infantile spasms, with onset usually

Table 9.3. Some causes of epilepsy

Metabolic causes:	Hypoglycaemia, hypomagnesaemia, fluid and electrolyte disturbances, acute intermittent porphyria, amino-acid disorders.
Trauma:	Head injuries, especially penetrating wounds and birth injuries.
Neurological causes:	Tumours, cerebrovascular accidents, degenerative and storage disorders, demyelinating diseases, Sturge–Weber and other malformations, tuberose-sclerosis. Infections, e.g. cytomegalovirus, toxoplamosis, meningitis, cysticercosis, syphilis.
Drug withdrawal:	Especially alcohol and the barbiturates.
Vitamin deficiency:	Pyridoxine.
Poisons:	Lead, strychnine.
Temperature:	Fever.

between 3 and 8 months, there is a characteristic patterns of fits with sudden brief flexion or extension spasms of varying severity. This disorder has a variety of causes in spite of a characteristic EEG of hypsarrhythmia. Idiopathic epilepsy usually starts around the age of 3 or later and is the commonest form of epilepsy until adult life, when tumours and cerebrovascular disease become prominent causes.

Head injury is a common cause of epilepsy, which is most likely to develop if the dura is penetrated, and if the injury is severe producing a post-traumatic amnesia of more than 24 hours. It usually results in both generalized and focal seizures, and in 50% of the patients who develop post-traumatic epilepsy the first fit does not occur until a year or more after injury.

Of particular interest has been the discovery that a specific pathological lesion, namely mesial temporal sclerosis, is found in some patients with epilepsy, especially complex partial seizures. It is often unilateral, and specifically there is sclerosis of hippocampus and related structures, with neuronal loss and increased glial elements. In that many patients who develop this lesion have a history of febrile convulsions in childhood, and that similar lesions have been produced in primates by experimentally provoking seizures, it has been suggested that the lesions themselves are the result of damage to the temporal lobe, which occurs during anoxic episodes at vulnerable periods.[393] The difficulties of the idiopathic-symptomatic dichotomy are here again noted, since it is presumably those children with a lowered seizure threshold who are the ones most likely to develop the febrile convulsions. The resulting structural damage then leads to an even greater chance of the development of complex partial seizures in adult life.

In attempting to understand how primary pathologies interact with other factors in the pathogenesis of epilepsy, Meldrum discussed neurochemical and cytological mechanisms.[393] Pathological processes such as ischaemia or hypoxia may destroy neurones whose neurotransmitters are primarily inhibitory, which results in a lowering of the seizure threshold. Of interest is the observation that action myoclonus in patients who have suffered hypoxic brain damage responds to 5-HTP administration, and that the patients most responsive are the ones who have low 5-HIAA in the CSF.[394] Deficits in serotonin activity have also been noted in other forms of epilepsy, and manipulation of monoamine turnover alters the seizure threshold in animals. In particular increasing the activity of dopamine or GABA within the central nervous system is anti-epileptic.[395]

Although the actual triggering mechanism for the majority of seizures is unknown, various processes have been suggested, including 'stress', alcohol withdrawal, lack of sleep, and fevers. In susceptible patients seizures may be provoked by such techniques as hyperventilation, or by administration of drugs that lower the seizure thresholds. There are a group of patients who suffer from reflex epilepsy where seizures are triggered by environmental actions or events such as flashing lights, reading, and noise.

The mirror focus describes a secondary focus of epileptic activity derived in the contralateral hemisphere from a primary focus. Kindling is a phenomenon in which repeated sub-threshold electrical stimulation leads to subsequent development of seizure activity. Both are experimental procedures that have relevance for human epilepsy.

DIFFERENTIAL DIAGNOSIS

In many cases the diagnosis of epilepsy, based mainly on the history and clinical description of the attacks, is not difficult, and is readily supported by EEG confirmation. However, there are patients, especially amongst those seen at specialist referral centres, where diagnosis is extremely difficult, and where a primary psychiatric diagnosis is amongst the differential diagnostic possibilities. Betts, in a survey of patients diagnosed as having epilepsy admitted to psychiatric hospitals in one area, found that 20% did not have epilepsy. Although some had a seizure at one time, it was often secondary to drug withdrawal or intoxication. A number of other patients presented with alternative psychiatric problems.[396]

Hysteria presenting as epilepsy can be most difficult to diagnose, especially since it sometimes occurs in patients who also have epilepsy. The diagnosis rests on the clinical description of the attack and on the taking of a good psychiatric history. Patients with abnormal illness behaviour are more likely to have family or past personal history of psychiatric illness, to have elements of the hysterical personality, and to be sexually immature. Careful documentation of the events surrounding seizures will often reveal that they occur in a setting of interpersonal stress, rarely occur when the patient is alone, and usually do not occur at night. Incontinence and self-injury do not rule out the diagnosis of abnormal illness behaviour. Many patients on psychiatric examination will be found to have current psychiatric illness, especially depression, and the discovery of convincing 'secondary gain' can clinch the diagnosis. Neurological examination may reveal anaesthetic patches and other signs indicative of hysteria.

The attacks themselves have a dramatic quality but often, especially if the patients also have epilepsy, on observation may resemble almost entirely an epileptic attack. Henry and Woodruff[397] have recently reported that in epileptic seizures deviation of the eyes is constant, whereas in hysteria resembling epilepsy the eyes always deviate to the ground, even when the patient is turned from one side to another. Recent advances in the use of telemetry can be useful in differential diagnosis. The patient is viewed by closed-circuit television while the EEG is monitored and transmitted to a receiver where it is recorded. Simultaneous reproduction of the EEG tracing and the patient's behaviour can then be observed at leisure, and by storing the information on videotape can be reassessed as many times as is necessary.[398] An alternative way of attempting to dissociate epilepsy from other forms of seizures is to use biochemical assessments, and recently the measurements of anterior pituitary hormones has been advocated. Patients with generalized tonic–clonic seizures show large increases in their prolactin levels 15–25 minutes following an attack, such changes not being observed in patients with abnormal illness behaviour.[399]

Hysteroepilepsy was the term used by Charcot to refer to patients in whom hysteria was present in combination with epilepsy. He felt that there was an affinity between the two disorders and referred to them both as neuroses. Although many of the patients he described would now be regarded as having complex partial seizures, the evidence that patients with organic brain disease are more susceptible to develop abnormal illness behaviour, and that patients with some forms of psychiatric illness have increased electroencephalographic abnormalities and a lowered seizure threshold, raises the possibility of a common underlying pathogenesis in at least some cases.

Panic attacks occur in patients with a prior history of anxiety neurosis and are often noted in the setting of stress. Although patients complain of epigastric discomfort, there is never a clearly defined sensation that rises to the throat as it does in patients who have the aura of complex partial seizures. The feeling is much more diffuse in panic attacks and spreads to involve the whole body. Hyperventilation, tachycardia, sweating and other manifestations of anxiety will often be reported by the patient. Loss of consciousness may occur, but this does not imply that the patient has had an epileptic seizure. However, there are a sub-group of patients who hyperventilate and, because of a lowered seizure threshold, may go on to have a generalized seizure.

With panic attacks the onset is often gradual with growing dysphoria, and after the attack, which terminates slowly, feelings of apprehension still exist. Some patients have episodes of depersonalization, or *déjà vu* experiences which may be misinterpreted as auras of complex partial seizures. Careful attention to their time on onset, length, and accompanying features will, however, usually enable them to be distinguished from epileptic manifestations. These episodes respond well to minor tranquillizers and poorly to conventional anticonvulsants.

Rage attacks may occur as ictal events but are extremely rare. Aggression may occur post-ictally, especially if a confused patient is forcibly contained, but often this is poorly directed and the patient is actually in more danger of harming himself than others. Fenton, in a survey of epileptic patients in prison, was able to find only two patients out of 158 whose crime was probably committed during a seizure, and no increase in crimes of violence in epileptic populations when compared to controls.[390]

Fugue states are prolonged episodes of amnesia associated with wandering that can occur with a variety of pathologies including psychiatric illness. The amnesia lasts hours, weeks or even years, and if related to psychiatric illness usually occurs in the setting of escape from difficult or intolerable circumstances.[224] Unlike epileptic automatisms which are briefer, patients remain able to manipulate their environments successfully and, while acting appropriately, fail to draw attention from others. A guide to the differential diagnosis of this and other problems discussed in this section is shown in Table 9.4.

INTER-ICTAL PSYCHIATRIC DISORDERS

The psychiatric disturbances associated with epilepsy are conveniently divided into peri-ictal and inter-ictal. The peri-ictal disturbances have been discussed

Table 9.4. The differential diagnosis of non-epileptic fits

	Epilepsy	Hysteria	Panic attacks	Rage attacks	Fugue states
Onset	Sudden	Sudden or gradual	Sudden: precipitating event	Sudden	Sudden
Duration	Minutes	Minutes or hours	Minutes or hours	Minutes	Hours or days
Termination	Sudden	Gradual or sudden: no confusion	Gradual	Gradual	Gradual
Accompanying features	Often preceding brief aura; incontinence; self-injury; eye deviation constant. Neurological reflex changes.	Bizarre pattern to fits, talking, secondary gain. Eye deviation to the ground stigmata	Preceding dysphoria	Preceding dysphoria. Co-ordinated and directed aggression.	Often depressive illness or other psychiatric disorder. Behaviour well-integrated.
Post-attack behaviour	Sleepy	Sometimes sleepy	Often dysphoria	Dysphoria	Amnesia
EEG	Usually abnormal	Usually normal	Usually normal	Usually normal	Usually normal

above and include pre-ictal mood changes, ictal auras and post-ictal confusional states. The inter-ictal disturbances have been more clearly defined in recent years. The history of the relationship between psychiatric disturbances and epilepsy has been summarized by Guerrant and others.[400] They defined four periods of thought which are delineated in Table 9.5. The period of epileptic deterioration, which assumed that all epileptics deteriorated because they had seizures, gave way to the period of the epileptic character, in which it was felt that the epilepsy and the mental changes were commonly associated since both were due to the same underlying neuropathological disorder. Specific character changes became described and all was blamed on a bad heredity.

Table 9.5. History of personality changes in epilepsy (after Guerrant et al.[400])

Period of epileptic deterioration	(–1900)
Period of the epileptic character	(1900–1930)
Period of normality	(1930–)
Period of psychomotor peculiarity	(1930–)

More recently, two conflicting views are concurrently held. The first is that the majority of epileptic patients are perfectly normal and that any abnormality that exists is secondary to brain damage, a result of seizures, psychosocial influences or anticonvulsant drug toxicity. The alternative view is that patients with complex partial seizures are more inclined to have psychiatric disturbances than other epileptic patients, as a result of temporal lobe dysfunction. A major problem in interpretation of the studies carried out in this field is that until recent times the classification of both psychiatric disorder and epilepsy has been inadequate, and that selected populations have been analysed. Neurologists have therefore emphasized the lack of psychiatric disorder in their patients, whereas psychiatrists have emphasized the association. More recent studies, however, do allow further assessment of these problems to be made.

PSYCHIATRIC ILLNESS IN EPILEPTIC PATIENTS

There are now a number of studies on unselected patients that demonstrate an increased incidence of psychiatric illness in epileptic populations. These, summarized in Table 9.6, indicate that the increased incidence occurs in adults as well as in children, and that it is having epilepsy, rather than a chronic disorder *per se*, that is associated with psychopathology.[401-6] Rutter,[405] in a study of unselected children on the Isle of Wight, noted the prevalence of deviant behaviour to be four times higher in patients with uncomplicated epilepsy compared with the general population. This was two to three times higher than in those with physical disorders not involving the brain.

Several of these studies indicated a higher incidence of abnormality in patients with 'temporal lobe epilepsy'. With the exception of certain personality changes[404] and organic brain syndromes no particular diagnostic category was

Table 9.6. Studies of unselected populations of epileptic patients[401-6]

Author	Population*	Incidence of psychiatric disorder	Control group
Henderson (1953)	Schoolchildren (C)	12%	—
Juul-Jensen (1964)	General population (A)	35%§	—
Pond and Bidwell (1959)	General practice study (A & C)	29%§	
Gudmundsson (1966)	Iceland survey (A)	52%§	—
Rutter et al. (1970)	Isle of Wight study (C)	28.6%§	6.6%
Mellor et al. (1973)	Unselected schoolchildren (C)	27.0%	15%

* A adults, C children.
§ Highest in complex partial seizures.

highlighted, generally patients with epilepsy suffering from the same psychiatric disorders as patients without epilepsy.

PERSONALITY DISORDER AND EPILEPSY

A number of specific personality types have been described in the literature as being closely interlinked with epilepsy. Pond suggested that patients with 'petit mal epilepsy' tended to be more neurotic and passive than others.[407] Specific personality patterns have in recent years been associated with complex partial seizures. As already noted, two views coexist about this relationship, one of which suggests that there is a specific personality disturbance which may be attributed to 'psychomotor epilepsy'. This view has been challenged on the grounds that most investigations had sampling bias, EEG evaluation problems, and used inadequate rating scales, and several studies failed to demonstrate differences between patients with temporal lobe abnormalities and others.[408] The majority of negative studies have come from the USA, with the exception of a recent attempt to assess a small number of epileptic patients and medical controls using the PSE.[409] Guerrant,[400] in a controlled study of the psychiatric status of 32 adult patients with psychomotor epilepsy, 26 with idiopathic grand mal epilepsy, and 26 non-epileptic patients with chronic psychiatric illness, found no difference between the three groups, although the incidence of psychiatric disorder was 90% in all three, and some excess of personality disorder was noted in the two epileptic groups. Small et al.[410] studied 50 epileptic patients with either psychomotor epilepsy or generalized epilepsy, and used neurological clinical examinations, the MMPI, the WAIS and the Rorschach tests. They found no differences in the psychiatric diagnoses, personality rating scales, or psychometric scores, with the exception that temporal lobe patients tended to score higher on some of the WAIS sub-tests. In a replication study, with the addition of another 50 cases from a psychiatric clinic, again the results were statistically negative. However, in these studies patients with temporal lobe abnormalities had more delusions, hallucinations and abnormal thought processes than the non-temporal lobe group. Stevens, in two more studies on patients attending neurology clinics, reported negative findings statistically, although again in her studies patients in the temporal lobe group scored higher on the paranoia, depression, and schizophrenia sub-scales of the MMPI.[411]

Supporters of the concept of the epileptic personality, the idea that 'chronic sufferers from temporal lobe seizures commonly show irritability, impulsiveness and bad temper . . . egocentricity, perseveration and religiosity . . . and a sensitive suspiciousness which may lead to frank paranoid attitudes . . .',[412] have a large number of anecdotal reports to depend on, and some recent studies. Ervin et al. examined 42 patients with temporal lobe epilepsy and reported 29 has having 'episodic symptoms such as sudden affective changes, sudden alterations in consciousness and hallucinations . . . characteristically the group was distinguished by loosely organized and immature patterns of adaptation . . .'.[413] Ounsted *et al.*[414] in a careful study of 100 children with temporal lobe epilepsy drew attention to the hyperkinetic behaviour of this group. Rutter *et al.*[405] also reported much more psychiatric disability associated with temporal lobe epilepsy in children than with other forms. Stores[415] investigated sex and laterality differences in children in relation to behaviour changes in temporal lobe epilepsy, and found that most disturbance occurred in males with left-sided foci. Rodin *et al.*,[416] in an age, sex and IQ-matched study of 78 patients with temporal lobe epilepsy noted that the latter were more difficult to treat, had more paranoia and depression, and more abnormal MMPI scores than those with other forms of epilepsy. Clinically they had more 'psychotic tendencies', and the most abnormal scores were noted in patients who had more than one seizure type, i.e. complex partial seizures which were also generalized. Bear and Fedio[417] designed their own rating scale taking traits from the literature suggested to exist in temporal lobe epileptic patients: 48 patients were compared, 15 with right temporal lobe abnormalities, 12 with left temporal lobe abnormalities, and a control group without epilepsy. They concluded 'Humourless sobriety, dependence, and circumstantiality most strongly characterize the epileptic sample.' Right-sided patients were more often described as showing elation, and left-sided patients had more anger, paranoia and dependence. Other authors have described a particular triad of changes in patients with temporal lobe epilepsy of hyper-religiosity, hypergraphia and hyposexuality.[200] While these results do not confirm that a particular 'epileptic personality' exists, they indicate that patients with temporal lobe lesions are more likely to have psychiatric disabilities, especially if they have more than one seizure type or the EEG disturbances are left sided. Specifically high ratings for paranoia, schizophrenia, and affective changes emerge in adults, and over-activity, anxiety, and aggression in children. It has been suggested 'the pairing of periodic changes in limbic activity, with temporarily coincident events in the external world, lead to altered modes of learning about external events . . .'.[417] Differences in behaviour therefore noted in patients with temporal lobe epilepsy may represent an organic psychosyndrome, dependent upon continuing dysfunction within the limbic system. It is further suggested that the chronic dysfunction somehow enhances cortical limbic connections bringing about 'functional hyperconnection leading to a suffusion of experience with emotional colouration'.[417]

PSYCHOSIS AND EPILEPSY

The relationship between epilepsy and psychosis has evoked as much discussion as that between personality disorder and epilepsy. A major problem has been the definition of psychosis and the selection issue with regard to the patients studied. Earlier writers such as Morel and Falret drew attention to the relationship between epilepsy and psychosis, in particular brief episodes of altered consciousness associated with hallucinations and delusions. Morel introduced the term 'larval epilepsy' in which the epileptic fit was masked and the patient exhibited changes in behaviour instead (Ref. 418, p.318). Hughlings Jackson reasserted the relationship with the statement that: 'Epilepsy is the cause of insanity in 6% of insane persons' (Ref. 387, Vol. 1, p.119), although again he was concentrating primarily on acute episodes of illness. This relationship between ictal events and psychosis has now been more clearly delineated as mentioned above. However, the concept that epilepsy may be related to more prolonged forms of psychiatric disturbance, and in particular that disorders such as schizophrenia may represent an inter-ictal complication, has only become crystallized more recently. The available literature was well-reviewed by Davison and Bagley.[318] They concluded that three relationships between psychosis and epilepsy exist, all of which are tenable. These are: (a) that they are coincidental; (b) that they have an affinity; and (c) that they have an antagonism.

The first relationship seems obvious in that for any group of patients where two disorders exist there will be a small number in which they occur together by chance. However, that they are not all coincidental was demonstrated by Slater and Beard.[419] Estimating the expected frequency of new cases of epilepsy and schizophrenia in the London area to be 4 to 5 per year, but finding 69 'easily', they concluded on statistical grounds that: 'Patients suffering from epilepsy develop schizophrenia-like psychoses with a much greater than chance expectation . . . .'.

Although at first sight the other two hypotheses, namely the antagonism and the affinity concepts, would seem to be incompatible, the possibility that the epilepsy and the schizophrenia-like symptoms are both manifestations of the same underlying disturbance of cerebral function has received considerable support from recent neurophysiological and biochemical findings.

The antagonism concept

Although Von Meduna had based the idea of convulsive therapy on clinical observations that seizures were effective in alleviating some psychiatric symptoms, and several authors had clinically described cases in which a psychosis resolved with an epileptic seizure, it was the studies of Landolt that led to a closer neurophysiological understanding of these observations.[420] Recording changes in EEGs both during pre-seizure dysphoric episodes, and during limited periods of frank psychosis lasting sometimes days or weeks, he noted improvement of epileptic activity during these episodes with 'forced normalization of the EEG'. Landolt suggested that similar changes could be produced by anticonvulsant drugs. At the end of the psychotic episode the EEGs returned to being abnormal showing epileptic activity, most of these patients having temporal lobe abnormalities. Similar phenomena were observed and recorded by others such as Dongier,[421] who concluded that the attacks in which there was normalization were longer than those where normalization did not occur. It is clear that these events are closely interlinked with neurophysiological mechanisms, but that they do not refer to the chronic inter-ictal psychoses.

The affinity concept

The increased frequency of psychotic patients in epileptic populations receives mention from several authors. In Gudmundsson's survey of epilepsy in Iceland, 5.5% of the men and 9.1% of the women were psychotic.[404] In addition there are several studies indicating an increased prevalence of epilepsy in psychotic patients. Kraepelin commented on this in his original studies. Yde et al.[422] noted the rate of epilepsy in 715 schizophrenics was twice that of the general population. Gruhle in the 1930s, and then Hill, and Pond in the 1950s give accounts of psychotic states in epileptic patients that closely resembled schizophrenia. Nearly all patients had temporal lobe lesions.[412, 423, 424] Ervin et al., in a survey of 31 patients with clinical epilepsy presenting as psychomotor seizures alone or in combination with others, reported that 90% were schizophrenics.[413] The diagnosis was made on clinical grounds using the criteria of Bleuler. Rodin, using similar criteria, examined six cases and suggested that 'schizophrenia-like symptomatology can be discerned to a varying degree in all of them . . . .'.[425]

One of the most comprehensive studies was that of Slater,[419, 426] who examined 69 cases and described four groups: one of 11 patients with short-lived confusional episodes in the course of their chronic psychoses; a second of 46 patients who had chronic paranoid states; a third of eight patients with hebephrenic schizophrenia; and a fourth, smaller group, that had petit mal epilepsy. A large number of these cases gave a history compatible with some accident or trauma which was responsible for their epilepsy. Clinically Slater stated: 'There was not one of the cardinal symptoms of schizophrenia (not) at some time exhibited by these patients', although catatonic pictures were rare. Some differences were noted between the presentation of these patients and schizophrenia in non-epileptic patients. In particular there was virtual absence of premorbid schizoid traits; maintenance of a good affective response and rapport; negative family history of psychiatric disorder; and a predominance of paranoid presentations. The mean difference between the age of onset of the epilepsy and that of the psychosis was 14 years. Eighty percent of his patients had temporal lobe epilepsy, and of 56 who had an air-encephalogram, 39 showed abnormalities, mainly of an atrophic process. In some cases this was confined to the temporal hornes, although in others a more generalized abnormality was detected. Of seven patients he described with 'centrencephalic epilepsy', the presenting picture was predominantly hebephrenic.

In contrast to the psychoses directly related to the ictus discussed above, in most of these patients the onset was insidious with a gradual appearance of delusions. Some patients, however, developed their illness in an episodic way following recurrent acute psychotic episodes. No relationship was found between the total fit frequency or drug treatment and the psychotic illness, although it was noted that 25% of the patients showed a decline in fit frequency as the psychosis became apparent, another manifestation of antagonism.

Flor-Henry[427] in a retrospective study of patients diagnosed as having schizophrenic-like psychosis and temporal lobe epilepsy, found that, compared to an epileptic control group, the psychotics had either a dominant hemisphere focus, if the disorder was unilateral or bilateral foci. Alternatively, in a group that had manic-depressive psychosis there was a tendency for the epilepsy to affect the non-dominant hemisphere. Again, there was an association between infrequent seizures and the psychosis. He concluded: 'that not only temporal lobe epilepsy predisposes to psychosis, but that it is especially responsible for the schizophrenic manifestations if the dominant hemisphere is involved'. Bruens[428] collected 19 patients with epilepsy and psychosis, 16 of whom had a chronic illness. There was a much higher incidence of temporal lobe epilepsy (84%), especially with bilateral lesions. The majority of the temporal lobe epileptic patients had paranoid symptoms but, unlike Salter and Flor-Henry, he felt that while the clinical picture was schizophreniform-like, in reality it failed to fulfil the strict criteria for the diagnosis of schizophrenia.

From the above, it can be concluded that there is an increased association between epilepsy and psychosis. The psychoses are either short-lived or chronic. The former are associated with a variety of EEG patterns and often with disturbance of consciousness (see Table 9.7), although in some the phenomenon of 'forced normalization' is seen. The psychoses when present often have schizophrenic-like symptomatology. Chronic psychosis is associated with epilepsy, particularly complex partial seizures, which some authors suggest also resembles schizophrenia phenomenologically. It is often paranoid in nature, and is more common with left-sided or bilateral foci than with right-sided lesions, and is more likely to occur when the number of seizures is diminishing.

Several mechanisms have been suggested to explain these findings, in particular the high association between temporal lobe lesions and psychosis. With regard to the normalization phenomenon it seems probable that a neurophysiological explanation exists to account for the coincident expression of psychosis with normalizing of the EEG. The facts that electrophysiologically abnormal activity may be detected in medial temporal structures in patients with psychotic illness (see below), and that stimulation of these regions is associated with depression of cortical activity suggest that some underlying biochemical process may be responsible for altering patterns of expression of abnormal electrical activity. Alteration of dopamine activity is one possibility, since dopaminergic compounds are both anti-epileptic and psychotogenic.[429]

With regard to the chronic psychoses, some, especially the Continental authors, suggest that the psychosis is a reaction to having epilepsy. This fails to account for the localization of the site of abnormality mainly to the temporal

Table 9.7. On the relationship between psychoses and epilepsy

		Disturbance of conciousness	EEG: most common disturbance
Episodic	Post-ictal automatism	+	Slow waves
	Petit mal states	+	3 per/sec. spike and wave
	Complex partial seizure states	+	Bilateral temporal lobe abnormality
	Confusional states	+	Generalized abnormality
	Psycho-organic episodes	+	Very abnormal EEG with slow dysrhythmia
	Forced normalization states	–	Normal
Chronic	Paranoid states	–	Temporal lobe abnormalities
	Schizophrenic-like states	–	Temporal lobe abnormalities (left side)
	Manic-depressive states	–	Temporal lobe abnormalities

lobes, and the laterality findings. Others have suggested that the epilepsy itself causes the psychosis, or that the epilepsy and the psychosis both have the same underlying pathogenesis,[427] although most authors agree that it is disturbances of the limbic system that are responsible for both the ictal manifestations and the psychosis. The comments of Symonds are pertinent. He referred to 'an epileptic disorder of function' suggesting that 'epileptic seizures and epileptiform discharge in the EEG are epiphenomena. They may be regarded as occasional expressions of a fundamental and continuous disorder of neuronal function . . . (it) . . . may be present continuously but at peaks at which seizures are likely to occur.'[430] He went on to suggest that it was the disorderly activity of the temporal lobe neurones, especially those undestroyed by pathology, that was the cause both of the seizures and the psychosis. While this would not account for the fact that the psychosis tends to come on a number of years after the epilepsy has started, or for the reciprocal relationship in some patients in the chronic psychotic group of the psychosis and the seizures, newer observations, in particular related to the phenomenon of kindling, may provide a neurological and experimental link to explain the gradual development of behaviour changes in patients with chronic limbic system epilepsy.

ELECTROPHYSIOLOGICAL CHANGES IN PATIENTS WITH SCHIZOPHRENIA — NON-EPILEPTIC

A number of EEG abnormalities have been reported in patients with schizophrenia. Hill observed abnormal EEGs in 33 of 80 schizophrenics; the changes ranged from 'non-specific' abnormalities to paroxysmal slow and fast activity with low-voltage spikes.[431] Some of the patterns were indistinguishable from those seen in epileptic patterns, and there was a particular association with catatonic schizophrenia. In addition, catatonic schizophrenic patients have a low seizure threshold, and in insulin coma therapy those schizophrenic patients that recovered were more likely to have a clinical seizure during treatment. Landolt reported that in non-catatonic schizophrenics the acute phases of the illness are associated with normalization of the EEG.[420] Since these early studies, the majority of reports confirm an increase in EEG abnormalities in schizophrenic patients. Of more interest, however, are the reports of Heath, replicated by others,[20] using implanted depth electrodes in psychotic patients. They demonstrated that the psychotic state was associated with spike and slow-wave recordings, in particular in the septal-accumbens region, which were not detected by conventional surface electrodes. Using the same techniques they also confirmed that in epileptic patients inter-ictal EEG abnormalities are observed in the deep temporal nuclei (hippocampus and amygdala), and that as the epileptic-like activity increased the emotional state changed. In that the location and appearance of the spikes reported by Heath resemble kindled spikes observed in experimental animals, further evidence is provided for the idea that changes related to kindling in the mesolimbic system may occur in the psychosis related to epilepsy.

EPILEPSY AND DETERIORATION OF COGNITIVE FUNCTION

Early authors concentrated more on disturbances of intellect than on psychotic manifestations in epilepsy. They commonly stressed that changes in memory occurred, which later proceeded to intellectual deterioration and dementia. Lennox (Ref. 432, p.664) suggested that cognitive deterioration was not universal in epileptic patients, but that when it occurred it was related to one of five factors. These were: (1) genetic influence; (2) organic abnormality of the brain acquired prior to the onset of seizures; (3) the epilepsy itself; (4) psychosocial isolation; and (5) sedative anticonvulsant drug toxicity.

Generally most studies indicate that non-institutionalized epileptic populations have a normal or near-normal distribution of the IQ with some skewing at the lower end of the scale; that patients with generalized tonic-clonic seizures tend to have lower IQ scores than those with partial seizures; that in children a relationship exists between disturbed behaviour and a low IQ. More specifically, relationships have been defined between brain damage and low IQ, although the contribution of the fit frequency to this remains controversial. Clinically, abnormal EEG patterns, especially clearly defined episodes of spike-wave activity, interfere with cognitive testing, and early onset epilepsy, hypsarrhythmia, and prolonged tonic–clonic seizures have all been related to intellectual deterioration. The effect of anticonvulsant drugs on cognitive function has been little studied, but the available evidence suggests that there is an influence, and drugs such as phenytoin (Epanutin) are more likely to produce cognitive deficits, than others such as carbamazepine (Tegretol).[433] In particular, progressive deterioration of intellectual function has been described in patients who have unrecognized anticonvulsant drug intoxication, especially with phenytoin (Epanutin). Some authors report that this is irreversible, although withdrawal of the phenytoin (Epanutin) in many cases will lead to an amelioration of the clinical picture.[433, 434]

Progressive deterioration of intellectual function is also seen in patients whose epilepsy is related to a progressive neuropathological process, such as a leucodystrophy in children, or cerebrovascular disease in adults. Other known causes include continuous sub-clinical seizures, or normal pressure hydrocephalus as a consequence of repeated head trauma. The possibility that in some patients a chronic viral slow encephalitis is occurring cannot be dismissed.

Diagnosing some of these conditions can be extremely difficult and may require full neurological assessment in an in-patient setting. Anticonvulsant drug toxicity in particular may produce a classical picture of dementia sometimes associated with focal neurological signs and dyskinesias in association with a raised CSF protein. This may lead to dismissal of the possibility that the drug is responsible for the clinical state, particularly since this form of toxicity has been described at so-called therapeutic anticonvulsant levels.

OTHER PSYCHIATRIC DISORDERS IN EPILEPSY

The commonest psychiatric illness in epileptic patients is depression. Transient depressive moods have been described as part of prodromata or as an ictal symptom. However, nearly one-third of patients with psychiatric problems in epilepsy have inter-ictal depression usually showing the features of 'endogenous depression', and a decline in the frequency of epileptic fits prior to the hospitalization for treatment of depression has been observed.[396] The depression may fluctuate in severity, and is reported to be commoner in patients with non-dominant temporal lobe lesions.[427] Suicide is a major problem, especially self-poisoning with anticonvulsant drugs.

The neuroses are reported with increased frequency in epilepsy, as are neurotic traits in childhood.[82] Pond and Bidwell demonstrated that more than half of the mentally disturbed patients in their study had neurotic symptoms.[402]

The relationship between epilepsy and sexual disorders had been much discussed. Hyposexuality, with diminished libido or impotence, has been related to temporal lobe epilepsy, and amelioration of these symptoms with hypersexuality has been noted after control of the seizures or temporal lobectomy.[435, 436] There are scattered reports of ictal sexual arousal, as well as documented cases of fetishism and transvestism associated with temporal lobe abnormalities.[437, 438]

THE INVESTIGATION OF EPILEPSY

Apart from the investigation of young children who have fits, where specialized investigations are required, out-patient examination of patients initially may determine whether or not a patient has epilepsy, and if so whether the epilepsy is due to a focal cause. To answer the first question it is important to take a good history and to carry out a full neurological and psychiatric assessment. Usually in uncomplicated cases the history is clearly suggestive of epilepsy, the clinical neurological examination being negative. Blood tests, including serology, and routine haematology are needed, and plain skull x-ray and EEG are usually requested at this stage. The former occasionally gives invaluable help in making a diagnosis for example of meningiomas, intracranial calcifications, or raised intracranial pressure. The latter may provide evidence of an electrical dysrhythmia which could help confirm a clinical diagnosis. The suggestion of focal epilepsy will require further exploration and the technique of choice now is the CT scan although some would recommend that all patients with possible epilepsy should have this. The finding of intracranial pathology requires further investigation under the appropriate specialist, using more sophisticated radiological techniques. Doubt over the epileptic nature of fits, and the possibility that they may be a form of abnormal illness behaviour, requires further psychiatric exploration and if necessary admission to a specialized unit where observation and telemetry may be carried out. If there is uncertainty about a diagnosis it is far better to forestall a diagnosis of epilepsy, with all the social and treatment implications that it carries, in favour of exploring alternative possibilities.

TREATMENT

The mainstay of treatment in epilepsy is anticonvulsant drugs. Recent advances, including serum level monitoring, the introduction of several newer drugs, and understanding of the pharmacology of these drugs, has led to marked improvements in management. In addition, patients with psychiatric disabilities require special consideration. The management of abnormal illness behaviour is discussed in Chapter 5.

Anticonvulsant drugs

Some of the available anticonvulsant drugs, their dose ranges, and half-lives are given in Table 9.8. Phenytoin (Epanutin) is highly bound to plasma protein and cleared from the plasma by hepatic metabolism. Widely varying serum levels are noted amongst different patients on the same dose, and the drug is handled by 'zero order' kinetics such that the enzyme that metabolizes it is saturable, and reaches its maximal action in the therapeutic range. This leads to a non-linear relationship between the dose and the serum level, and since there is only a small margin between its therapeutic and toxic levels, intoxication can readily be precipitated.[439] Examples of relationships between dose and serum levels with this drug are shown in Figure 9.2. It can be seen in some patients that small increases in oral dose can lead to marked increases in levels.

Primidone (Mysoline) is partially converted to phenobarbitone, and although it seems probable that primidone itself exerts independent anticonvulsant activity, this has never been clearly demonstrated. Phenytoin (Epanutin), phenobarbitone and primidone (Mysoline) all influence folate metabolism and have been associated with folic acid deficiency. Carbamazepine (Tegretol) is structurally related to the tricyclic antidepressants; sodium valproate (Epilim) is a GABA agonist; and clonazepam (Rivotril) is a benzodiazepine. The actual mode of action of the anticonvulsant drugs is unknown, although some alter the metabolism of monoamines and GABA. In particular, increases in 5-HT metabolism have been shown with clonazepam (Rivotril), diazepam (Valium), and phenytoin (Epanutin). Raised 5-HIAA levels in the CSF are seen in treated epileptic patients, especially those showing intoxication.[440]

The side-effects of anticonvulsant drugs are legion. While acute toxic effects have been recognizes for a long time, chronic effects, especially subtle ones on behaviour and cognitive function, have not been widely discussed until recently (see Table 9.9).[433, 441, 442] Neuropsychiatric side effects, in particular of phenytoin, include the production of an encephalopathy with deterioration of IQ, changes in behaviour such as apathy and depression, and occasionally dyskinesias and hyperactivity. Irritability in children is a well-known side-effect of phenobarbitone. It has been suggested that some of the newer anticonvulsants, such as carbamazepine (Tegretol) and sodium valproate

186

Table 9.8. Some anticonvulsant drugs

Name	Half-life (in hours)	Recommended serum levels (μmol/l)	Indications
Phenytoin (Epanutin)	—	40–100	Generalized seizures: simple or complex partial seizures.
Phenobarbitone	36 (Children) 140 (Adults)	60–180	Generalized or simple partial seizures.
Carbamazepine (Tegretol)	8–45	16–40	Generalized seizures. Simple or complex partial seizures.
Ethosuximide (Zarontin)	30–100	300–700	'Petit mal' epilepsy.
Sodium Valporate (Epilim)	10–15	—	'Petit mal': generalized seizures: myclonic epilepsy. Simple or complex partial seizures.
Sulthiame (Ospolot)	—	—	Complex partial seizures.
Clonazepam (Rivotril)	20–40	—	Myoclonic epilepsy
Primidone (Mysoline)	3–12	—	Generalized: complex or simple partial seizures.

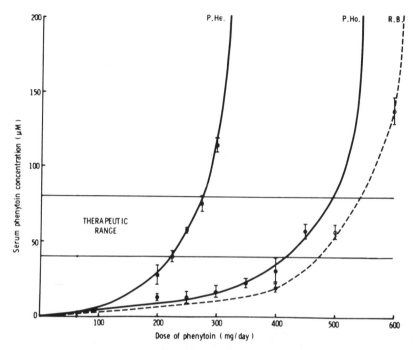

Figure 9.2. Relationship between phenytoin dose and serum levels (from Richens)[439]. Dose/serum level relationship for phenytoin in three patients in whom steady-state concentrations were measured at several doses of the drug. Each point represents the mean ± S.D. of 3–7 separate estimations. The curves were fitted by computer using the Michaelis–Menten equation. The therapeutic range suggested by Buchthal *et al.* (1960) has been drawn in to illustrate the steepness of the relationship within this range.
Note: $4\,\mu M = 1\,\mu g/ml$

(Epilim), are less likely to induce these side-effects, in particular the neuropsychiatric disabilities. Sodium valproate (Epilim) has been reported to produce a reversible alopecia and carbamazepine (Tegretol) has been associated with water intoxication, although the mechanism of this is unclear.

Interactions between anticonvulsants and other drugs, or between anti-convulsants themselves, present problems in management. Some of the established interactions of the former kind are shown in Table 9.10. The interactions with psychotropic drugs have been poorly worked out, although there is some evidence that antidepressants and major tranquillizers may increase phenytoin levels, and that phenytoin itself may lower antidepressant levels. Sulthiame (Ospolot) increases phenytoin levels, carbamazepine (Tegretol) and the benzodiazepines lower phenytoin levels; and sodium valproate (Epilim) can raise serum phenobarbitone and lower serum phenytoin.

Choice of drugs in epilepsy requires the balancing of several factors. One of these is the seizure pattern. It is clear that for petit mal epilepsy the drugs of

Table 9.9. Chronic toxic effects of some anticonvulsant drugs (from Reynolds[433, 441, 442])

Nervous system	Cerebellar atrophy (?) Peripheral neuropathy Encephalopathy Other mental symptoms
Haemopoietic system	Folic acid deficiency Neonatal coagulation defects
Skeletal system	Metabolic bone disease Vitamin D deficiency
Connective tissue	Gum hypertrophy Facial skin changes Wound healing Dupytren's contracture Other
Skin	Hirsutism Pigmentation Acne
Liver	Enzyme induction
Endocrine system	Pituitary-adrenal Thyroid-parathyroid Hyperglycaemia (diabetogenic)
Other metabolic disorders	Vitamin B_6 deficiency (?) Heavy metals
Immunological disorders	Lymphotoxicity Lymphadenopathy Systemic lupus erythaematosus; antinuclear antibodies Immunoglobulin changes (?) Immunosuppression

choice are ethosuximide (Zarontin) or sodium valproate (Epilim). For generalized seizures and partial seizures there is a wider choice, although phenytoin (Epanutin), carbamazepine (Tegretol), primidone (Mysoline) and phenobarbitone have been the most widely used. There is little evidence that any one of these drugs is better at controlling the seizures than any other, although in practice phenytoin (Epanutin) is still the most widely used in the UK, although in the Scandinavian countries carbamazepine (Tegretol) is the drug of first choice. Phenytoin (Epanutin) is unsuitable for a number of patients in view of its metabolism and side-effects. The latter, especially hirsuteness, gum hypertrophy and acne with coarsening of features, suggests that it is not the first drug of choice for children or adolescent girls. The possibility that teratogenic effects occur with some anticonvulsants has been raised, and phenytoin (Epanutin) in particular has been associated with an above-normal

Table 9.10. Anticonvulsant drug interactions (from Richens[439])

1. *Interference with the handling of antiepileptic drugs*
   (*a*)   Drugs which elevate phenytoin levels:

   Sulthiame   Dicoumarol
   Pheneturide   Disulfiram
   Isoniazid   Phenyramidol
   Chloramphenicol

   (*b*)   Drugs which lower phenytoin levels:

   Diazepam   Carbamazepine
   Chlordiazepoxide   Ethanol
   Clonazepam

2. *Drugs whose effects are known to be reduced by antiepileptic therapy*

   Griseofulvin   Nortriptyline
   Warfarin and coumarins   Diazepam
   Cortisol and dexamethasone   Doxycycline
   Contraceptive pill   Digitoxin
   Vitamin D   Metyrapone
   Phenylbutazone and antipyrine   Quinine

risk for cleft palate and a variety of skeletal abnormalities.[443] It is not general however to stop or change medication in well-controlled epileptic patients during pregnancy, although if it is clinically possible it is wise not to start anticonvulsants during this time, especially during the first trimester. Since serum levels of phenytoin and phenobarbitone tend to fall in pregnancy, these need to be monitored if the control of the epilepsy is proving difficult.

Other drugs sometimes used in the management of epilepsy include the benzodiazepines such as clonazepam (Rivotril) and nitrazepam (Mogadon), and pheneturide (Benuride), acetazolamide (Diamox), amphetamines and steroids.

Whichever drug is finally chosen, there is growing evidence that one drug is better than two, and if it is possible, polytherapy should be avoided. Shorvon et al.[444] achieved complete control in nearly 80% of new patients with either phenytoin (Epanutin) or carbamazepine (Tegretol), using serum level adjustments to achieve optimum levels. The addition of a second drug in the cases not controlled seemed to make little difference to the seizure frequency. Although management of the chronic treatment-resistant patient is clearly different, there is growing evidence that in this population too, polypharmacy may be unncessary for many.

Dosage varies with each individual although generally it is wise to start with a small dose and increase gradually until satisfactory control over seizures occurs. Many anticonvulsants can be given on a once-daily or twice-daily dose regime, and compliance may be enhanced by this prescription. Recently it has become usual to request serum level estimations in the management of epilepsy. While it is not essential to measure these at every visit, and some doubt is now cast on the early findings of a clear relationship between serum levels and side-effects, requests for serum levels are found to be especially useful in the following situations:

(a) where there is doubt about the patient taking medication;

(b) where occult toxicity is suspected;

(c) where drug interactions are suspected, and the epilepsy is becoming unstable;

(d) in toxicated patients who are on several drugs, or in a patient intoxicated on a small dose of a drug;

(e) in patients with some predisposition or disease, such as hepatic or renal disease, that may influence drug metabolism and make control difficult;

(f) where seizures are continuing, in spite of apparently adequate doses of anticonvulsant medications.

There is little value at present in requesting serum levels of either serum sodium valproate or primidone, since interpretation of the findings is extremely difficult.

Drug therapy in neuropsychiatric problems

Although anticonvulsant drugs are not the only cause of neuropsychiatric disability in patients with epilepsy, the recognition of possible side-effects from these drugs is important, if only that they are potentially reversible. Carbamazepine (Tegretol) probably has psychotropic properties in some patients,[433] and there are numerous reports of beneficial changes in cognitive abilities, personality, or mood when epileptic patients are given this drug instead of some alternatives. The changeover, if required, is most effectively carried out slowly by adding carbamazepine (Tegretol) to the existing regime and withdrawing the alternative drugs *pari passu*. For many patients with psychiatric disability, especially if their attacks are also inadequately controlled, this is preferable to adding psychotropic drugs to the existing regime. Improvement in the mental state is often accompanied by an improvement in the fits, and such a change should always be considered in patients with progressive dementia of unexplained aetiology. If, however, the clinical condition suggests that alteration of therapy is unwise, then psychotropic drugs can be used in addition to the anticonvulsants. Most of the non-MAOI antidepressants and the major tranquillizers are convulsant and there is a danger of increasing seizure frequency with them. Amitriptyline and clomipramine are the most seizurogenic and should be avoided whereas some newer antidepressants, such as nomifensine (Merital) may lead to little alteration of the seizure threshold and are to be preferred.[445] Generally the butyrophenones, such as haloperidol (Haldol) and pimozide (Orap), are less associated with precipitation of seizures than the other major tranquillizers, although evidence on this point is limited. Whichever drug is chosen, polypharmacy should be avoided, dose should be increased slowly, and serum anticonvulsant levels checked, especially if a further deterioration in behaviour is noted.

Management of psychoses presents particular difficulties especially if normalization of the EEG is associated with deterioration of behaviour. If the psychosis is directly related to epileptic activity, then of course a better control of the seizures is indicated. If not, then a balance between anticonvulsant drugs, major tranquillizers, fits and psychosis has to be aimed for. If the seizures are under good control, and the main problem is the psychosis, good effects can sometimes be achieved by lowering of the anticonvulsant dosage. ECT is not contra-indicated in this population, especially if the mood disturbance is paramount, and intramuscular phenothiazines may be useful in the management of long-term problems.

Other aspects of treatment

In addition to anticonvulsant drugs, a variety of other techniques have been employed in the management of epilepsy. Some of these, such as the ketogenic diet, were of value before drugs were widely used, but may still be useful in the occasional patient. Biofeedback has recently been introduced as a possible therapy in which the patient 'feeds back' to himself his EEG. It is claimed that by increasing the frequency of certain EEG patterns (12–14 c/s) the fits decline, although double-blind controlled trials have not yet been conducted. An older variant of a similar technique is conditioning, in which some patients have trained themselves by a variety of techniques to suppress their seizures.

Surgery may be contemplated, especially in cases of clearly focal epilepsy that is intractable with other forms of treatment. Of particular relevance is the operation of temporal lobectomy for unilateral temporal lobe epilepsy. Falconer et al.[446, 447] studied 100 patients who underwent temporal lobectomy, and noted improvement in seizures in 80% of them. Significant social adjustment was also noted, especially with an increased capacity to work, and improved interpersonal relationships. The best results were achieved in patients with mesial temporal sclerosis. Patients with psychosis were found to have more hamatomas on neuropathological examination, and did badly in spite of improvement in their seizure control. Post-operative depression and psychosis is a complication of surgery, and suicide a risk.

Other operative procedures used occasionally in epilepsy include hemispherectomy, section of the corpus callosum, cerebellar stimulation and the stereotactic placement of lesions in a number of sites within the limbic system, basal ganglia and connecting pathways.

Psychosocial aspects of the management of epilepsy have often been neglected. It is clear that the epileptic patient has a large number of difficulties to cope with, not the least having epileptic seizures. Although chronic and continuing, the burden of epilepsy often comes to the surface at certain times. Some of these are outlined in Table 9.11. The initial impact of making a diagnosis may be very severe, especially if a child is involved, and attention and care need to be directed both towards the patient and the parents. Some parents develop quite irrational beliefs about the cause of epilepsy in their child, which can be a great problem in future management.[448] Educational

Table 9.11. Events during which crises arise in epilepsy

1. Diagnosis
2. Education
3. Puberty
4. Occupation
5. Marriage
6. Parenthood
7. Death of parents

needs are of vital importance, and although the trend is towards educating more children within the established school system, for some, special schools will be required. Adolescence is frequently dogged by problems. Overprotective parents find their child's attempts to gain independence difficult to cope with, and support is required at these times often for the whole family. Compliance can become a major difficulty at this stage, and not being able to drive a car is a source of frustration for anyone, but for the adolescent, whose friends all can drive, it can be devastating.

Occupational abilities need to be assessed. Some jobs are not available for people with epilepsy, and many employers are not happy to employ epileptic patients. Referral to the Disablement Resettlement Officer or social worker or both will enable structured and organized help in this field, which avoids a source of continuing frustration and disappointment. Often patients have little idea of how to set about finding jobs themselves, and in particular are unaware of the training schemes that may be available. In patients who have a job, failure to do well at it is often related less to fits, and more to personality problems or psychiatric disability which may be amenable to treatment. Marriage and parenthood often raise again the patient's dependence–independence conflicts, but in addition brings further worries about rejection from the spouse on account of fits, or fear of passing on epilepsy to their children. Difficulties, including loss of libido, may need special counselling or therapy. At all times patients with epilepsy should have access to professional people who understand their difficulties and are willing to give them time in solving their problems. The relationship of stress to seizures may need clarification, and subtle changes in the patient's life-style that diminish stress may diminish seizures. Specialized psychotherapy is rarely indicated, but should be available if the situation demands it. Group psychotherapy, both of parents and of patients, is a successful alternative if it can be arranged. Hospital admission may be needed from time to time, particularly for acute crises, especially where overt psychiatric illness develops that cannot be managed alternatively. A vicious circle of increasing psychiatric disability, leading to increased fits, leading to increased psychiatric disability is well-known, and sometimes requires emergency admission. Particularly difficult cases may benefit from admission to a specialized centre, such as the Chalfont Centre for Epilepsy, for more long-term reassessment and rehabilitation.

SLEEP DISORDERS

A number of separate stages of sleep are now recognized, identifiable by their electroencephalographic patterns. Orthodox sleep, or non-rapid eye movement sleep (N-REM), is accompanied by slow waves with superimposed bursts of low-voltage 13–15 c/s activity, referred to as sleep spindles. Four stages are recognized, referred to as Stages I to IV, through which the drowsy subject proceeds to sleep. In Stage II, K-complexes (slow-wave transients) and spindles are seen on a background of low-voltage, mixed frequency EEG activity. In Stage III the background is even slower and in Stage IV high-amplitude, slow-wave activity dominates the recording. Stages III and IV, in which K-complexes and sleep spindles are seen, is sometimes referred to as slow-wave sleep or delta-wave sleep.

In paradoxical sleep (REM), there is a fast cortical E.E.G. activity similar to that seen in the waking state, associated with disappearance of muscular tone and the appearance of rapid eye movements. During a night's sleep the REM activity occurs in four to six periods lasting up to 30 minutes, approximately 90 minutes apart. The first one occurs about 90 minutes after the beginning of sleep, and the total REM time for an average adult is 20–25% of the total sleep. During REM sleep, heart rate, blood pressure, and respiration become variable, showing mean increases over the N-REM periods, and cerebral blood flow is increased. Dreaming is the subjective equivalent of REM sleep, and patients awoken during N-REM sleep often report that they are 'thinking'.

Deprivation of REM sleep leads to REM subsequently appearing at shorter intervals (REM pressure), and to REM rebound with increased amounts of REM activity on subsequent nights' sleep.[449] Jouvet has assembled arguments in favour of the two different types of sleep being regulated by separate mechanisms.[450] It is now thought that REM sleep is activated by pontine activity, since coagulation of the pontine reticular formation leads to disappearance of REM activity, whereas typical EEG patterns of wakefulness and slow-wave sleep persist. Coagulation studies also indicate that the locus coeruleus is involved. Destruction of the serotonin containing raphe nuclei leads to insomnia, and increasing serotonin synthesis promotes REM sleep.

Sleep disturbances are common in neuropsychiatric illnesses.[449] In depression there are longer waking periods, decreased slow-wave sleep and decreased total sleep time. Early morning waking is characteristic of certain forms of depression and in manic illness there is reduced sleep time, again with early morning waking. Improvement in the sleep pattern is usually associated with clinical improvement. In schizophrenia there is often delayed sleep onset, decreased REM time, decreased Stage IV sleep and a failure of REM rebound after experimental deprivation. Insomnia is common in anorexia nervosa. In organic brain syndromes sleep is disordered, especially with lesions of the midbrain or hypothalamus. Von Economo[451] suggested, on the basis of his observations, that lesions in the anterior hypothalamus were responsible for insomnia. Hypersomnia has been noted following hypothalamic, thalamic, mesencephalic, pontine and medullary lesions.[452] Metabolic abnormalities, and cranial irradiation are also known to produce disturbance of sleep patterns.

A number of psychotropic drugs influence sleep. Tricyclic antidepressants, particularly clomipramine (Anafranil), suppress REM sleep. Tryptophan (Pacitron) and reserpine increase it. Monoamine-oxidase inhibitors, especially phenelzine (Nardil) in larger doses, almost abolish REM sleep. Barbiturates and phenothiazines, atropine and amphetamines also reduce REM time. Although with some, such as the barbiturates, the REM time tends to recover after a few days on treatment, with others such as the MAOI drugs, REM suppression can continue for many months. Following withdrawal of drugs that suppress REM sleep, rebound is usually observed. In contrast to many of the psychotropic drugs, the benzodiazepines tend not to interfere with REM sleep.

Sleep-walking, most commonly seen in children, occurs in slow-wave sleep and presents as purposeless behaviour which may continue for up to 30 or 40 minutes, for which there is usually amnesia. Night terrors, which although commoner in children may occur in adults, usually are experienced early in the night in Stage III or IV sleep. In many cases they are accompanied by intense autonomic discharge and sometimes sleep-walking, and in children may last up to 20 minutes with only partial amnesia. In contrast nightmares occur during REM sleep, recall is usually vivid, and the accompanying autonomic changes are less.[449]

There are a number of primary sleep disorders described. *Gelineau's syndrome* comprises narcolepsy, cataplexy, sleep paralysis and hypnogogic or hypnopompic hallucinations. Narcolepsy is defined as brief but unavoidable attacks of sleep that occur during waking hours; in cataplexy attacks of loss of muscle tone and movement occur with laughing or strong emotion. Narcolepsy usually starts between the ages of 15 and 35 and may precede other symptoms of Gelineau's syndrome by a number of years. In some cases family members are affected, and the inheritance conforms to that of an autosomal dominant gene.[453] A similar picture has been described following several CNS disorders including multiple sclerosis, encephalitis, head injury, meningiomas, tumours of the third ventricle, and epilepsy.[454] The sleep periods last for about 15 minutes, although they may be prolonged, and after them patients awake feeling refreshed. The episode itself may consist of N-REM sleep, although in the presence of the other symptoms of Gelineau's syndrome, the sleep pattern of the narcoleptic attack is usually REM sleep. Nocturnal sleep in narcoleptic patients is also seen to be disturbed, with REM patterns occurring immediately on going to sleep. A quarter of patients have periods, lasing minutes or hours, of automatic behaviour, for which there is subsequent amnesia.

Narcolepsy alone, or the full complement of Gelineau's syndrome, is seen in only a small number of patients, the majority showing the combination of narcolepsy and cataplexy. The disorder is associated with considerable psychiatric morbidity. Pond,[455] in a study of eight cases, noted common character traits including narcissism, lack of energy and passivity. In all the married patients sexual maladjustment was obvious, especially premature ejaculation and frigidity. Smith[456] noted a number of cases in the literature in which paranoid psychoses developed, and described two further cases, one clearly schizophrenic. Sours[457] suggested that the personality of the narcoleptic patient was passive–aggressive, and a large number showed overt psychopathology. Ten of 75 patients studied developed 'frank schizophrenic reactions', three of whom were receiving dexedrine. More recently Roy[458] examined 20 patients clinically and with rating scales to assess their psychiatric status. Ten had a personal history of psychiatric abnormality, and eight had recognizable psychiatric illness at interview. One was depressive, one had a schizophreniform psychosis, and five had personality disorders and marital problems. Two of ten men, and all of the women, had sexual dysfunction, nine of the women being frigid for many years. The EPI scores, however, were within the normal range.

In view of such morbidity, and the known link between monoamines and both psychiatric disability and sleep disturbance, a number of investigators have tried to assess monoamine metabolism in narcoleptic patients. However, no consistent abnormality to-date has yet been detected. Parkes et al.[459] report diminished mean HVA in the CSF of their patients, but normal 5-HIAA, 5-HT, and tryptophan levels. CSF aspartate was also reported to be low, the interpretation of which was uncertain, but the low HVA was thought to be related to diminished locomotor activity.

Treatment is usually with amphetamine or methylphenidate (Ritalin). Clormipramine (Anafranil) and clonazepam (Rivotril) are helpful for the cataplexy and sleep paralysis, which usually do not respond to amphetamines.

In disorders characterized by hypersomnia there is excessive diurnal sleepiness, and the patient is not refreshed by short episodes of sleep. The *Kleine–Levin syndrome* has been fully documented by Critchley[460]. The characteristic features are recurrent hypersomnia and over-eating, which can last for days or even weeks. He described 11 cases and documented 15 others from the literature. Onset was between 10 and 44 years, and nearly all were males. Premorbid personality was said to be normal. Each attack occurred with a periodicity of approximately 6 months, the symptoms developing abruptly or gradually with mounting malaise, tiredness and headache. During attacks patients were irritable, showed unrest, were aggressive when disturbed, and appeared agitated and were hyperactive with fidgeting. Occasionally visual or auditory hallucinations were reported, and difficulty in thinking, disorientation, and incongruous speech were not uncommon. Feelings of depression and elation were also described. The over-eating was referred to as hyperphagia, in which patients ate food placed in front of them, rather than morbid hunger. During attacks, for which there may be partial or total amnesia, the EEG was variable showing mainly non-REM sleep, but between attacks the EEG was normal. A variant of this syndrome, not associated with megaphagia, has been reported to occur in association with menstruation.

During the hypersomnia there was an abnormal increase in the CSF 5-HIAA, suggesting altered neurotransmission.[461]

The *Pickwickian variant* of hypersomnia consists of frequent short episodes of spontaneous sleep with apnoea, hypercapnia, and obesity. The patient's night sleep pattern is interrupted by long apnoeic episodes terminated by irregular snorting. A similar disorder has been described in non-obese subjects with respiratory tract obstruction due to deformities. Clomipramine (Anafranil) may help some of these patients, although in severe case tracheostomy is indicated.[449]

Roth *et al.*[462] described *hypersomnia with sleep drunkenness*. Patients reported deep sleep, and difficulty in coming to complete wakefulness, accompanied by confusion, disorientation, poor motor co-ordination, slowness and repeated return to the sleep state. EEG changes were not characteristic. The majority of patients had diurnal hypersomnia, and there was a high incidence of headaches and migraine, depression, and neurotic symptoms in their patients.

Hypersomnia has also been described in epilepsy, drug intoxications, hypothyroidism and as a symptom of abnormal illness behaviour. Recurring drowsiness at puberty has been described in girls, and attributed to hysteria.[460]

CHAPTER 10

Movement Disorders

The relationship between movement disorders and psychiatric illness is an important one. First, psychiatric disorders are accompanied by some change in movement, which should form part of the clinical description. This varies from the more gross changes of catatonia, to the more subtle fine tremors of an anxiety state. Some disorders, in particular schizophrenia, are associated with a variety of abnormal movements which may lead to diagnostic confusion. Further understanding of the pathogenesis of the movement abnormalities may provide important information about the associated psychiatric disturbance.

Secondly, abnormal movements are noted in a number of patients following psychotropic drug therapy. These occur particularly with the antipsychotic major tranquillizers, but have also been described with some other drugs. Often unrecognized, they can be misdiagnosed as hysteria, or be mistaken for the worsening of psychiatric illness. When severe they can be disabling and distressing. Prevention and management of these complications of therapy is therefore important if it is at all possible.

Thirdly, there are a number of movement disorders which manifest initially, or during the course of their progress, some form of psychiatric illness. In particular the relationship between Parkinson's disease and its variants, and Huntington's chorea, to psychiatric illness are of great relevance, since recent understanding of abnormal neurochemical mechanisms in these conditions may provide insight into the development of the psychopathology. Certain neurotransmitters, in particular dopamine and GABA, seem to be of importance to both movement disorders and psychiatric illness. Clinical links between movement abnormalities and psychopathology are therefore of central importance in neuropsychiatry.

MOVEMENT DISORDERS IN PSYCHIATRIC PATIENTS

Griesinger commented: 'We observe, in most of the insane, slight inconsiderable disorders of muscular movement . . . .' (Ref. 4, p.104). He went on to describe a number of observations such as changes of voice tone, increased or decreased muscular activity, and rigidity. He continued: '. . . of far greater significance are . . . the persistent automatic grimacing, strabismus originating during the disease . . . painful convulsions of the muscles of the neck — those confused convulsive movements of the extremities which cause the patient often to walk irregularly or to progress in short leaps . . . their continuance usually indicates a transition to the state of incurability. A constant trembling, grinding of the teeth, chorea-like movements in adult lunatics, automatic circular movements, walking backwards, and likewise, at least in the majority of cases, symptoms of the development of serious organic disease of the brain: although in accordance . . . with certain observations . . . we must admit the possibility of the production of the phenomena from simple nervous irritation or from temporary palpable disease.'

At the time that he was writing, the classification schemes that we use today were not available, but his descriptions indicate the spectrum of movements recorded, and suggest that they were not necessarily only confined to patients that we would now recognize as having progressive neurological illness. Since his time, a number of other authors have commented on such movement disorders in psychiatric patients although accounts since the introduction of the major tranquillizers are open to obvious criticism. In depression, there is diminution of motor activity with vacant facial expression, diminished blinking and speech rate, and motionless, sometimes stiff, limbs. The angle of the mouth is drawn down, the muscles of the forehead are in constant contraction, and the eye gaze is down with diminished eye-to-eye contact. In stupor, the patient's activity is reduced to a minimum with, however, the ability to react to external stimuli. In agitated depression, restlessness is observed with increased central and peripheral movements, jerking of the limbs and trunk, repetitive, often stereotyped, movements of the hands, the fingers of which may, for example, pick at the skin or be clenched together, or clench the arm of a chair. If severe, pacing may occur with the stereotypy of a caged animal. In the manic phase of a bipolar illness there is continuous overactivity with increased speech rate, gesticulations, and increased extensor posture as opposed to the universal flexor posture of depression. Grinding of the teeth, tics, increased blinking and stereotypies are also observed. In anxiety, there is often the increased occurrence of semi-purposeful movements such as coughing, scratching, stroking, and throat clearing, and an increase in tics, blinking and tremor.

Several authors have commented on the abnormal movements of schizophrenia (Ref. 7, pp. 180–4, 400–11, Ref. 174, p.118, Ref. 463, pp.79, 126, Ref. 464, p.105). Kraepelin noted increased tendon reflexes, clonus, tremor, stiffness and rigidity. Muscular spasms and 'spasmodic phenomena in the musculature of the face and of speech, which often occur . . . some of them resemble movements of expression, wrinkling of the forehead, distortion of the corners of the mouth, irregular movements of the tongue and lips, twisting of the eyes, opening them wide and shutting them tight . . . grimacing . . . smacking and clicking of the tongue, sudden sighing, laughing and clearing of the throat . . . . We observe in the lip muscles fine lightening-like or rhythmical twitchings, which in no way bear the stamp of voluntary movements. The same is the case in the tremor of the muscles of the mouth . . . . Several patients continually carried out peculiar sprawling, irregular, choreiform, outspreading movements, which I think I can best characterize by the expression "athetoid ataxia".' Kraepelin also commented on the states of excitement which were encountered in some patients noting 'impulsive actions and senseless movements'. The latter involved rhythmic repetitive movements with the patients often assuming odd postures. Bleuler confirmed these observations and defined further the stereotypies noted in schizophrenia, such as: 'rubbing the right hand over the left thumb for decades; continuous rubbing with the right hand over the middle of the breast; running the finger along all edges; tapping with the foot'. Such stereotypies persisted for many years in some patients, and if they ran together, occupied a great deal of the patient's time. Kraepelin, along with Griesinger, considered the development of such movements as a bad prognostic sign. Both authors commented on the motor disturbances of catatonia which included severe forms of akinesia, stupor, flexibilitas cerea, the assumption of unusual postures and drooling, or alternatively hyperkinesis in which continuous overactivity, with the patient performing strange acts, occurred. The latter included mannerisms, stereotypies, negativism, automatic behaviour to command and impulsivity. The akinetic forms may suddenly give way to catatonic excitement. In catalepsy patients would hold strange postures for weeks or months at a time. The limbs became rigid, or were waxy and flexible, and would remain in positions in which they were placed for long periods. More rarely, if patients began to carry out actions they would repeat them, being unable to stop.

Other authors have drawn attention to 'dementia praecox parkinsonoides' — a rare form of schizophrenia — and have commented on the markedly severe motor disturbances that develop in patients with schizophrenia shortly before they die.[465] Jones and Hunter[466] in a study of 111 schizophrenic patients who had been admitted to hospital before 1946, classified the abnormal movements seen into four groups: tremor, choreoathetosis, tics, and stereotypies; 45 of their patients had never received any drugs, 40% of which were reported as having abnormal movements, all types of movements being represented. Jones[467] studied the stereotypies and mannerisms of 13 schizophrenic patients and recorded the list of movements as shown in Table 10.1. No relationship was noted between these and the length of hospitalization or length of the illness. They were diminished by concentration, and such acts as counting or writing. All but one of the patients in this study were receiving major tranquillizers and withdrawal of the drugs tended to increase these particular movements. They were unable to find any 'psychological meaningful' connection related to them.

Table 10.1. Stereotypies and mannerisms in schizophrenic patients

Repetitive movements of part or whole of the limb
Walking backwards and forwards
Rocking
Repetition of a purposeful act
Biting and other repetitive movements of the jaw
Picking
Fingering the self
Fingering other objects
Touching the self with the tongue
Rubbing the self or external objects
Facial grimacing
Smiling
Frowning
Facial expressions of fear or embarrassment
Looking or turning away
Sitting curled in a foetal position
Standing in a rigid posture

The association of such abnormal movements with schizophrenia has led to several suggestions regarding the pathophysiology of schizophrenia. Griesinger commented: 'In mental disease, this motory side of the soul-life and the musculo-motory function are both altered in the same morbid manner' (Ref. 4, p.43). Kleist originally suggested that cortical lesions were related to such phenomena but later, in the light of new discoveries regarding the basal ganglia, emphasized the sub-cortical apparatus, especially the striatum.[34] In particular, research and observations on patients with encephalitis lethargica brought about this change of viewpoint. Thus, similar motor disturbances to those discussed above were observed in patients suffering from this form of encephalitis. The disease, secondary to epidemic viral influenza, led to a variety of neuropsychiatric symptoms, some of which resembled schizophrenia. The associated motor phenomena are shown in Table 10.2. Also shown for comparison are the motor disorders mentioned in connection with schizophrenia, and the similarities noted. Since the characteristic neuropathological changes observed in encephalitis lethargica were in the basal ganglia and the tegmental area of the mesencephalon,[468] it was suggested that alterations of activity in these regions were related both to post-encephalitic states, and schizophrenia. More recent evidence to support the view that disturbances of the basal ganglia occur in schizophrenia comes from observations of motor disorders following treatment with antipsychotic drugs that are known to alter CNS dopamine activity in particular in the nigrostriatal and mesolimbic systems. The fact that psychopathology and motor symptoms seem both related to the activity of similar neurotransmitters, and that the areas of the brain thought to be involved appear to be anatomically related, provides neurophysiological support for the clinical observations, and leads to further understanding of mechanisms of expression and behaviour.

Table 10.2. Comparison of movement abnormalities in schizophrenia, encephalitis and following alteration of dopamine activity

	Schizophrenia	Encephalitis	Dopamine stimulation	Dopamine blockade
Echolalia, echopraxia	+	+	+	
Stereotypy	+	+	+	
Mannerisms	+	+		
Tics	+	+	+	+
Choreiform movements	+	+	+	+
Torticollis	+	+		+
Hyperkinesis	+	+	+	+
Akinesia	+	+		+
Athetosis	+	+	+	
Myoclonic jerks	+	+	+	
Increased salivation	+	+		+
Increased muscle tone	+	+		+
Masked face	+	+		+
Tremor	+	+		+
Catatonia	+	+		+
Waxy flexibility	+	+		+

MOVEMENT DISORDERS SECONDARY TO TREATMENTS OF PSYCHIATRIC ILLNESS

Shortly after the introduction of major tranquillizers for the management of psychosis, abnormalities of movement were noted. These, loosely described as 'extrapyramidal', have now been more clearly defined and classified, and fall into two major groups (see Table 10.3). The acute onset disorders include acute dystonias, akathisia, akinesia Parkinsonism and the 'rabbit syndrome'. The chronic ones are mainly tardive dyskinesia. The latter term was specifically introduced to refer to movement disorders secondary to drug treatment that were delayed in onset. In a comprehensive study of 3775 patients treated with major tranquillizers, Ayd noted extrapyramidal disorders in 39%:[469] 21.2% had akathisia, 15.4% Parkinsonism, and 2.3% dystonia. The latter occurred earlier than the akathisia, and the Parkinsonism appeared

Table 10.3. Extrapyramidal effects of psychotropic drugs

Acute	Chronic
Dystonia	Tardive dyskinesia
Akathisia	
Akinesia	
Parkinsonism	
Rabbit syndrome	

later. He commented on the close similarity of the clinical presentation of these disorders to those seen in non-drug-induced extrapyramidal disease.

Acute dystonia

This condition usually appears within a few hours of starting the offending drug, although the onset may be delayed up to two or three days. In 90% of cases the onset is within 4½ days. Typically, the movements are unco-ordinated and spasmodic and may involve the body, the limbs, the head and neck. The jaws may be clenched tightly together or facial grimacing occur. Retrocollis, torticollis, antecollis or opisthotonos may be seen. Rarer presentations include oculogyric crises, facial distortions with puffing of the cheeks and 'schnauzkramp', respiratory abnormalities with dyspnoea, and gait disturbances. Oculogyric crises may begin with a fixed stare which later proceeds to eye deviation. In one variant the eyes perform circling movements which may be associated with increased blinking. Characteristically, repeated spasms of muscles occur with hypertonicity between the attacks. The spasms themselves are distressing and painful. These disorders are commoner in males between 5 to 45 years of age, and in younger patients the trunk and the limb involvement is greater than in older patients. The onset of the symptoms can be violent and abrupt, and they are sometimes mistaken for epileptic seizures, tetanus, or even meningitis. Unless recognized as a complication of drug therapy they may be diagnosed as 'hysterical'.

It is estimated that acute dystonias occur in 2½–5% of patients following routine administration of these drugs, although some of the more potent neuroleptics produce a higher incidence than this. The disorder is seen following the majority of major tranquillizers but has also been noted following propranolol. It has never been reported following reserpine or related drugs.

Treatment involves administration orally, i.m., or i.v. of anticholinergic drugs such as benztropine (Cogentin) or orphenadrine (Disipal). Diazepam (Valium) will also produce a therapeutic response.

The occurrence of such a reaction to a major tranquillizer is not a contraindication to further therapy, but if re-started the drug should either be given at lower doses, or prescribed in combination with an anticholinergic drug.

The mechanism of the production of the dystonia is as yet unclear but is thought to be related to the increased dopamine turnover that has been shown to occur following the administration of dopamine-blocking drugs. This paradoxical situation is thought to be due to the post-synaptic blockade diminishing feedback inhibition of the pre-synaptic cell, leading to an increased output of dopamine. This occurs transiently and is associated with an increased CSF HVA. The increased production of dopamine then stimulates dopamine receptors that are not blocked by the action of the drug, and thus leads to the dystonia. Why there should be a population of receptors not blocked is unclear, although one suggestion is that there may be two different types of dopamine receptor, each population being differentially affected by dopamine-blocking drugs.

Akinesia

The commonest movement disorder following the administration of major tranquillizers is akinesia. It occurs approximately 4 to 24 hours following administration of the drug, and it is so common that it is seldom recognized. It may lead to diagnostic difficulties. Thus the patient's spontaneous movements are reduced with minimal facial expression and reduced volitional behaviour. The patient may complain of fatigue. On examination muscle tone is not increased and the patient is thought to be sedated, a clinical picture which may be mistaken for the apathy of depression or schizophrenia. It is helped by lowering the dose of the tranquillizer, or by adding anticholinergic drugs. In that it can be reversed by the administration of L-dopa, and resembles a similar clinical pattern seen in Parkinson's disease, it is thought to be related to reduced dopamine activity in the nigrostriatal neuronal system.

Akathisia

This phenomenon is usually seen in the age range of 12 to 65, and unlike dystonia is often less acute in onset. The incidence rises with increasing length of treatment, 90% of affected patients developing symptoms within 75 days of starting their drugs. It is commoner in females. It presents as motor hyper-activity with restlessness, shifting posture, inability to stay still or sit down for more than a few moments. Patients may shuffle their legs or tap their feet, and it may be associated with additional movements such as chewing, tongue-rolling or finger-twisting. They complain of a subjective sense of discomfort and associated feelings of tension. Resemblance to agitation may clinically lead to a mistaken diagnosis of agitated depression, especially if there is an accompanying akinesia. It occurs in some 20% of patients treated with major tranquillizers, but has also been reported following reserpine. Treatment is by reduction of the drug dose, or by administration of either anticholinergic drugs or a benzodiazepine, such as diazepam (Valium).

Similar clinical pictures were reported in patients with post-encephalitic disorders, and are noted following L-dopa therapy in Parkinson's disease. It is thus thought that this disorder is related to abnormalities of dopamine transmission within the basal ganglia, although to-date there is no direct evidence for this.

Parkinsonism

This presents with increased muscular tone, rigidity, increased salivation, gait and posture disturbances, and a picture which is clinically identical to the idiopathic variety of Parkinson's disease. Tremor occurs later in the picture, and is less common than rigidity and akinesia. The Parkinsonism comes on gradually, although prior to the overt development of the clinical picture patients may complain of weakness and joint pains, often in the limbs that later develop rigidity. It occurs in a wider age range than the other acute syndromes (15–80), and females are more affected than males. About 90% of patients who develop Parkinsonism do so within the first 75 days of treatment. In some series, up to 60% of patients have Parkinsonian symptoms, although mostly it remains mild, and an inverse relationship between the occurrence of Parkinsonism and tardive dyskinesia has been reported.[470] It is also noted following the administration of reserpine and related drugs.

Although it has been suggested that anticholinergic drugs will reduce the incidence of Parkinsonism in patients on major tranquillizers, and they may well be useful when the disorder is established, the use of routine prophylactic anticholinergic drugs to prevent the occurrence of Parkinsonism is not justified. Not only may they in some patients exacerbate the motor disorder, but may also induce a toxic psychosis. In addition, anticholinergic drugs reduce the therapeutic efficiency of the antipsychotic drugs, possibly by interference with the absorption of the latter from the gastrointestinal tract. Reduction of the dose of the major tranquillizer may alleviate the Parkinsonism, and while the latter is reversible, in some patients it is noted to linger on for several months following discontinuation of the drugs. If the Parkinsonism is not treated, and the patient is maintained on the same dose of drugs, there is a tendency for the Parkinsonism to resolve over a period of time.

Because of the close similarity to idiopathic and post-encephalitic Parkinson's disease, the production of this clinical picture is thought to reflect dopamine blockade of neurones in the nigrostriatal pathway. The observations of increased familial incidence of Parkinson's disease in patients who develop the drug-induced disorder is further evidence for this.

The relationship of the antipsychotic effects of the drugs to their ability to induce Parkinsonism has been investigated with variable results. Thus, all the antipsychotic drugs seem to produce these symptoms with the exception of sulpiride, thioridazine (Melleril) and clozapine. The reasons for these exceptions are unclear, although inherent anticholinergic activity or action on only specific types of dopamine receptor has been suggested. Earlier reports implied that production of Parkinsonism was necessary for the antipsychotic response to occur, although later studies, and the introduction of newer antipsychotic drugs that did not produce Parkinsonism, have not confirmed these observations.[471]

Treatment is either with reduction of the dose of the antipsychotic drug, or by changing to an alternative drug such as thioridazine (Melleril) which has lower incidence of extrapyramidal side effects. Administration of anti-Parkinsonian agents such as benztropine (Cogentin) or orphenadrine (Disipal) can be carried out, although is perhaps best avoided.

A variant of the clinical pattern, sometimes associated with Parkinsonian features, is called 'the rabbit syndrome'. Rapid chewing-like movements of the lips occur, that resemble a rabbit chewing. Although some authors categorize this syndrome with tardive dyskinesia, these movements do not involve the tongue, are reversible, and are alleviated by anticholinergic drugs and therefore do not clinically or biochemically resemble the tardive dyskinesia syndrome.

Subacute syndromes

Although the akathisia and Parkinsonism referred to above often arise subacutely, a number of unusual motor disorders may be seen with these drugs that do not clearly fall into the existing classifications. Breugel's syndrome (see below) may occur and be confused with tardive dyskinesia or hysterical disorders. Catatonic reactions are also described with posturing, waxy flexibility, withdrawal, mutism and associated Parkinsonism. This may be misinterpreted as an exacerbation of, for example, an underlying schizophrenia, and lead to increased prescription of major tranquillizers. However, withdrawal of the medications in these cases will lead to a gradual disappearance of the symptoms.[472]

Tardive dyskinesia

This is a chronic disorder which occurs secondary to the administration of major tranquillizers, although similar clinical pictures occur in elderly patients who have not been on these drugs. Rarely, it has been reported in association with antihistamines, anticholinergic drugs, phenytoin, L-dopa, and the tricyclic antidepressants. Some of the main differences between the acute and chronic movement disorders related to drugs are shown in Table 10.4. Tardive dyskinesia usually occurs after at least 3 months' therapy, and its appearance is gradual. Often the first movements noted are following reduction in drug dosage. The characteristic feature is persistant abnormal muscular activity, which predominantly affects the tongue and peri-oral region. Typically, there is smacking of the lips, masticatory jaw movements and protrusion of the tongue, either singly or in combination, and there are often abnormal associated choreiform or athetoid movements in the limbs and occasionally the trunk. Blepharospasm, blinking, tics and brief eye deviations, hypo- or hypersalivation and laryngeal spasms are also noted.[473] More rarely, to-and-fro clonic movements of the spine in an anterior–posterior direction are seen, which occasionally are the only manifestations of the condition. In the early stages of the disorder the movements may be subtle, and only noted if, for example, the patient is asked to hold his mouth open, when abnormal tongue movements may be observed. There is difficulty in keeping the tongue protruded for more than a few seconds and continuous rhythmic movements

Table 10.4. Some differences between acute and chronic syndromes

Acute	Chronic
Cause distress	No distress (usually)
Reversible	Mainly irreversible
Respond to anticholinergic drugs	Worse with antiparkinsonian drugs
Improve with decrease dose of major tranquillizer	Worse with decrease of major tranquillizer
Age 5–80	Usually older than 30

of the tongue while it rests inside the mouth. Patients often dismiss mildly abnormal jaw movements as due to 'denture difficulty'.

In one study of patients in a geriatric nursing home, 2% of the patients not receiving major tranquillizers had such movement disorders, compared with nearly 40% of those being treated.[474] In a population of younger psychiatric patients receiving minimal exposure to major tranquillizers, there was no dyskinesia, compared with 16% in a heavily medicated age- and sex-matched population.[475] The disorder is reported more commonly in females, and there seems little doubt that the elderly are more susceptible than the young. The pattern of abnormalities is different in different age groups with a tendency for the peri-oral distribution to occur with advancing age. In younger patients the extremities are more often involved, with trunk involvement, strange postures and even ballistic movements leading to gait disturbances, rocking and rotatory pelvic motions. In children, a syndrome of choreiform movements similar to Huntington's chorea has been recorded associated with myoclonic jerks, posturing, and rocking movements of the body and head.[476]

Generally, in contrast to the acute disorders, these chronic movement disorders do not provoke distress. However, if severe they may lead to interference with eating, speaking and occasionally respiration; in younger patients particularly the posture and gait abnormalities may be severely disabling.

Unlike the acute syndromes, tardive dyskinesia does not improve with stopping the medication, and is made worse by this or by anticholinergic drugs. Although it is generally considered to be irreversible, this is probably not the case, and a gradual reduction in symptoms occurs in some patients over a number of months.

Clinically, these movements need to be distinguished from other varieties of drug-induced movement disorders discussed above. It is the time relationship to the drug intake, the lack of subjective distress and the clinical picture, in particular with the writhing, chewing movements and associated tongue abnormalities, that suggest the appropriate diagnosis. They also have to be distinguished from movement disorders associated with schizophrenia, and from similar pictures with a bucco-linguo-masticatory presentation seen in elderly patients not taking neuroleptic drugs. In these patients, the disorders may reflect some underlying neurological abnormality such as cerebral atrophy or arteriosclerosis. Other disorders in the differential diagnosis include post-encephalitic states, variants of torsion dystonia Breugel's syndrome, the Gilles de la Tourette syndrome, Wilson's disease and Huntington's chorea. The latter in particular may present with a similar clinical pattern, although usually there is less involvement of the peri-oral region with more involvement of the trunk and the extremeties.

The mechanism of the production of tardive dyskinesia is not clarified. Several authors have drawn attention to the relationship between underlying neurological disease and dyskinesia, suggesting that it may not occur in the absence of structural neuropathology. However, more recent studies have questioned this assumption.[477, 478] There does not seem to be a relationship to pre-existing movement disorders of schizophrenia, nor is tardive dyskinesia confined to populations with schizophrenia and is also seen in other groups, for example neurotic patients who receive these drugs. All of the phenothiazines, and the majority of the butyrophenones, have been implicated, with the exception to-date of pimozide (Orap). No consistent CSF abnormalities or neuropathological changes at post mortem have been described,[473] although several reports of microscopic changes in the substantia nigra have appeared.[479, 480] In that the disorder is seen mainly in association with dopamine-blocking drugs, and especially when the dose of the drug is reduced, it has been suggested that dopamine receptor supersensitivity is implicated. This is supported by observations that similar movements are seen following L-dopa therapy in Parkinson's disease and that L-dopa itself exacerbates the movements of tardive dyskinesia.[481] Unlike the situation with the acute dystonias, where increased turnover of dopamine is held responsible, here denervation receptor supersensitivity is thought the most likely explanation. Animal experiments have shown that destruction of the nigrostriatal neurones can lead to increased responsiveness in caudate neurones to dopamine agonists, and animal models of movement disorders, some of which are similar to tardive dyskinesia, have been developed by destruction of dopamine neurones with 6-hydroxydopamine and subsequent injection of dopamine agonists.[482] Whether such supersensitivity is associated with microstructural changes at the synapse which leads to irreversibility is unknown.

A large number of drugs have been used to treat tardive dyskinesia with variable success. Most studies have been carried out for a few weeks only, and in many cases they represent anecdotes or open studies (see Table 10.5). These drugs have mainly been used in an attempt to alter neuronal transmitter activity, in particular of dopamine and acetylcholine. Drugs that reduce dopamine by depletion, such as reserpine and tetrabenazine, often produce dramatic changes in the clinical picture, but also induce depression and Parkinsonism. However, development of the latter is not invariable, suggesting that the therapeutic effect is not simply due to the production of rigidity.[483] The major tranquillizers themselves will suppress the dyskinesia, and increasing the dose of existing regimes often leads to reduction of movements. Butyrophenones, in particular pimozide (Orap), have also been

Table 10.5. Drugs used in the treatment of tardive dyskinesia

Main neurotransmitter system	Drug
Dopamine	Phenothiazines
	Reserpine
	Tetrabenazine (Nitoman)
	Methyldopa (Aldomet)
	Thiopropazate (Dartalan)
	Haloperidol (Haldol), Pimozide (Orap), Clozapine (Loxapine)
	α-Methylparatyrosine
Acetylcholine	Neostigmine
	Physostigmine
	Dimethylaminoethanol (Deanol)
	Choline
	Lecithin
Serotonin	Cyproheptadine (Periactin)
GABA	Sodium valproate (Epilim)
	Baclofen (Lioresal)
OTHERS	Lithium
	L-Tryptophan
	Sodium Valporate (Epilim)

effectively used, although it is unclear how long such an effect lasts, and breakthrough may be expected after a number of months or even years.

Anticholinergic drugs usually exacerbate the dyskinesia, and so cholinergic agents, in particular physostigmine (Eserine), dimethylaminoethanol (Deanol), choline, and lecithin have all been used, but none have been consistently active in abolishing movements. Other drugs tried include lithium, minor tranquillizers, tryptophan and sodium valproate (Epilim). Prior to initiating therapy for tardive dyskinesia it is important to assess how far advanced and how disabling the condition really is. If it is in the early stages, then withdrawal of the major tranquillizers, if clinically possible, is better than adding other medications, and in all probability reversal of the dyskinesia will occur. If well-established, then treatment will be required only if the condition is disabling to the patient either socially or mechanically. In that the major tranquillizers are the drugs thought responsible for the disorder in the first place, use of similar drugs in management may seem illogical, and other drugs are to be preferred. In many cases a combination of the reduction of the dose of major tranquillizer and the addition of a small dose of reserpine has been recommended.[484] Gibson[485] has recently indicated that when patients are receiving intramuscular depot therapies, halving the dose leads to an initial worsening of the movements which is later followed by remission in some patients, although subsequent relapse may occur. In very severe cases, stereotactic surgery may be indicated and partial relief of symptoms has been reported following lesions in the region of the red nucleus.[486]

NEUROPSYCHIATRIC ASPECTS OF MOVEMENT DISORDERS

Parkinson's disease

Although descriptions of similar disorders existed prior to 1817, it was James Parkinson who clearly delineated this disorder of 'involuntary tremulous motion with lessened muscular power . . . with a propensity to bend the trunk foward and to pass from a walking to a running pace: the senses and intellects being uninjured.' (Ref. 487, p.1). Since this description a large number of neurological deficits have now been associated with the disorder, impairment of the 'senses and intellects' have been described, and specific therapies have been defined.

Parkinson's disease is a common disorder which slowly develops, starting usually in the 40 to 50 age range. As such, it is 'idiopathic', although secondary Parkinsonism is seen following arteriosclerotic disease, head injuries, encephalitis, and more rarely tumours, syphilis, manganese poisoning and carbon monoxide toxicity. Drug-induced Parkinsonism is extremely common and has been discussed above.

The main neurological features are outlined in Table 10.6. In post-encelphalitic patients the age of onset is usually younger, and there is more associated psychiatric disability, a higher incidence of autonomic disturbance, a greater tendency to oculogyric crises and a more greasy skin. The tremor of Parkinson's disease is classically a 4–8 cycles per second movement which is maximal at rest and increased by excitement or anxiety. It may involve any of the limbs or the head, jaw and tongue, and ceases during sleep. The muscular over-activity, leading to increased tone in agonists and antagonists, results in the characteristic 'lead-pipe rigidity' which, if there is associated tremor, produces 'cog-wheel rigidity'. Posture is one of flexion, with a festinant gait and an inability to control the centre of gravity which may lead to antero- or retropulsion.

Psychiatric symptoms

In contradiction to Parkinson's original statement, psychiatric disability has now been clearly defined in this disorder, although early concepts of specific personality types in such patients have now been discarded. Psychiatric disturbances have been noted in up to 90% of patients and these include depression, obsessional symptoms, psychoses, and changes in cognitive function.

Depression is reported to occur in 30–60% of patients.[488, 489] Robins[490] compared 45 patients with Parkinson's disease, not on L-dopa, with 45 age- and sex-matched chronically physically disabled patients using the Hamilton

Table 10.6. Some neurological characteristics of Parkinson's disease

---

Muscular rigidity
Mask-like faces
Tremor
Characteristic gait and posture
Hypokinesia
Slow monotonous speech
Palilalia
Salivation
Positive Glabellar tap
Blepharospasm, oculogyric crises, diminished blinking
Dysarthria
Impaired ocular convergence
Absence of associated movements on walking
Increased width of the palpebral fissure
Dysphagia
Low vital capacity
Seborrhoea
Orthostatic hypotension
Aches, pains and discomfort
Urinary abnormalities

Rating Scale. The Parkinson's disease patients had significantly higher depression scores, especially on items of suicide, work and interest, retardation, anxiety, somatic symptoms and loss of insight. In this study the physical disability of the studied patients did not correlate with the depression score. Mindham[491] in a study of 50 patients attending a neurological clinic noted 48% with affective symptoms, but in his study these did correlate with the severity of the disease. The relationship between the affective symptoms and the physical symptoms persisted during treatment, and patients showing improvement in the latter showed a decline in their depressive symptomatology.

In contrast to depression, manic-depressive psychoses and schizophreniform psychosis are held to be rare in Parkinson's disease. Apart from a recent report in which four cases of schizophrenia-like symptoms were reported to coexist with Parkinson's disease,[492] most authors can cite only single cases, or psychoses that developed in association with encephalitis, dementia, or secondary to anticholinergic or L-dopa therapy.

Cognitive deficit, which in its most severe form presents as dementia, is now also recognized in Parkinson's disease. Since neurosurgical ablation of the basal ganglia leads to deterioration, often transient, of psychometric performance,[493] and lesions of the striatonigral pathway result in impaired cognitive abilities,[21] it is likely that some of the abnormalities of sensory-motor co-ordination which are seen in Parkinson's disease are a reflection of basal ganglia disturbances. The hypokinesia presents as slowness in the initiation of movements and response to commands, not entirely dependent on muscular rigidity. Assessing the actual incidence of dementia is very difficult. Patients with diffuse cerebrovascular disease who have Parkinsonism will usually have a degree of dementia and some of these patients have been included in series of Parkinson's disease. Estimates, however, must be based on patients with clearly delineated idiopathic Parkinsonism. Distinction in life can be difficult and this, plus the lack of objective psychometric testing in many series, probably accounts for the large discrepancies reported. However, some irreversible decline in cognitive function has been reported in up to one-third of hospital patients with Parkinson's disease,[491] a higher incidence than in matched control samples. In one study of idiopathic Parkinsonism, 40% incidence of dementia was found and the degree of dementia was related to the severity and duration of the illness.[494] In contrast to some negative studies,[495] Loranger[496] in a study of 63 patients prior to L-dopa therapy noted verbal-performance discrepancies on the WAIS which were not explained by associated depression, motor disability, drugs, or surgery; 40 patients were re-examined 5 to 13 months after L-dopa therapy, and half of them had improvements in their I.Q. scores by 10 points or more. Again this was unrelated to physical improvement. Riklan[497, 498] also noted a variety of intellectual, cognitive and perceptual test deficits in Parkinson's disease which, while associated with the severity of the disease, were more related to the 'akinesia' than the rigidity. He confirmed that increases in arousal and activation occurred in patients on L-dopa therapy, and that these were associated with an improvement on psychological testing.

Differential diagnosis and variants

The picture of Parkinson's disease when established is almost unmistakeable. However, early recognition may be difficult, especially if presentation is without tremor and with mild non-specific complaints of muscle aches, pains, and stiffness. Presentation as an affective disorder is not uncommon, and the early clinical picture with hypokinesia may lead to a mistaken diagnosis of depression. *Benign essential tremor* may give rise to confusion. In this disorder there is often a positive family history, and it usually starts at an earlier age than Parkinsonism. The tremor does not subside with intention, there is no associated rigidity or posture change, and often patients suggest it responds to alcohol.

The association of Parkinsonism with severe autonomic insufficiency is referred to as the *Shy-Drager syndrome*. These patients develop severe orthostatic hypotension in association with impotence, incontinence, and anhidrosis.[499]

Progressive supranuclear palsy (the Steele–Richardson syndrome)[500] is characterized by Parkinsonism, which affects particularly the neck and trunk muscles, and is associated with dysarthria, dysphagia and paralysis of upward gaze. Lateral conjugate gaze later becomes affected. This disorder is associated with a dementia which has distinctive features, referred to as a subcortical dementia (see Chapter 7).

Other disorders which should be considered in the differential diagnosis include hepatolenticular degeneration (Wilson's disease), Huntington's chorea, the Creutzfeldt–Jacob disease, post-traumatic states, and post-anoxic syndromes.

Pathogenesis

There is no doubt now that the main neuropathological findings in Parkinson's disease reside in the basal ganglia. In particular, there is loss of pigmentation in the substantia nigra, with evidence of neuronal loss on microscopic examination. It is thought that the nigrostriatal pathway, predominantly inhibitory and dopaminergic, is damaged, leading to increased striatal activity. The normally high concentration of dopamine in the striatum is reduced in Parkinson's disease, and this deficit was thought to be the final cause in the production of the disorder. However, these ideas, while leading to the establishment of L-dopa therapy, have become increasingly criticized, in particular because other neurotransmitter abnormalities are now established in association with the disorder. Since anticholinergic drugs alleviate Parkinsonian symptoms, and there are high concentrations of acetylcholine in the striatum, it has been suggested that there is a balance between cholinergic and dopaminergic activity in the maintenance of motor behaviour. Other neurotransmitters and enzymes found to be abnormal in post-mortem studies include noradrenaline, serotonin, and glutamic acid decarboxylase.[501] It is clear that while dopamine plays an important role, it is not entirely responsible for the resultant clinical picture.[502]

Treatments

Prior to the introduction of L-dopa, the main therapies available were anticholinergic medication and neurosurgery. Charcot suggested atropine, and a number of related compounds are still used, including benzhexol (Artane), procyclidine (Kemadrin), orphenadrine (Disipal) and benztropine (Cogentin). These have most effect on the rigidity and little or no effect on tremor. L-dopa is now usually given in association with a decarboxylase inhibitor. Thus, L-dopa is systemically converted into dopamine and other catecholamines by the enzyme, dopa-decarboxylase. This results in unpleasant side-effects, and lowers the level of L-dopa available to enter the central nervous system. Peripheral blockade of the decarboxylase enzymes by an inhibitor, which itself does not cross the blood–brain barrier, means that the somatic side-effects are diminished, and more L-dopa is available to act centrally. Combinations of L-dopa and decarboxylase inhibitor that are available include Madopar and Sinemet. The main effects of this treatment are on the hypokinesia and rigidity. L-dopa itself has a half life of 3–4 hours, and there is considerable variability in the response of patients to the drug. In particular, patients with post-encephalitic disease may respond at lower doses than other patients, and side-effects may be severe. It is customary to increase the dose slowly and to obtain a balance between therapeutic response and side-effects. These medications are often used in combination with one or more of the other anti-Parkinsonian drugs, and it is thought that maximum benefit may sometimes not occur for up to 2 years after the start of therapy. Amantadine (Symmetrel) has also been used for treatment. It has fewer side-effects and produces improvement in most symptoms of the disease. The effect, however, is often short-lived. More recently bromocriptine (Parlodel), a dopamine receptor agonist, has been shown to be effective, especially in patients unable to tolerate L-dopa, and may be used in combination with the latter drug. The MAOI-β-enzyme inhibitor, deprenyl, may also be used with L-dopa in treatment.[503]

The on–off phenomenon refers to swings in response to L-dopa that may occur several times a day, often suddenly, in which the patient is disabled. It usually starts from 1 to 3 years after the initiation of L-dopa therapy and occurs in up to 40% of patients treated.[504] There are some suggestions that this disabling phenomenon is helped by bromocriptine (Parlodel) and deprenyl.

Stereotactic surgery is much less used now than it was previously. Operations were mainly aimed at the thalamus and globus pallidus, and the effect on tremor was often dramatic. Rigidity was also reduced but morbidity was high, particularly after bilateral operations, and included speech disorders, intellectual deterioration and emotional instability.

Side-effects of the drug treatment of Parkinson's disease are very common. The anticholinergic drugs produce nausea, dry mouth, blurred vision, and an acute organic brain syndrome with hallucinations and delusions. Amantadine may cause livedo reticularis, oedema and seizures. Of major interest, however, has been the side-effects of L-dopa therapy. In addition to nausea and other gastrointestinal symptoms, it produces abnormal movements including choreoathetotic movements, tics, akathisia and restlessness, dystonias and dyskinesias. Elation, depression, delusions, hallucinations and schizophreniform states in the setting of clear consciousness have also been reported, in addition to toxic organic brain syndromes. Mindham *et al.*[505] followed patients on L-dopa therapy for 6 months and found that 55% of them at some time became clinically depressed. Half of these patients had a history of prior affective illness. A control group who received other treatments, such as anticholinergic drugs, had much less in the way of psychiatric disability. They concluded that affective disorders are particularly common following L-dopa therapy, especially in patients with a history of depressive illness. In contrast to these clear results, others have reported significant reductions of depressive symptoms with L-dopa.[506]

Bromocriptine (Parlodel) is very prone to produce toxic side-effects, including nausea, vomiting, dizziness, fatigue, lethargy, and in particular organic brain syndromes with hallucinations and delusions. Psychiatric disturbances are said to be more frequent than with L-dopa, and as with the latter, an increase in abnormal movements is also noted. More unusual are reports of increased redness and temperature of the skin.

Treatment of the neuropsychiatric side-effects themselves can be difficult and require reduction of the anti-Parkinsonian drugs, and associated administration of psychotropic drugs or ECT. The antidepressant nomifensine (Merital), with its inherent dopamine agonist activity, may be particularly useful for the depression, and of the major tranquillizers, thioridazine (Melleril) may least exacerbate the underlying Parkinson's disease. A course of ECT will often benefit the affective disturbance as well as bring about improvement of the motor disability.

Huntington's chorea

Huntington's original description of this disorder placed emphasis on its hereditary nature, its onset in adult life, and the tendency to insanity and suicide that occurred with it.[507] It is now known to be inherited as a Mendelian dominant disorder with almost complete penetrance. It occurs world-wide with a prevalence of 4–7 per 100 000 and affects both sexes equally, although there seems to be a predominance of patrilinear descent. The average age of onset is between 35 and 42, although presentation in childhood is not uncommon, occurring in 10–20% of cases.[508] Clinically it is characterized by abnormal choreiform movements, although early movements may resemble restlessness and fidgetiness. Many patients show tics, facial dyskinesias, lip-pouting, and tongue protrusion. Often the first movements are orofacial or in the hands and neck, but as the disease progresses the limbs and trunk become more involved. Rigidity may occur and finally gross movements are seen leading to ataxia, loss of balance, and confinement to chair or bed. The movements are made worse by anxiety, can be controlled for a time by effort, and are lessened in sleep, although in some patients the movements continue throughout the night, a feature almost unique to this disorder. Speech may be affected and the facial expression eventually comes to resemble that of vacuous apathy.

The psychiatric disturbances recorded with Huntington's chorea are listed in Table 10.7. While in the majority of cases these occur after the onset of the chorea, in about one-third the reverse is the case. The early symptoms include irritability, emotional lability and increased excitability. Relatives complain that patients are more and more difficult to live with and personality changes are noted, including irresponsible and often promiscuous behaviour, untidiness, inefficiency at work, and loss of interest in the home or family life.[508] Alcoholism is also frequently commented on.

The depression in Huntington's chorea is characterized by psychotic features, particularly with persecutory delusions, and unipolar depressive swings are often recorded prior to the onset of the choreiform movements. A high frequency of suicide or attempted suicide has been reported, in some patients even before they have knowledge that they or someone in their family has Huntington's chorea.[509]

Table 10.7. Psychopathology of Huntington's chorea[508-15]

Study		Origin	Sample size	Schizophrenia	Paranoid states	Depressive states	Manic states	Dementia
Brothers	1964	Tasmania	155	20 (12.9)	15 (9.7)	13 (8.9)	4 (2.6)	103 (66.5)
McHugh	1975	USA	8	2 (25.0)	— (—)	5 (62.5)	2 (25.0)	8 (100)
Dewhurst	1969	UK	92	7 (7.6)	— (—)	42 (45.6)	2 (2.2)	83 (90.2)
James et al.	1969*	USA	18	5 (27.7)	1 (5.5)	2 (11.1)	— (—)	— (—)
Oliver	1970*	UK	100	12 (12.0)	— (—)	35 (35.0)	— (—)	15 (15.0)
Minski	1938	UK	66	4 (6.1)	3 (4.5)	11 (16.7)	1 (1.5)	42 (63.6)
Heathfield	1967	UK	80	9 (11.2)	5 (6.3)	10 (12.5)	4 (5.0)	78 (97.5)
Bolt	1970	UK	334	8 (2.4)	50 (15.0)	28 (8.4)	2 (0.6)	234 (70.0)
TOTAL			853	67 (7.9)	74 (8.6)	146 (17.1)	15 (1.7)	563 (66.0)

* Early signs

The relationship to schizophrenia is important but not well-documented. Table 10.7, taken from studies conducted throughout the Western world, indicates the percentage of psychopathology in populations of patients with Huntington's chorea.[508-15] Psychotic states, in particular schizophrenia, occur with a frequency of 16.5%. Dewhurst and Oliver[511] reported the presenting features on admission to a mental hospital of over 100 patients with Huntington's chorea: 50% of their sample first presented with a psychiatric syndrome, and of 92 who received a psychiatric diagnosis, 8% were diagnosed as schizophrenic, and 15% were having hallucinations of which the majority were auditory. Brothers[508] reported that schizophrenia was the most common psychiatric reaction to occur prior to the onset of chorea, and that the hebephrenic variety was commoner than the paranoid. A number of his series were admitted to hospital with a diagnosis of schizophrenia, some several years before the onset of the chorea. In only two of the cases was schizophrenia also present in the family. Bolt[510] reported paranoid delusions in 33% of patients. In one patient who had psychosis preceding chorea, the interval before the appearance of the latter was 19 years. A total of eight patients had illnesses resembling hebephrenic or simple schizophrenia, and there was no evidence that this psychosis was present in the families of the patients. Her conclusion was that: 'It is improbable that a relatively high proportion of patients suffering from Huntington's chorea should by chance also suffer from one of the functional psychoses'.

The most frequent psychiatric disorder present is dementia, and some 50–70% of patients show signs shortly after the chorea is manifest. Gradual development of dementia eventually occurs in almost all cases, although single case studies do suggest that it can be absent, this being a familial trait. The dementia itself varies considerably from case to case in respect of the rate of progress, the stage of the disease in which it becomes apparent, and the severity. There does not seem to be a relationship between the severity of the chorea and the degree of dementia. Memory difficulties often appear first, followed by a loss of judgement and insight. Although some authors suggest that the dementia has no particular features that distinguish it from other presenile dementias, there is now growing evidence that the pattern is different from the more typical 'cortical' dementias such as Alzheimer's disease. Aminoff et al.[516] studied 11 patients, using sub-tests of the WAIS and memory tests, and while all their patients showed intellectual deterioration, the pattern was similar to that occurring normally with age. No selective immediate memory impairment was recorded, and they commented on the difference between their findings and the pattern of intellectual change commonly seen in presenile dementias. McHugh and Folstein[514] carried out a detailed study of eight patients all of whom suffered from some degree of dementia. They reported early changes in the capacity of patients to think about problems either at home or at work, and that problem-solving became more difficult. Later, a decline in performance scores on the WAIS became apparent, and a verbal-performance deficit appeared. At this stage memory difficulties were reported. Patients were often orientated for time and place, but performed badly tasks that required attention and concentration, for example 'Serial Sevens'. They were unable to repeat parts of well-known stories or to do carry-over subtractions. In particular, they commented on several aspects of cognitive function that were specifically spared in Huntington's chorea. Thus, the Huntington's patients did not develop aphasia, neglect, cortical blindness, alexia, apraxia and agnosia, which are common, for example, in Alzheimer's disease. The memory deficit was not typical of that seen in Korsakoff's syndrome. They commented in particular on the appearance of the severe apathetic state of patients, which affected their intellectual performance, giving to an observer the appearance of a much worse decline in abilities in their daily affairs than would be thought likely from formal intellectual testing. In the late stages, their patients showed a marked progression of this apathy to complete inertia, resembling the picture of akinetic mutism. They suggested that this pattern of dementia resembled subcortical dementia. Caine et al.[517] have recently reported on the cognitive abilities of 18 patients with Huntington's chorea using the WAIS, a specific parietal lobe test battery, and projection tests. They found an inability to plan, organize, sequence and recall factual material, and suggested that patients lose their finely detailed memories of things. Patients were often overwhelmed by too much information, requesting a slower presentation of the data. Although some deficits in performance were noted on the parietal lobe battery, in particular errors in stick figure and block figure construction, other aspects of this battery were unimpaired. They suggested that this pattern of abnormality was very similar to that seen in patients with frontal lobe syndromes, with loss of 'cortical executive function'.

Variants and differential diagnosis

Some 5% of patients with Huntington's chorea present as the juvenile type with marked rigidity, cerebellar ataxia, dystonic posturing, abnormal eye movements, and an increased incidence of epilepsy. In these patients there is a relative absence of choreiform movements. The Westphal variant refers to an adult form with rigidity and hypokinesia.

The differential diagnosis includes Sydenham's chorea, Wilson's disease, and other choreiform disorders, in particular movement disorders secondary to major tranquillizer therapy. Tardive dyskinesia clinically may resemble Huntington's chorea in its early stages, and diagnostic difficulty is even greater in that some patients with Huntington's chorea would have been given major tranquillizers for their behaviour disorders. Diagnosis is usually based on a careful history, familial incidence, and additional techniques such as electroencephalography, where low-voltage waves are often reported, and CT scanning, which shows destruction of the basal ganglia associated with atrophy.

Pathology

It has been known for a number of years that the major macroscopic changes in Huntington's chorea occur in the corpus striatum, although ventricular dilatation and cortical atrophy also occur. Atrophy is marked in the caudate and putamen, which are usually reduced to half of their normal size.

Recently, attention has been focused on biochemical changes that occur in this disorder. As with Parkinson's disease, it was initially thought that dopamine might be involved, especially since the movements are diminished by dopamine–blocking drugs. Although the overall concentration of brain dopamine appears to be normal in choreic brains, the CSF HVA concentration is low.[518] The atrophy present means there is a decrease of some 50% in the total dopamine content of the striatum, although relative to other neurotransmitters dopamine actually is in excess. Recent work has shown that in the substantia nigra, caudate, putamen and globus pallidus there is a decrease of the enzyme glutamic acid decarboxylase (GAD), and GABA. Deficits in the cholinergic system have also recently been recorded, although the significance of this, and the relationship to the GABA abnormality is not understood.[519]

Treatment and prevention

To-date there are no specific treatments for Huntington's chorea. The abnormal neurotransmitter abnormalities described have given some hope that replacement therapy may be available as has been the case for Parkinson's disease. However, to-date all treatments that influence GABA mechanisms, such as Baclofen (lioresal) or sodium valproate (Epilim) have been unhelpful. Other treatments tried include dimethylaminoethanol (Deanol) and physostigmine (Eserine), which influence cholinergic activity. It is known that the chorea can be controlled to some extent using tetrabenazine (Nitoman), the phenothiazines, and butyrophenones. Where indicated, treatment for psychiatric disorders, such as antidepressants, minor tranquillizers and ECT, should be initiated.

Genetic counselling is very important, and information can be made available to families through the 'Association to Combat Huntington's Chorea'. Relatives of established patients require a considerable degree of support, not only on account of the changed behaviour of one member of their family, but also because of the possible development of the disease in themselves. A number of possible mechanisms for predicting the later development of the disease have been suggested, including the induction of abnormal movements by a challenge with L-dopa, electroencephalographic abnormalities, abnormal fibroblast growth in tissue culture, abnormal neuro-otological and neuro-ophthalmological testing, and thumb opposition tests, although the predictive value of these is as yet unknown. The only follow-up studies pertain to the electroencephalographic data which were collected in 1948. The predictions were correct in less than 50% of the cases, and clinically this is of no value.[520, 521]

Hepato-lenticular degeneration (Wilson's disease)

This disorder was first delineated by Kinnier Wilson. The characteristic features he described were 'generalized tremor, dysarthria and dysphagia, muscular rigidity and hypertonicity, emaciation, spasmodic contractions, emotionalism.'[522] In addition, the associated liver cirrhosis is now well-defined, and is present to a variable extent dependent on the age of presentation. Wilson's disease is inherited as an autosomal recessive trait, the median age of onset being around 12 years old. Before 10 the presentation is predominantly hepatic with jaundice, malaise, weight loss, etc., whereas after it is mainly neurological.[523]

The neurological presentation initially is with fine tremor of the hands, exacerbated by excitement and relieved by relaxation. Unlike other extrapyramidal tremors, it is increased by movement and can be absent at rest. It does not involve the head or trunk until a later stage in the disease. The onset of tremor is shortly followed by a slurring dysarthria, and a variety of neurological signs including rigidity, loss of facial expression, ataxia, increased salivation and postural abnormalities. In some patients, episodic spasms of bizarre movements or dystonia may be superimposed, during which abnormal postures may be maintained for hours (Ref. 524, p.302). When such spasms are relieved, attempts to speak, or further movements, may result in renewed spasm and posturing. All the abnormal movements in this disorder disappear during sleep.

A major characteristic of Wilson's disease is the Kayser–Fleischer ring. This is a green-brown ring seen around the cornea and is due to pigment forming in Descemet's membrane. At first this abnormal pigment is deposited at the top and bottom of the cornea but as the disorder progresses it surrounds it to complete a circle. It is best visualized by examining the eye obliquely from above, or with a slit-lamp microscope.[523]

The earliest psychiatric disturbances are increased restlessness, and as the disorder progresses, euphoria, lability of affect, and dementia with impaired comprehension, memory difficulties and poor judgement, occur. The facial expression is said to be characteristic, with retraction of the upper lips, drooling of saliva, and a facial grin. A relationship of Wilson's disease to psychosis has been reported, which usually occurs in patients with late-onset disorder. Davison and Bagley[318] reviewed 520 case reports of Wilson's disease, noting eight acceptable and 11 doubtful cases of schizophrenia. They felt this prevalence was in excess of that found in the general population, and noted the relative absence of a family history of schizophrenia in these cases. Beard[525] considered the clinical picture was typical of schizophrenia, although he was unable to confirm any increased association.

The main pathological findings are a multilobular cirrhosis of the liver, and changes in the brain which are marked in the putamen, caudate nucleus and globus pallidus. However, changes are also seen in the cerebral cortex. It is now known that in Wilson's disease there are abnormal accumulations of copper in the affected areas. This occurs because caeruloplasmin — the copper-carrying plasma protein — is markedly reduced. This has led to biochemical criteria for the diagnosis of the disorder in that copper excretion in the urine is usually elevated, and serum copper and caeruloplasmin are low. Rarely it is necessary to do a liver biopsy to confirm the diagnosis.

Treatment is with the chelating agent penicillamine (Distamine) which promotes copper excretion. In that it has a number of unpleasant side-effects including the nephrotic syndrome, skin rashes and haematological disorders, its use requires careful monitoring so that its therapeutic and toxic effects can be balanced. Slow improvement in the neurological symptoms may be expected, although if treatment is delayed, irreversible central nervous system damage will occur. L-dopa may be a useful adjunct to therapy, especially in patients who respond poorly to penicillamine.

Sydenham's chorea

This disorder is characterized by choreiform movements that occur following infection in childhood, usually with rheumatic fever. It presents between the ages of 5 and 20, but may occur in pregnancy or be precipitated by taking oral contraceptives. It first manifests as clumsiness with fidgetiness and restlessness, before the chorea itself becomes apparent. Eye-rolling, head-turning, tongue protrusion, and bizarre orofacial movements may occur, and in severe cases speech, eating, and swallowing may be affected. The upper and lower limbs are also affected by choreiform activity. The movements are exacerbated by anxiety, but disappear during sleep. Affective disturbance and behaviour abnormalities are often reported in the course of the illness, and patients may appear depressed, emotionally labile, or even present pictures of mania and schizophrenia.[526, 527] Sequelae include personality change, neurosis, and possibly schizophreniform psychosis.[528] Because of the presentation, the disorder often initially receives a diagnosis of 'hysterical'. At autopsy, changes in the basal ganglia have been described, although cortical damage has also been noted. It is distinguished from Huntington's chorea primarily by the younger age of onset, and the absence of a family history of chorea.

Dystonia

Although this term is used to refer to a specific symptom of abnormal muscle contraction, it is in addition used to describe a group of disorders also referred to as *dystonia musculorum deformans* or *torsion dystonia*. As originally described it was an hereditary, progressive disorder, beginning in the second or third decade, characterized by spasms of the flexor muscles of the limbs and the spinal muscles. Other involuntary movements such as tics or choreoathetoid movements were superimposed (Ref. 524, p.302). It may occur spontaneously, but is also seen secondary to a number of CNS disorders such as encephalitis lethargica, Wilson's disease, anoxia, as a complication of phenothiazine drug therapy, or as a symptom of Huntington's chorea or the

Lesch–Nyhan syndrome. Dystonic movements usually begin in the extremities, especially in the legs. In the variety in which the head is twisted to one side, the term *torticollis* is used. If the head is brought forward or pulled backward it is referred to as *antecollis* or *retrocollis* respectively.

The hereditary form of the disorder is commoner in the Ashkenazim Jews, although it is autosomal recessive in this population, as opposed to the hereditary form in non-Jews in which an autosomal dominant inheritance is found.[529] The disorder is usually progressive, the abnormal posture spreading to involve various parts of the body, speech, and swallowing, although in each individual patient the course is variable. The later the onset of the disorder, the more benign the course, and the more it is likely to be confined to one segment of the body (focal dystonia). In a follow-up study of 72 patients Marsden *et al.*[530] found that generalized dystonia developed in 85% with an age of onset of under 10; in 60% with an onset between 11 and 20; and in only 40% with an onset after 20. The disorder, if it began in the legs, which was more common under the age of 10, carried to a worse prognosis, whereas the later-onset variety tended to start in the arms and axial muscles, the legs rarely being affected.

Dystonic spasms may initially occur in association with movement, and diminish with rest, and are exacerbated by stress. Rhythmic spasms of variable intensity occur, which may sometimes even resemble a tremor.[531]

Eldridge reviewed the anecdotal studies of dystonia musculorum deformans which suggested an apparent high intelligence in these patients, especially in those with the recessive type of inheritance.[529] Controlled studies have confirmed such reports.[532]

A number of different patterns of segmental dystonia are described. These usually occur in patients with no hereditary predisposition, although a family member may have had an alternative dystonic expression. The commonest is spasmodic torticollis, but others include blepharospasm, writer's cramp and oromandibular dyskinesia. It has been argued that they are all manifestations of torsion dystonia, probably related to disease processes in the basal ganglia.[531]

Spasmodic torticollis

In this disorder dystonic movements lead to deviation of the head to one side, or occasionally in the antero-posterior direction. It begins insidiously in the fourth or fifth decade with jerking of the head and muscle spasms. The latter may be quite painful. As the disorder progresses the spasms become longer and eventually the head is persistently held in an abnormal position. Cervical spondylosis may result from these abnormalities of posture, leading to further pain and discomfort. The movements are exacerbated by stress and tension but disappear in sleep. The prognosis is poor, and no treatments are consistently successful, although spontaneous remissions do occur.

Early writers suggested the disorder had a psychiatric basis. Tibbetts[533] in a study of over 100 cases was able to divide them into two main groups, which he called 'typical' and 'atypical'. The distinguishing features of the latter were an earlier age of onset, neurotic traits were likely to be present, and there were fewer complaints of pain. Evidence of dystonia elsewhere was rare, significant past psychiatric histories were present in one-third, and a disturbed marital state found at onset in three-quarters. The inference from this study was that the 'typical' group was linked to neurological pathology. However, nearly one-half of that group also had neurotic personalities, and abnormal mental states were frequently present at the onset of the disorder. In particular, significantly more of the 'typical' group developed depression, which was mainly 'endogenous' in type. Cockburn[534] studied the premorbid personalities of 55 patients with this disorder by retrospective completion of the EPI, and assessment of childhood neurotic complaints. When compared with matched controls no difference was noted, and the patient's scores were within the normal range for the English population. There was however a non-significant excess of anxiety reported in the patients. Other workers have reported inability to recognize unpleasant components of their emotional experience, repression and more obsessional traits in patients than in normals, with significant maladjustments in life-style, and severe sexual and marital disharmony.[535]

Writer's cramp

In this condition, spasm of the fingers, hand, arm and sometimes shoulder girdle occur during writing. It is present only with writing, and leads to the sufferer to hold his pen in an abnormal fashion, often then taking up writing with the other hand. Subsequent development of the cramp in that hand is not uncommon. The spasms are often associated with aches and pains in the affected arm, and occasionally are accompanied by tremor. It is related to a variety of other occupational cramps, including musician's cramp, typist's cramp, tailor's cramp, etc., in which the performance of skilled, fine movements becomes difficult or impossible.

Writer's cramp is more prevalent in males and usually occurs in the third or fourth decade. In many patients other dystonic features are noted in the history, or develop subsequently. It tends to be a chronic disorder with fluctuations in severity, although spontaneous remissions are recorded. Crisp and Moldofsky,[536] in a detailed study of seven patients, noted unresolved ambivalence over writing with resentment at having to write. Parental loss preceded the development of the symptoms in two patients, and the personality of the sufferers was described as 'tense, striving, sensitive, conscientious, precise, emotionally over-controlled . . . with a need to help others . . . .'. Citing psychophysiological observations that some patients, when angry, react with increased muscle tension in the arm, they suggested that some form of psychophysiological predisposition may interact with emotional conflict, especially in the setting of a need to write in frustrating but unavoidable circumstances, to produce the clinical picture. Other explanations are that writer's cramp and other occupational cramps are manifestations of dystonia, in which the initial muscle spasms appear with the most skilled and over-learned actions.[531]

A variety of treatments have been employed: orthopaedic, neurological and psychiatric, with little consistent success. Crisp and Moldofsky used relaxation, retraining and psychotherapy in combination and noted that all but one of their group improved. Biofeedback techniques may offer a useful alternative.[537]

Blepharospasm–oromandibular-dystonia syndrome (Breugel's syndrome) [538]

This syndrome, in which prolonged spasms of the jaw and mouth occur, often in association with blepharospasm, is to be distinguished from the chewing-like movements of tardive dyskinesia (see Figure 10.1). Although similar clinical pictures have been noted in basal ganglia disorders, or as a side-effect of major tranquillizer therapy, an idiopathic variety has been described by Marsden. Females are more frequently affected than males, and the onset is usually in the sixth decade. Blepharospasm may occur on its own and lead to blindness lasting for several minutes. The dystonia leads to prolonged contractions of the jaw muscles, forcing the teeth together or alternatively

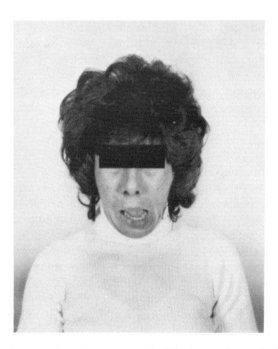

Figure 10.1. A patient showing the movements of the jaw and mouth characteristic of blepharospasm–oromandibular-dystonia syndrome

pulling the mouth open. These last up to a minute and, if severe, lead to difficulties with speaking, eating, and sometimes jaw dislocation. Tongue protrusion, lip-pouting, and occasionally dystonic postures elsewhere in the body may be noted. In a number of patients, depressive symptoms are reported before the onset of the muscular symptoms.

A variety of treatments have been tried, mainly psychotropic drugs which alter neurotransmitter function, but the symptoms are often recalcitrant. Any accompanying depression is treated with antidepressants, although this may make the movement disorder worse. The pathogenesis is unknown, but it has been suggested that it is a manifestation of torsion dystonia, and because of the relationship to dopamine-blocking drugs, that abnormalities of dopamine activity are in some way involved.

Gilles de la Tourette syndrome

The first case report of this disorder was by Itard in 1825. He described a 26-year-old female who developed symptoms at the age of 7, who, on account of coprolalia and echolalia, spent most of her life in seclusion. This case, along with eight others was reported by Gilles de la Tourette in 1885.[539] Since his descriptions, over 500 cases have been published and the symptomatology well described. Shapiro et al. (Ref. 540, pp.254–5) suggest that the criteria for diagnosis include:

(1) age of onset between 2 and 15 years;
(2) multiple, rapid, stereotypic, and involuntary muscular and verbal tics;
(3) fluctuating clinical course; symptoms wax, wane, and slowly change;
(4) voluntary effort can always reduce or completely control symptoms for brief periods and occasionally for prolonged periods, but results in subsequent tension and ultimate increase in discharged symptomatology;
(5) non-anxious concentration or preoccupation is associated with decrease in symptoms, and a variety of psychosocial situational factors may be associated with an increase or decrease in symptoms;
(6) symptoms always disappear during sleep;
(7) the illness is life-long and chronic.

In addition, confirmatory signs include coprolalia, copropraxia, echolalia, echopraxia, and palilalia. Frequent accompaniments of the disorder are a history of hyperactivity or perceptual problems in childhood, abnormal non-specific electroencephalograms, soft signs of neurological abnormality and subtle signs of organic dysfunction on psychological testing. Coprolalia occurs in some 50% of patients, but movements simple or complicated are universal, the latter including jumping, squatting, skipping, hitting, touching, dancing, echo movements, and startle reactions. Vocal tics, apart from coprolalia, include hisses, barks, grunts, snorts, sniffs, coughs, unintelligible sounds, clicking, lip smacking, spitting, and echo phenomena. There is a sub-group of patients that have symptoms resembling focal dystonia. A family history of tics is often obtained.

Shapiro,[541] in a study of 33 patients with Gilles de la Tourette syndrome, noted a higher incidence of males, and an average age of onset of 7.4 years. The first symptom was highly variable but was often eye blinking, and when past and present symptoms were cumulated, simple movements were reported in all patients, the majority of them showing eye blinking or head twitches, followed by shoulder shrugs, arm jerks and facial grimaces. The lower limbs and torso were less commonly involved.

Gilles de la Tourette syndrome may be mistaken for Sydenham's chorea, and it is not uncommon for patients diagnosed later to have been given an earlier diagnosis of chorea. The sequelae of encephalitis lethargica include tics and coprolalia (*klasomania*), and tic-like movements may be seen in other neuropsychiatric disorders such as Huntington's chorea, the Lesch–Nyhan syndrome, myoclonic epilepsy and schizophrenia. In addition there are a number of tic disorders that do not progress to the full picture of Gilles de la Tourette syndrome which include acute, simple or transient tics of childhood, chronic simple tics, and persistent simple or multiple tics of childhood or adolescence which, while initially indistinguishable from the Gilles de la Tourette syndrome, spontaneously remit during adolescence.[540]

The aetiology of Gilles de la Tourette syndrome is unknown. Initially Gilles de la Tourette suggested the disorder was allied to some other unusual disorders of movement including myriachit, latah, and 'the Jumpers of Maine'. This is now considered to be the case. These other conditions, in which a variety of unusual movements occur, often in response to startle, are now referred to as 'culture-bound neuroses', and in latah, tics are not seen.[542]

Corbett[543] compared patients with Gilles de la Tourette syndrome with those having simple or multiple body tics. Apart from a tendency for patients with Gilles de la Tourette syndrome to be more severely affected later in adolescence, little difference was noted in family history, associated psychiatric symptoms, or frequency of brain damage between the groups. The conclusion was that the Gilles de la Tourette syndrome represented the more severe end of the spectrum of tic syndromes.

Explanations for the tics vary from early psychoanalytic speculations involving repression, to theories of the behaviour therapists who suggest that they are conditioned avoidance responses. Shapiro *et al.* (Ref. 540, pp.364–7) described the Gilles de la Tourette syndrome as 'an organic disease of the central nervous system'. This approach fails to emphasize the close inter-relationship between movement disorders and psychopathology outlined here, and is essentially dualistic. The Gilles de la Tourette syndrome is a functional disorder in the original sense of the word (see page 3), in which occasionally overt structural brain damage is noted. Of 6 cases that have come to post-mortem to-date, three have been normal, and three have shown changes, two of which may have affected the corpus striatum. The high incidence of electro-encephalographic abnormalities, the relationship with similar phenomena noted after encephalitis, and the history of disturbed behaviour in childhood, all indicate a relationship of the syndrome to disturbed neuronal mechanisms.

Successful treatment with major tranquillizers suggests a relationship to abnormal dopamine mechanisms, further supported by observations of exacerbation of tics with L-dopa and amphetamine (Ref. 540, pp.206–10). In treatment haloperidol (Haldol) and pimozide (Orap) appear the most useful psychotropic drugs, although in some patients phenothiazines, or antidepressants, especially clomipramine (Anafranil), can benefit. In addition, behaviour therapy, psychotherapy, and hypnosis have all had their advocates. In one follow-up study[544] coprolalia indicated a poorer prognosis, and was related to high psychiatric morbidity, especially affective illness. Bruun *et al.*[545] followed up 80 patients after an average of nearly 3 years. Two patients had committed suicide, and among 78 remaining there were only four in complete spontaneous remission.

ABNORMAL MOVEMENT DISORDERS AND PSYCHIATRY

Although it is thought that most of the important movement disorders referred to above are related to basal ganglia disorders, the search for clearly-defined structural lesions in post-mortem specimens of many has been remarkably unrewarding. However, observations of movement disorders, similar to the idiopathic varieties, which follow L-dopa therapy, or prescription of drugs that block dopamine receptors, suggest at least that a functional disturbance of dopamine mechanisms occurs in these states.

Many of these disorders respond poorly to treatment, and patients often find them extremely distressing; as a result, by the time presentation to a psychiatrist occurs, the movement disorders and psychopathology have become closely interlinked. Examination of patients at this stage leads to the suggestion that the psychiatric disability is 'secondary' to the movement disorders, and that any depression is 'reactive'. Nevertheless, the frequent occurrence of the first abnormal movements in the setting of stress, the frequent history of a depressive illness ante-dating the symptoms, the frequent reporting of obsessionality and emotional over-control in the personality style of these patients, and the knowledge that both psychiatric illness and movement disorders are in some way related to disturbances of neuro-transmitter, and in particular monoamine function, all suggest that the links between the two are more complicated than this.

The interaction with psychiatric illness cannot be ignored, either at the theoretical or the clinical level. Earlier authors often diagnosed these patients as 'hysterical', and even today many patients with clearly-defined extrapyramidal movement disorders go undiagnosed for a number of years. The evidence that movement disorders were hysterical has always been slender, but the clinical presentation can be confusing. In particular such a variety of unusual movements occur, which fluctuate with place and time, and some very unusual attributes are noted, such as the 'geste antagoniste' in dystonia musculorum deformans, in which the patient appears to maintain a rigidly fixed posture, but a gentle touch from the examiner's finger to oppose the dystonia will allow movement of the body part with ease. Similarly it has been noted that patients with movement disorders which affect gait, walk forward with difficulty, but can often walk backwards normally. However, it has to be emphasized that diagnosis of symptoms as hysterical requires positive clinical features, as well as the incongruent neurological ones as discussed in Chapter 5. This confusion may be minimized if it is accepted that movement disorders do not present with the relatively well-defined focal symptomatology that traditional neurology looks for. They are primarily functional disorders.

CHAPTER 11

Organic Treatments

PSYCHOTROPIC DRUGS

Although certain compounds that influence behaviour have been known for many centuries, it is only since the introduction of chlorpromazine in 1952 and then shortly afterwards the antidepressants, that the full potential of psychopharmacotherapy has become recognized. At present many physicians still fail to understand fully the impact of the notion that it is possible to induce changes in behaviour by medications which influence brain chemistry, and there are still a few who believe that the effect of all such drugs is no more than placebo. It is becoming clearer that different classes of drugs alter the metabolism of different chemical systems, and that some clinically diagnosed disorders respond better to one class of drugs than another. The theoretical ideas about how these compounds work are compatible with some of the findings quoted earlier, which have related to the pathogenesis of the various psychiatric disorders. While there is no absolute right or wrong way to prescribe psychotropic drugs, and many of the drugs available have several chemical actions, and thus have a scatter of clinical effects, including the therapeutic ones, it is suggested that there are logical and illogical ways to prescribe.

Psychopharmacology

After the administration of a drug orally it is absorbed from the gastrointestinal tract and passed to the liver via the portal system. In the liver metabolism may occur, usually by oxidation, reduction, hydrolysis, or conjugation. Metabolism through the liver is referred to as 'first pass' metabolism. The metabolites of the major drugs, especially those produced by oxidation and conjugation, tend to be inactive, although some metabolites are as active, or even more active, than the parent compound. Drugs given intramuscularly avoid this 'first pass' effect.

A number of drugs increase the activity of the enzymes responsible for the metabolism either of themselves (auto-induction) or other drugs. Barbiturates, phenytoin, primidone and steroids have been particularly implicated in this process, but the enzyme-inducing properties of the psychotropic drugs have been relatively little studied. It is known that chlorpromazine has the ability to induce its own metabolism.

The majority of the psychotropic drugs are secondary or tertiary amines and weak bases, and are absorbed better from the duodenum than the stomach. They are lipid-soluble and thus taken up by the brain, and are highly protein-bound. The half-life of a drug refers to the time taken for it to decrease in its concentration in the plasma by 50%. The quicker the metabolism, the shorter the half-life. Clinically knowledge of the half-life is useful, since it is recommended that the dose interval in prescription is equivalent to that of the half-life. The steady state is the situation in which serum level of a drug reaches a plateau, and excretion is in balance with intake; approximately the time of four half-lives is required to reach this situation following the commencement of treatment. Factors that influence drug metabolism include genetics, age, diet, coexistent medications, and coexistent disease, especially of the liver, kidney, and heart.

Antidepressant drugs

These fall naturally into two classes, the monoamine oxidase inhibitors (MAOI) and the non-monoamine oxidase inhibitors (non-MAOI). The former can again be subdivided into the hydrazines and the non-hydrazines; the latter into tricyclic and non-tricyclic sub-classes.

(a) MAOI antidepressants

These drugs act by inhibition of monoamine oxidase, the enzyme responsible for the intraneuronal degradation of the monoamines. The hydrazine derivatives include isocarboxazid (Marplan), nialamide (Niamid) and phenelzine (Nardil). The non-hydrazine group includes tranylcypromine (Parnate) which chemically resembles amphetamine, and pargyline (Eutonyl). The structure of some of the MAOI antidepressants is shown in Figure 11.1, and their dose range and tablet size in Table 11.1. It is suggested that they act by inhibiting the breakdown of the catecholamines and serotonin, thus increasing the amount available in any neuronal system. Following administration, brain levels of noradrenaline, serotonin, and dopamine are raised, and an increase in spontaneous motor activity has been recorded in a variety of animals. It is now known that there are at least two monoamine oxidase enzyme systems within the central nervous system, and each of them is preferentially inhibited by a different drug. Current terminology labels the two enzymes as A and B. The A enzyme is sensitive to clorgyline and metabolizes both serotonin and noradrenaline, whereas the B enzyme is inhibited by deprenyl, and has as its substrates phenylethylamine and tryptamine.

Tranylcypromine (Parnate)

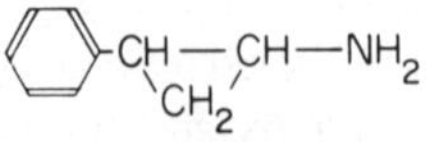

(Amphetamine)

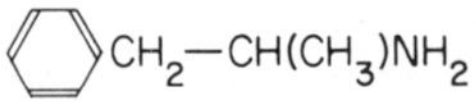

Phenelzine (Nardil)

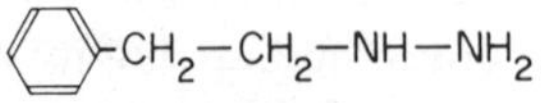

Isocarboxazid (Marplan)

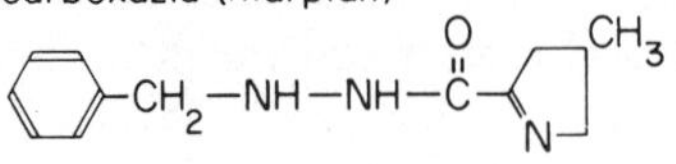

Iproniazid (Marsilid)

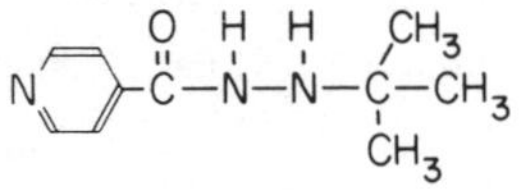

Nialamide (Niamid)

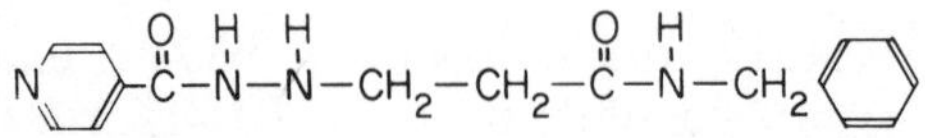

Figure 11.1. The structures of some MAOI antidepressant drugs

Tyramine and dopamine are substrates for both of the MAO enzymes. The relevance of this distinction for clinical practice is as yet unclear, and perhaps of more importance in prescribing is the acetylator status of the patient. Thus these drugs, metabolized by acetylation, will be broken down more quickly in a patient who is a fast acetylator, as opposed to someone who is a slow acetylator. It has been suggested but not confirmed that the clinical improvement following treatment is better in slow acetylators, and this is thought to be dependent upon the different rate of metabolism.[546] In that the acetylator status is genetically determined, patients with relatives who have responded to MAOIs are themselves also likely to respond.

Table 11.1. Some MAOI drugs and their dose ranges

	Tablet size (mg)	Daily dose (mg)
Hydrazines		
Isocarboxazid (Marplan)	10	10–60
Phenelzine (Nardil)	15	30–90
Non-hydrazines		
Tranylcypromine (Parnate)	10	30–60

A number of studies have indicated that the clinical effectiveness of the MAOI drugs is greater than placebo, and it has been suggested that tranylcypromine (Parnate) and iproniazid (Marsilid) are the most effective, followed by phenelzine (Nardil), and that isocarboxazid (Marplan) and nialamide (Niamid) are the least effective.[547] Although originally these drugs were avoided because of fear of adverse reactions, it is clear that recently they are being used with increasing frequency. There is growing opinion that they are better for 'atypical depressions', which include depression combined with anxiety, somatic depressions, and phobic anxiety states, especially agoraphobia. They may be particularly useful in the phobic anxiety-depersonalization syndrome. Their value in more severe typical depression, in which non-MAOI antidepressants are indicated is limited. Tyrer[548] suggested that the clinical features most commonly associated with a good response include hypochondriasis, somatic anxiety, irritability, agoraphobia and social phobias, and anergia and a poor result is associated with guilt, depressed mood, ideas of reference and nihilistic delusions.

Following administration, there is sometimes a delay before a clinical response is achieved, which may be days or even weeks, although the delay with the non-hydrazine drugs is less than with the hydrazine group. These compounds suppress REM sleep, and the onset of clinical improvement coincides with this change in sleep pattern. Larger doses lead to quicker REM suppressions and earlier remission of symptoms.

It is customary to start with doses in the medium range, and then increase after 1 or 2 weeks depending on the patient's response. Once treatment is started it may continue for several years if necessary. One of the limitations of the drugs is interaction with foodstuffs and other drugs. The reaction with food is now known to be due to tyramine, although some other amines such as L-dopa or tyrosine may also be involved. Tyramine is formed by degradation of protein-containing food, and acts as a pressor by releasing noradrenaline from noradrenergic endings into the circulatory system. If MAO is inhibited, tyramine's pharmacological effects are potentiated. A list of some of the interacting substances is given in Table 11.2. The reactions seem commonest with tranylcypromine (Parnate). Generally patients do not find it difficult to avoid these substances, although alcohol can be a problem. While some would suggest that alcohol should be avoided altogether, since the alcohol itself is not responsible for the reaction, only specific drinks need to be avoided, and moderation is of course recommended. This adverse reaction, when it occurs, consists of headaches, sweating, nausea, vomiting, and a rise in blood pressure that may lead to intracranial bleeding. The reported fatalities have almost always been associated with cheese.

MAOI drugs may be combined with tricyclic or other antidepressants in certain clinical situations. Although this form of therapy can lead to unwanted effects, especially hypotension, used carefully it can be very useful, especially in the resistant depressions. It is suggested that the two drugs should either be started simultaneously, or the non-MAOI antidepressant started

Table 11.2. Substances that may interact with MAOI drugs

Cheese — especially matured (not including cottage cheese or cream cheese)
Marmite, Bovril and other protein extracts (not including Bisto)
Pickled herring, liver, game food, broad beans (whole)
Yoghurt
Alcoholic drinks: especially chianti, beer and red wine (excluding spirits)
Drugs: amphetamine; fenfluramine (Ponderax); ephedrine, phenylpropanolamine, pethidine and other narcotics, antihypertensives, tricyclic antidepressants*; cocaine, barbiturates and general anaesthetics, antihistamines, L-dopa, insulin and anti-hypoglycaemic drugs.

---

*See text.

first, and the MAOI added later. The dosage of both should initially be lower than usual, and built up gradually. If there is a fear that the patient may react adversely because of, for example, age, then the patient should be initially admitted to hospital and monitored especially for blood pressure changes. It has been suggested that amitriptyline and trimipramine are safer in combination with the MAOIs than imipramine;[549] interactions with some of the newer non-MAOI drugs have not been evaluated.

Apart from the hyper- and hypotensive reactions, other side-effects of the MAOIs include tremor, weakness, dizziness, hyperreflexia, irritability, ataxia, impotence, hypotension, micturition problems, sweating, hyperpyrexia, rashes, and, rarely, convulsions. The drugs are contraindicated in liver disease, congestive heart failure, and following cerebrovascular accidents. The hypertensive complications described above respond to α-adrenergic blocking drugs, such as phentolamine (Rogitine) or chlorpromazine (Largactil).

(b) Non-MAOI antidepressants

The first of these to be synthesized and used was imipramine, followed shortly thereafter by amitriptyline. These two antidepressants are probably still the most widely used. The early members of this group were all variations of the tricyclic nucleus, but more recently drugs have been developed which have a non-tricyclic structure. The form of some of these compounds is shown in Figure 11.2. The tricyclic drugs are thought to act by inhibition of monoamine uptake into the presynaptic neurone, thus enhancing the availability of the monoamines within the synaptic cleft. It has been shown that different drugs have predominant actions on different monoamine systems. Generally, drugs which are tertiary amines have more effect on 5-HT uptake, and secondary amines more on catecholamine uptake. The non-tricyclic non-MAOI anti-depressants may have an entirely different mode of action. Nomifensine (Merital) has a dopamine agonist action, and maprotiline (Ludiomil) has no effect on 5-HT systems but acts primarily on catecholaminergic uptake. L-tryptophan (Optimax, Pacitron) is thought to act as a precursor to serotonin. The situation with flupenthixol (Fluanxol) is uncertain. Although it has

TRICYCLIC:

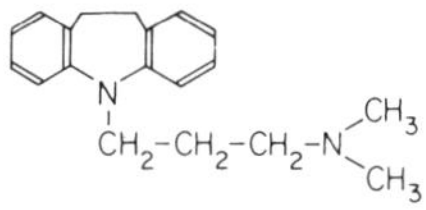

Imipramine (Tofranil)

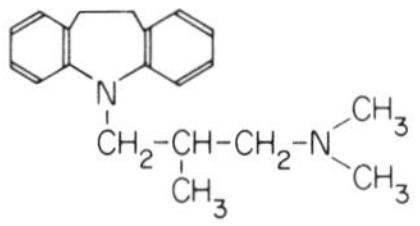

Trimipramine (Surmontil)

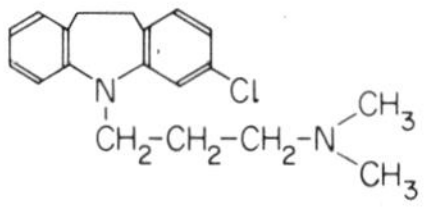

Clomipramine (Anafranil)

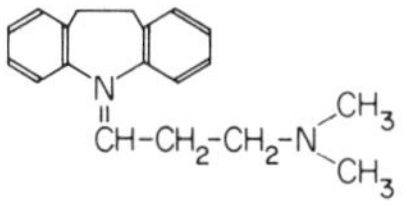

Amitriptyline (Triptyzol)

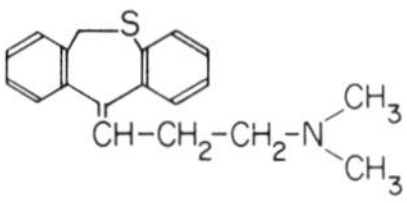

Dothiepin (Prothiaden)

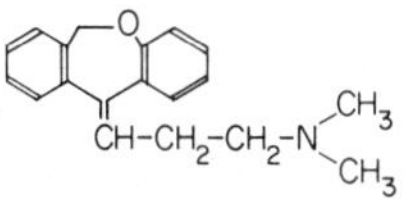

Doxepin (Sinequam)

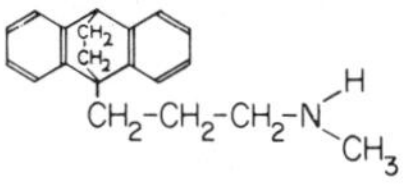

Maprotiline (Ludiomil)

Others include:

Nortriptyline (Aventyl)

Protriptyline (Concordin)

NON-TRICYCLIC:

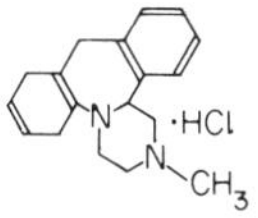

Mianserin (Bolvidon)

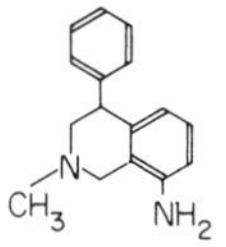

Nomifensine (Merital)

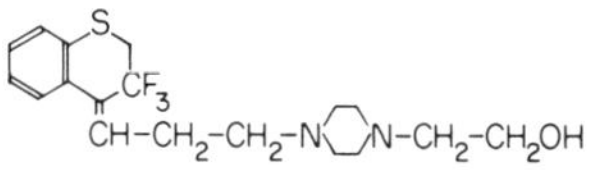

Flupenthixol (Fluanxol)

Others include:

L-Tryptophan (Optimax, Pacitron)

Viloxazine (Vivalan)

Iprindole (Prondol)

Figure 11.2. The structures of some non-MAOI antidepressant drugs

undoubted antidepressant action, this seems to occur with only small doses, larger doses being antipsychotic. While the latter action is related to its dopamine-blocking potential, the reasons for its antidepressant action are as yet unknown. X-ray crystallography has revealed complementary spatial relationships between some of the antidepressants and noradrenaline, indicating a possible mechanism whereby the inhibition of uptake activity occurs at the molecular level. Alteration of structure, for example by addition of methyl groups to the side chain, leads to a different configuration and interaction with the indole nucleus.[550]

Clinically there are now a number of trials which indicate that these drugs are superior to placebo in action, and it is now customary to compare new antidepresants with a tricyclic reference compound. As such it is not possible to indicate superiority of the newer drugs over the more established antidepressants, since to produce significant differences would require very large numbers of patients, which is impracticable in a clinical trial. However, the non-MAOI antidepressants differ considerably in their side-effects, and different drugs may thus be suited to quite different groups of patients. Major differences lie in their sedative properties, which are often due to antihistaminic action, and in their anticholinergic properties. Table 11.3 shows a spectrum of the effects of various antidepressants in blocking the re-uptake of the monoamines, and their antihistaminic and anticholinergic properties.

Table 11.3. Some properties of the non-MAOI antidepressants

	NA	5-HT	DA	AH	AC
Nomifensine	+	−	+	−	−
Mianserin	−	−	−	+	−
Viloxazine	+	−	±	−	−
Maprotiline	+ +	−	±	+	−
Imipramine	+	+	±	+	+
Amtriptyline	+ +	+	±	+	+ +
Chlorimipramine	+	+ +	±	+	±
L-Tryptophan	−	−	−	−	−
Flupenthixol	−	−	−	±	−

*NA, inhibition of noradrenaline uptake; 5-HT, inhibition of serotonin uptake; DA, inhibition of dopamine uptake; AH, antihistaminic; AC, anticholinergic.

The drugs that have sedative properties include amitriptyline (Tryptizol), trimipramine (Surmontil), sinequan (Doxepin), clomipramine (Anafranil) and mianserin (Bolvidon). Less sedative are imipramine (Tofranil) and maprotiline (Ludiomil), and least sedative are nomifensine (Merital), protriptyline (Concordin) and flupenthixol (Fluanxol). Anticholinergic effects are greatest with the tricyclic drugs and least with newer drugs, such as nomifensine (Merital) and mianserin (Bolvidon). The clinical implications are that patients with depression requiring sedation because of anxiety, agitation or insomnia need more sedative drugs, whereas those with retardation and less agitation require the least sedative drugs. If the insomnia is prominent then the whole of the dose prescribed should be given at night-time, and thus maximum sedation is obtained without the need for additional hypnotic medication. Some patients, especially the elderly or those with heart or urinary problems, are unable to tolerate anticholinergic compounds and thus drugs with high anticholinergic activity need to be avoided. The effect of some of the antidepressants on heart rate and atrioventricular conduction times have indicated a spectrum of cardiotoxicity of the antidepressant drugs, the tricyclic drugs being more toxic than the non-tricyclic ones.[551, 552] Some of the anti-depressants, especially protriptyline (Concordin), flupenthixol (Fluanxol) and nomifensine (Merital) in some patients have mild alerting properties. Therapeutically this may be useful, although if agitation or anxiety are present it may lead to an initial worsening of the symptoms and insomnia.

Nearly all the non-MAOI antidepressants lower the seizure threshold and may precipitate seizures. Not all do to the same extent, however, and a spectrum of epileptogenic activity has been suggested (see Figure 11.3).[445] The mechanism of this side-effect is not understood, although it may be due to interference with monoamine or GABA activity. In that patients with organic neurological disease may have a lowered seizure threshold, use of the tricyclic drugs in such cases seems illogical. Some of the special precautions required in the management of epileptic patients are discussed in Chapter 9.

Nomifensine (Merital), alone of these antidepressant drugs currently available, has dopamine agonist properties. This makes it the antidepressant of choice in conditions such as Parkinson's disease, alternatives being drugs that are also highly anticholinergic.

Choice of non-MAOI antidepressants is therefore related to the clinical pattern of the depression, and particular attention needs to be paid to age, accompanying anxiety or agitation, insomnia, and other medical diagnoses. It is important to take from the patient a drug history, and to find out if any close relative has had a depressive illness, and if so to what drug they may have responded. If a patient has been reliably treated before on a particular antidepressant and suffered few side-effects from it, it is logical to start the patient on the same preparation, unless there are now medical contra-indications. Potential suicide risk may be one such reason. One advantage of the newer antidepressants, such as flupenthixol (Fluanxol), nomifensine (Merital), and mianserin (Bolvidon), is that they are less hazardous when patients take overdoses.

The dosage of some of the drugs is shown in Table 11.4. It will depend upon the drug used, patient tolerance, and associated medical problems and speed of response required. While in some patients large doses may be used immediately, it is wise, especially if there is a suggestion of lowered seizure threshold or cardiac problems, to start on lower doses and build up levels slowly over 1 or 2 weeks. The response may be delayed, however, and if an earlier response is deemed necessary flupenthixol (Fluanxol) seems to have a more rapid onset of action than the majority of the other antidepressants, and

236

NON-M.A.O.I. ANTIDEPRESSANTS AND EPILEPSY

(CLINICAL & EXPERIMENTAL STUDIES)

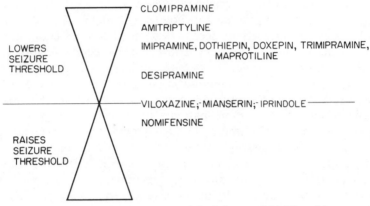

Figure 11.3. Spectrum of convulsant potential of the non-MAOI antidepressant drugs

Table 11.4. Dose of the non-MAOI antidepressants

	Tablet strength (mg)	Daily dose (mg)
Amitriptyline (Triptizol)	10, 25	50–200
Impramine (Tofranil)	10, 25	50–200
Protryptyline (Concordin)	5, 10	15–60
Trimiprimine (Surmontil)	10, 25, 50	50–200
Nomifensine (Merital)	25	50–200
Mianserin (Bolvidon)	10, 30	10–60
Viloxazine (Vivalan)	50	10–400
Maprotiline (Ludiomil)	10, 25, 50, 75, 150	50–200
L-Tryptophan (Pacitron; Optimax)	500	2000–6000
Flupenthixol (Fluanxol)	0.5	1.0–3.0
Clomipramine (Anafranil)	10, 25, 50	50–200
Dothiepin (Prothiaden)	25, 75	50–200
Doxepin (Sinequam)	10, 25, 50, 75	50–200

may be useful initially. Although in general, polypharmacy should be avoided, a combination of flupenthixol (Fluanxol) in the day-time, and a more sedative antidepressant at night-time is often successful. Other combinations that are sometimes used include L-tryptophan (Optimax; Pacitron) in combination with clomipramine (Anafranil), both of which are serotoninergic and therefore complementary. MAOI drugs may be combined with L-tryptophan, and a combination of non-MAOI and MAOI therapy is discussed above. Some preparations are available that combine antidepressants with phenothiazines, such as Triptafen-DA, which contains amitriptyline and perphenazine, or Motival, which is fluphenazine and nortriptyline. Generally such combinations are best avoided, and if tranquillizing action is required in addition to the antidepressant, then it is best in the first instance to use an antidepressant with sedative potential. If antipsychotic activity is required then a major tranquillizer may be given as a separate preparation.

Sometimes it is necessary to give higher doses than those quoted in Table 11.4. In general, the tricyclic antidepressants have long half-lives and can be given once daily, and as indicated, night-time is best from the point of view of unwanted side-effects, and compliance. Once started, antidepressants should be continued, in the absence of severe side-effects, for 6 to 12 months.

Recently, techniques have become available to measure serum antidepressant levels with relative ease. This is usually done with gas-liquid chromatography, although other methods include radioimmunoassay, and mass spectrometry. The drugs following absorption are metabolized by methylation and hydroxylation in the liver before passing into the circulation, where they are strongly bound to protein, about 10% remaining unbound. In measurement both free and total levels can be estimated, although most research to-date has looked at total levels. Plasma levels estimations indicate that between individuals, variation in levels on the same dose of drug is wide, and in patients day-to-day variation is 15–20%.[533] Studies of the relationship between these levels and the clinical efficiency have led to conflicting results. One problem is that many of these drugs break down to the desmethylated metabolites, which are active compounds. For example, desmethylimipramine appears rapidly in the plasma following an oral dose of imipramine, and in patients on chronic treatment represents the major active metabolite. Some authors have claimed that a therapeutic window exists, such that levels below or above this window lead to poor results. While at present there is no consensus of opinion, and it may well be that each of the drugs behaves in a different way, what does appear is that generally high levels of the drug lead to more side-effects, and patients with low levels respond poorly. Interaction studies between the tricyclic antidepressants and other drugs indicate that barbiturates lower, and major tranquillizers raise the serum levels of antidepressants, which effects occur mainly by altering the activity of metabolizing enzymes in the liver.

There are a large number of side-effects associated with these drugs shown in Table 11.5. Some of them occur commonly and are usually quite tolerable, such as a dry mouth; others are much rarer and extremely discomforting, such as the dyskinesias. Some may be used therapeutically, such as the hypnotic effects. Interaction of the antidepressants with other therapeutic drugs can be a problem, in particular interference of the tricyclic antidepressants with antihypertensive therapy has been noted with bethanidine (Esbatal), debrisoquine (Declinax) and guanethidine (Ismelin). It is important to note that non-specific electrocardiographic changes may occur, which include T-wave changes, prolonged Q–T intervals and depressed S–T segments. Overdose with these drugs frequently leads to cardiac complications, hypotension, seizures and coma. Management of these must include careful cardiac monitoring and the administration of anti-arrhythmic drugs if

Table 11.5. Some side-effects of non-MAOI antidepressant drugs

Sedation
Dry mouth
Palpitations and tachycardia — changes on ECG
Visual difficulties
Postural hypotension
Nausea and vomiting, heartburn
Constipation
Glaucoma
Urinary retention, impotence, delayed ejaculation
Paralytic ileus
Galactorrhoea
Sweating
Tremor
Convulsions
Ataxia
Dyskinesia
Induction of Delirium
Agitation; transient hypomania; acute depersonalization; induction of psychosis;
    aggression
Jaundice (cholestatic)
Weight gain

indicated. Physostigmine (0.5–1.0 mg i.m., repeated as necessary) has been recommended for the reversal of the anticholinergic effects. In view of the possibility of death from seizures, the administration of anticonvulsants other than barbiturates is sometimes used in management.

Major tranquillizers

These drugs fall naturally into four groups: phenothiazines, butyrophenones, thioxanthines, and others. The phenothiazines are based on the tricyclic nucleus, in which different configurations of the side chain lead to alteration of their properties. Three sub-groups are recognized: those with an aliphatic side chain, such as chlorpromazine (Largactil); those with a piperidine side chain, such as thioridazine (Melleril); and those with piperazine side chains, such as trifluoperazine (Stelazine). Representatives of these and their structural relationships are shown in Figure 11.4. The butyrophenones and related drugs, such as pimozide (Orap), are distinguished from the pheno-thiazines by their configuration (see Figure 11.5). Included in this group are fluspiriline and penfluridol, both of which are long-acting oral preparations. The thioxanthines have a structure which is similar to the phenothiazine nucleus, and include chlorprothixine, thiothixine (Navane) and flupenthixol (Depixol). Other major tranquillizers include molindone, the rauwolfia alkaloids, such as reserpine and tetrabenazine (Nitoman), oxypertine (Integrin), loxepine, sulpiride, and clozapine (Leponex) (see Table 11.6).

The distinguishing characteristics of all these compounds is that they are

Nucleus :

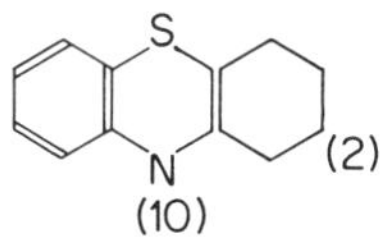

(10)   (2)

Aliphatic side-chain: e.g. Chlorpromazine (Largactil)

$$(10) -CH_2-CH_2-CH_2-N(CH_3)_2$$
$$(2) -Cl$$

Piperidine side-chain: e.g.   Thioridazine (Melleril)

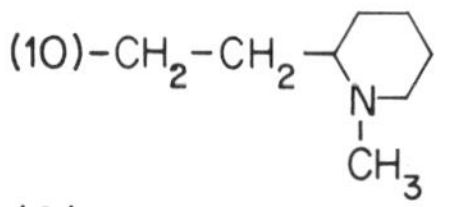

$(10)-CH_2-CH_2$

CH_3

$(2)   -S-CH_3$

Other examples: Pericyazine (Neulactil)

Piperazine side-chain: e.g.   Trifluoperazine (Stelazine)

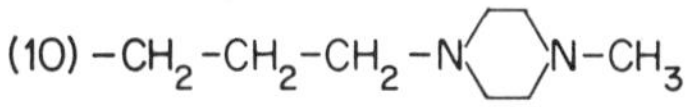

$$(10) -CH_2-CH_2-CH_2-N \overline{\quad} N-CH_3$$

Other examples: Perphenazine (Fentazin)

Fluphenazine (Moditen)

Thiopropazate (Dartalan)

Figure 11.4. Structures of the phenothiazine compounds

Haloperidol (Haldol)

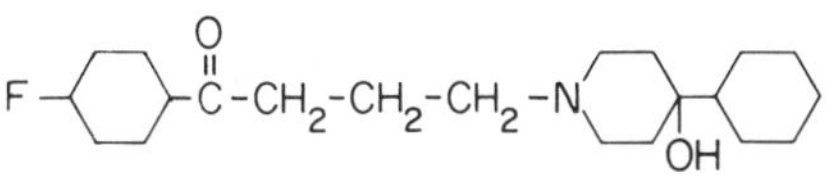

Related drugs: Pimozide (Orap)

Penfluridol

Fluspiriline (Redeptin)

Figure 11.5. Structure of the butyrophenones

antipsychotic, they evoke extrapyramidal symptoms of various types, and their effect is related to their potential for blocking the dopamine receptor. Several laboratory techniques have now been developed to assess the latter. These include the ability of drugs to inhibit apomorphine-induced behaviour

240

Table 11.6. Divisions among the major tranquillizers

Phenothiazines:	(a) Aliphatic
	(b) Piperidine
	(c) Piperazine
Butyrophenones:	Haloperidol (Haldol)
	Pimozide (Orap)
	Fluspiriline (Redeptin)
	Penfluridol*
	Benperidol (Anquil)
Thioxanthines:	Thiothixine (Navane)
	Flupenthixol (Depixol)
	Chlorprothixine (Taractan)
	Clopenthixol (Clopixol)

Molindone*
Sulpiride*
Clozapine*
Reserpine (Serpasil)
Tetrabenazine (Nitoman)
Loxapine*
Oxypertine (Integrin)

*Not available in the UK.

changes in animals; to increase the turnover of HVA in various brain areas, such as the corpus striatum or the nucleus accumbens; to block stimulation of dopamine-sensitive adenylate-cyclase; and to displace receptor binding with H^3-dopamine or H^3-spiroperidol at post-synaptic dopamine receptor sites. With few exceptions the ability of these drugs to block the receptor correlates directly with their clinical antipsychotic action. In addition, since they readily produce extrapyramidal side-effects, it is suggested that the antipsychotic potential may be due to this blockade in the mesolimbic or mesocortical dopamine systems, whereas the motor effects are related to effects on the nigrostriatal system. There are three drugs that have minimal extrapyramidal side-effects, namely sulpiride, clozapine (Leponex), and thioridazine (Melleril). These seem to act mainly on limbic structures, and less at the striatum, and two of them (clozapine and thioridazine) have inherent anticholinergic potential which may counteract the development of any Parkinsonism.

There has been growing interest in the substituted benzamide drugs, which include tiapride and sulpiride. In general these compounds, derived from metoclopramide, act like dopamine receptor antagonists, but tiapride seems to act more on the caudate system, and sulpiride more on the mesolimbic system. In consequence, tiapride seems to block dyskinesias, for example L-dopa-induced dyskinesias, but is not clearly antipsychotic, whereas sulpiride is antipsychotic, and exerts little or no effect in experimental models of motor dysfunction.

As with the antidepressants, the major tranquillizers possess antihistaminic and anticholinergic properties, giving rise to a variety of side-effects.

Chlorpromazine (Largactil) and thioridazine (Melleril) are strong α-adrenergic blocking agents. All except thioridazine (Melleril) are anti-emetic. The difference between the drugs in relation to their hypnotic potential is shown in Figure 11.6. If sedation is required on account of agitation or anxiety, then drugs such as chlorpromazine (Largactil) are preferred. In apathetic psychotic patients, in contrast, drugs such as pimozide (Orap) or perphenazine (Fentazin) may be more logical. Extrapyramidal side-effects will be less with thioridazine (Melleril) than with haloperidol (Haldol; Serenace), and if the patient complains of anticholinergic side-effects, drugs with minimal anticholinergic action, such as haloperidol (Haldol; Serenace), are indicated.

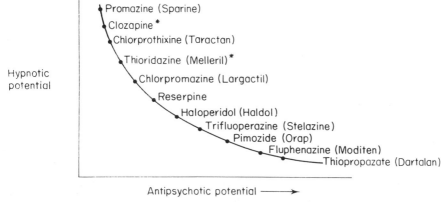

Figure 11.6. The hypnotic and antipsychotic potential of the major tranquillizers. Those marked with an asterisk have strong anticholinergic properties

Chlorpromazine is easily absorbed and metabolized in the liver, and after an oral dose the peak plasma level occurs at 1½–3 hours. Some metabolites, such as the sulphoxide, have little pharmacological activity, while others, such as the hydroxy derivatives, are much more potent. Protein binding is strong. The drug preferentially accumulates in the brain, such that the brain:plasma concentration is about 5:1. After termination of therapy, excretion of the drug, or one of its metabolites, may continue for up to several months. Haloperidol is less rapidly absorbed after an oral dose, maximal concentrations occurring around 5 hours. It is over 90% bound and does not induce its own metabolism.

The dosage of major tranquillizers has to be titrated for individual patients against symptoms, and in some cases very large doses are required. With drugs that have α-adrenergic blocking potential, such as chlorpromazine (Largactil), such doses may lower blood pressure, and monitoring of the latter may be required. It is usual to start patients on oral medications, but since the half-lives of these drugs are often short, once a day medication is often difficult, and twice daily regimes are indicated. Following control with oral therapy, especially if the patient has schizophrenia, a change to an intramuscular preparation is often preferred. The available preparations are shown in Table 11.7

with their approximate dose ranges. It is usual to give a test dose to ensure that no untoward reaction occurs, before commencing therapy on full intramuscular doses. There is little evidence that any one of these preparations is superior therapeutically to the others, although extrapyramidal symptoms are reported to be less with flupenthixol (Depixol).[554]

Table 11.7. Available I.M. preparations of the major tranquillizers

Fluphenazine	Decanoate	(Modecate)	25 mg	2–4 weekly
Flupenthixol	Decanoate	(Depixol)	20–40 mg	2–4 weekly
Fluspiriline		(Redeptin)	2–20 mg	1–2 weeks

In schizophrenia, once treatment has been started, it should be continued indefinitely. Usually this will mean regular injections with an intramuscular preparation, supplemented where necessary with oral medication. Although factors other than the medication affect relapse in schizophrenia, it appears that nearly all patients get some protection by continued therapy. 'Drug holidays', for example not taking drugs at weekends or stopping for several weeks at regular intervals, are thought by some to be useful, although the effects of this have not been evaluated. As a rule, polypharmacy should be avoided, and a large dose of one drug is preferred to smaller doses of two. However, some patients seem to respond better on a combination of, for example, a phenothiazine and a butyrophenone. Commonly, major tranquillizers are combined with anti-Parkinsonian drugs, but since some major tranquillizers, such as thioridazine (Melleril), have inherent anticholinergic activity, this is often not necessary. Recent studies have shown that the anticholinergic drugs, by delaying gastric emptying and absorption from the gastrointestinal tract, lower plasma levels of the major tranquillizers and diminish therapeutic potential. In addition it has not been conclusively shown that they actually diminish the reported incidence of extrapyramidal effects.

In some cases it is necessary to tranquillize patients rapidly, and large i.m. or i.v. doses may be indicated. A regime may include haloperidol (Haldol; Serenace) 10–20 mg every 30 to 60 minutes, following an initial loading dose of 10–30 mg i.m. Changeover to oral therapy should be done as soon as possible. Side-effects such as acute dystonias are rare, and with haloperidol (Haldol; Serenace) severe blood pressure changes are not noted.

The side-effects of the major tranquillizers are similar to those listed for the antidepressants in Table 11.5. More particularly encountered are the extrapyramidal problems which include acute dystonias, akinesia, akathisia, Parkinsonism, and tardive dyskinesia (see Chapter 10). Agranulocytosis, due to a direct toxic effect of phenothiazines on bone marrow, sometimes occurs, and depression of the white cell count is often encountered. Photosensitivity is a problem with chlorpromazine, and can lead to skin eruptions on exposure to sunlight, or a pattern of contact dermatitis. Retinal pigmentation has occasionally been described with thioridazine (Melleril). It has been suggested that a severe depressive illness may occur in some schizophrenic patients when treated with intramuscular preparations.[555] The exact relationship between the medication and the depression is unclear, since post-psychotic depression is a recognized clinical entity irrespective of whether such treatment has been given. However, when depression occurs in these situations it responds to antidepressants, or if necessary ECT. Occasionally catatonic reactions, with posturing, waxy flexibility, withdrawal, and regression have been reported. This has gradual onset and may be confused with a deterioration of a psychosis.[472]

In addition to the use of major tranquillizers in schizophrenia, they are used in the management of manic-depressive illness, and in patients with organic brain syndromes — acute or chronic — where behaviour has become unmanageable by other means. They have also been used in alcohol or other drug withdrawal states, although their potential to lower the seizure threshold is a problem. More recently their use in depression and in some neurotic illness has been advocated. Flupenthixol (Fluanxol) is an antidepressant, and similar action has been ascribed to some other thioxanthenes such as chlorprothixine (Taractan). This effect is observed only with small doses. Since flupenthixol is marketed as an i.m. preparation (Depixol) it may find use in the management of resistant depression, and in patients whose compliance is low. Fluspiriline (Redeptin) 2 mg i.m. weekly may be useful in the management of severe chronic neuroses, especially where there is a prominent anxiety component in the symptoms. Pimozide (Orap) has been used successfully in patients suffering from monosymptomatic hypochondriacal delusions.[556] These patients, with personality well retained, develop a delusion about some particular part of their body (dysmorphophobia), and frequently present to specialists such as dermatologists or plastic surgeons.

Minor tranquillizers

This category of drugs includes three main groups; barbiturates, benzodiazepines, and others. As such they are the most widely used drugs in psychiatry. They have in common sedative and anticonvulsant properties, but differ in a number of respects, as indicated in Table 11.8. The barbiturates include phenobarbitone (Luminal), butobarbitone (Soneryl), and amylobarbitone (Amytal). They are rapidly absorbed from the gastrointestinal tract, are powerful inducers of hepatic enzymes, and the duration of their clinical action

Table 11.8. Properties of the three main groups of minor tranquillizers

	Barbiturates	Benzodiazepines	Meprobamate
Tranquillizing	+	+	+
Anticonvulsant	+	+	+
Muscle relaxant	±	+	+
Suicide potential	+	−	+
Addictive potential	+	±	+

is approximately 8 hours. They are sedative and anxiolytic, but have a generalized depressant effect on the brain, which, amongst other things, leads to respiratory depression, which is especially dangerous if an overdose is taken. Their enzyme induction effects leads to adverse interactions with other drugs, such as the coumarin anticoagulants.

The benzodiazepines have a common structure, but differ with respect to their metabolites (Table 11.9). They range from the more hypnotic, such as flurazepam (Dalmane), nitrazepam (Mogadon), and temazepam (Normison) to the less hypnotic, such as diazepam (Valium), chlordiazepoxide (Librium), lorazepam (Ativan), clobazam (Frisium), oxazepam (Serenid-D) and chlorazepate (Tranxene). These lesser hypnotic compounds, however, do possess hypnotic properties if the dose is increased sufficiently. With the exception of lorazepam (Ativan) and oxazepam (Serenid-D), they have long half-lives and can be given on a once daily dosage. The hypnotic ones are used primarily as night-time sedatives, the others in the management of anxiety states, muscle tension states, and spasticity. Clonazepam (Rivotril) is a benzodiazepine which appears to be more specific in its effects on the 5-HT system, and is used in the management of epilepsy. The position of diazepam (Valium) in this condition has yet to be fully evaluated, although its use intravenously in status epilepticus is well-substantiated.

Table 11.9. Some benzodiazepines and their metabolites

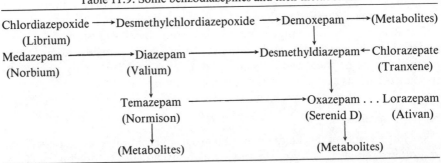

Following oral doses, diazepam (Valium) is more rapidly absorbed than chlordiazepoxide (Librium). In contrast to the barbiturates, benzodiazepines act chiefly on the limbic system and respiratory depression is therefore less of a problem. The mode of action is unclear. Their effect on monoamine turnover is uncertain, but they do influence GABA pathways by enhancing transmission in GABA-ergic neurones. Recently, specific benzodiazepine receptor sites have been discovered, especially in the cerebral cortex, cerebellar cortex, limbic system, and basal ganglia.[557, 558]

After overdose, if a benzodiazepine is taken alone, death rarely results. Tolerance is less likely to occur with the benzodiazepines than with the other minor tranquillizers, although dependence has been described, and withdrawal symptoms occur when they are stopped in patients who have been on them for some time. Release of aggression has been reported both in animals and humans. Both barbiturates and the benzodiazepines seem liable to provoke depression in a number of patients, although this has never been subjected to a formal study.

Other minor tranquillizers include meprobamate (Equanil) which is absorbed rapidly, and induces its own metabolism with a half-life of about 12 hours. It is approximately halfway between the barbiturates and the benzodiazepines in terms of producing tolerance, sedation, and cortical depression. Other hypnotics sometimes used include chloral hydrate, dichloral-phenazone (Welldorm), glutethamide (Doriden), paraldehyde, chlormethiazole (Heminevrin) and a combination of methaqualone and diphenhydramine (Mandrax).

Of the anxiolytic drugs, the benzodiazepines are the drugs of choice. There is little evidence that, of those available, any one is preferable to another, but clinically some patients just prefer a particular compound. Lorazepam (Ativan) seems especially useful for patients with non-epileptic fits and muscle tension states. There is little reason to prescribe barbiturates or meprobamate, and recently there has been a tendency to remove patients from barbiturates, even if they have been on them for 20 or 30 years. In some cases complete withdrawal is impossible without producing severe and often prolonged psychiatric symptomatology.

With regard to the hypnotics, the benzodiazepines are again drugs of choice. They produce little change in the regular sleep pattern, except for some loss of slow-wave sleep.

The dosage of drugs used is based mainly on clinical judgement, and for tranquillization once daily or twice daily regimes are recommended. Although some tolerance to all these drugs, including the benzodiazepines, may occur, some people get a clinical effect from the minor tranquillizers for many years. It is important that they should not be continued longer than is necessary, but when withdrawal is undertaken, medication should be stopped slowly rather than rapidly.

Side-effects, other than those already mentioned, include drowsiness, interference with cognitive performance, and withdrawal seizures. Major and important side-effects, such as respiratory and circulatory failure, are usually confined to overdoses, and are seen mainly with the barbiturates.

β-adrenergic blockers

Although initially introduced for the management of cardiovascular disorders, the β-blocking drugs have recently become widely used in psychiatric conditions. They block β-adrenergic receptors in the sympathetic nervous system, acting therefore as catecholamine antagonists. Structurally they resemble the catecholamines (see Figure 11.7), and their mode of inhibition is competitive. As a consequence of β-blockade they decrease the heart rate, lower the blood pressure and may cause bronchial constriction. The site of action of these drugs in psychiatric disorders is not clear. While there is evidence for central adrenergic systems, and β-adrenergic receptors have been identified in the limbic system and neocortex,[559] the possibility that their action is primarily on peripheral receptors has been raised. Thus anxiety symptoms most helped by these drugs are somatic ones, such as palpitations, sweating, and diarrhoea, and some of the β-blockers, such as practolol, have little ability to cross the blood–brain barrier, but appear to be effective anxiolytics.[560, 561]

The decision as to whether to use these drugs as opposed to minor tranquillizers in anxiety states rests on several considerations. Firstly, β-blockers are contra-indicated in some patients where β-blockade is likely to affect other medical conditions, especially respiratory and cardiac disorders. Secondly, they are poorly tolerated by some people, and can induce quite severe malaise and lethargy which, if unrecognized, may be taken for further symptoms of the underlying psychiatric disturbance. Thirdly, if they are of value, the patients most likely to benefit seem to be those with mainly somatic symptoms of anxiety. In one trial comparing diazepam (Valium) with propranolol (Inderal) and placebo, while both active drugs were preferred to the placebo, diazepam (Valium) was more effective in anxiety relief in a group of patients without somatic symptoms.[560] It is possible to combine a minor tranquillizer with a β-blocker if necessary.

The dose varies with each patient, but generally less is required in the treatment of anxiety states than in treating disorders such as hypertension. Most patients with anxiety symptoms who will respond, do so to under 120 mg daily. These drugs have been used in other neuropsychiatric disorders apart from anxiety. Schizophrenia has been reported to respond successfully to large doses (750–3000 mg daily),[562] although further confirmation of this needs to be obtained from trials. They have also been used in Parkinson's disease, benign familial tremor, drug-induced tremor, migraine and tension headaches.

Side-effects include fatigue, lethargy, insomnia, depression, hallucinations and hypotension. Patients with a tendency to asthma or cardiac failure may respond adversely, and they should be avoided in such conditions.

Lithium

Lithium carbonate was first introduced in the treatment of manic illness in 1949, and in recent years has become the drug of first choice in the management of the manic phase of manic-depressive psychosis. Following ingestion it is absorbed rapidly, peak concentrations occurring 1–2 hours later, and the half-life is approximately 24 hours. It is mainly excreted in the urine, and thus patients with renal disease readily become intoxicated. Since it is reabsorbed with sodium into the proximal renal tubules, any drug that leads to a negative sodium balance, such as a diuretic, will lead to increased retention of lithium, as may alteration of the diet, heavy sweating and diseases that reduce sodium intake. Its mode of action is unknown, but it reduces the sodium content of various parts of the brain; increases 5-HT synthesis and noradrenaline turnover; and increases platelet 5-HT uptake.

Although the main indication is in the prophylactic management of bipolar manic-depressive illnesses, recently it has become acknowledged as useful for the management of recurrent unipolar depressive illness. In both, the drug may be used in the treatment of the acute illness, especially mania, when it is started in combination with a major tranquillizer. Other uses include the treatment of recurrent aggressive disorders, migraine, cluster headaches and alcoholism, although its value in these conditions is poorly evaluated. In one double-blind study of prisoners, there was significantly less aggressive and threatening behaviour reported when lithium was compared to placebo.[563]

Table 11.10. Toxic effects of lithium

Neuropsychiatric	Drowsiness
	Confusion
	Psychomotor retardation
	Restlessness
	Stupor
	Headache
	Weakness
	Tremor
	Ataxia
	Choreoathetoid movements
	Dysarthria
	Blurred vision
	Seizures
	Dizziness, vertigo
	Impaired short-term memory and concentration
Gastrointestinal	Anorexia, nausea, vomiting
	Diarrhoea
	Dry mouth, metallic taste
	Weight gain
Renal	Microtubular lesions
	Impairment of renal concentrating capacity
Cardiovascular	Low blood pressure
	ECG changes
Endocrine	Myxoedema
	Hyperthyroidism
Other	Polyuria and polydipsia
	Glycosuria
	Rashes

Lithium has a large number of toxic effects, which are listed in Table 11.10, and are minimized by regular monitoring of the serum lithium levels. It is suggested that the therapeutic non-toxic range for the drug is 0.6–1.5 μmol per litre, although variations for individual patients are recognized. Some respond at much lower levels, others develop toxicity at such levels, and still others require levels above 1.5 μmol per litre to obtain benefit. Although monitoring is carried out weekly at first, when stable levels are reached 3-monthly assessments are acceptable. Patients with cardiac or renal disease, or in other situations that may interfere with the clearance of lithium, will obviously need more regular monitoring, and prior to starting therapy, urea and electrolytes

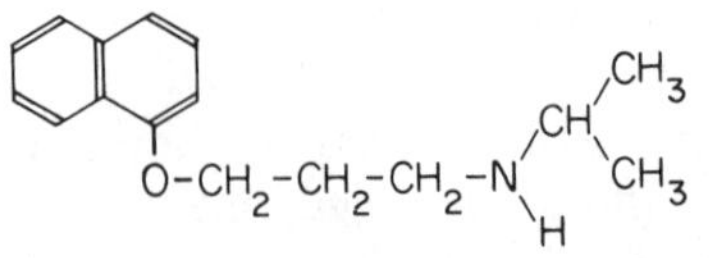

Propranolol (Inderal)

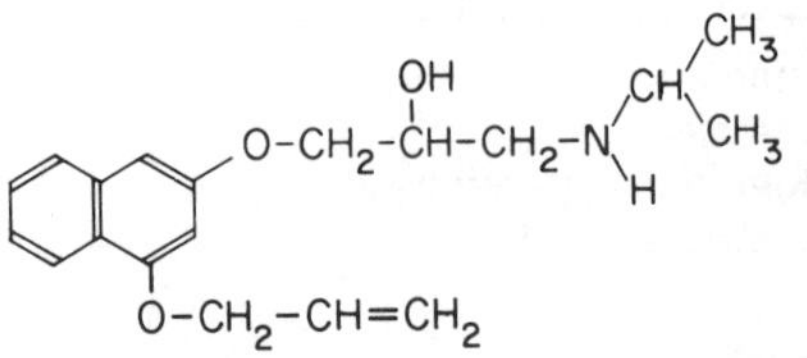

Oxyprenolol (Trasicor)

Figure 11.7. Structures of some β-blocking drugs

should be checked, in addition to thyroid and renal function. Although a teratogenic effect of lithium in humans has not been demonstrated, there are reports of a higher incidence of congenital malformations in babies born to mothers who take lithium, and it should probably be discontinued during pregnancy if it is at all possible. The commonest side-effects of chronic treatment are polyuria with polydypsia, tremor, weight gain, and hypothyroidism. Gastrointestinal symptoms often are seen immediately on ingestion of the drug, which may be lessened by the use of sustained release preparations, or taking the drug with an alkali such as milk. Impending toxicity is heralded by vomiting, diarrhoea, tremor, ataxia and drowsiness.[564] Severe intoxication often leads to neurological signs such as hyperactive reflexes, seizures and tremors, which may sometimes be unilateral, and be interpreted as an alternative neurological illness. If toxicity results in coma, dialysis should be considered, especially if clearance is in any way delayed. On stopping the drug the serum concentration of lithium usually falls by about a half each day. During treatment, transitory abnormalities of thyroid function may appear, including an increased serum TSH and a lowered triiodothyronine and thyroxine. This does not require treatment, but if myxoedema develops, and it is necessary to continue the lithium treatment, then additional thyroxine therapy will be required.

Available preparations of lithium contain lithium carbonate (Camcolit); delayed release preparations can be taken once a day (Phasal; Priadel). In acute mania the starting dose is usually 600–900 mg daily, which is then increased until serum levels are satisfactory. In less urgent situations smaller doses are started, and the dose gradually increased until control is achieved. Once therapy is started, especially in bipolar affective illness, treatment will need to be continued for possibly several years.

Convulsive therapy

Although alternative methods of inducing a convulsion are available (e.g. flurothyl) the most commonly used method in clinical practice is electro-convulsive therapy (ECT). This treatment was originally introduced by Cerletti, following the observations of Von Meduna of an antagonism between epilepsy and psychosis.[565] Originally the treatment was thought to be most useful for schizophrenia, although now the main indication is depressive illness. The use of general anaesthetics with muscular relaxation, and the increasing popularity of non-dominant unilateral ECT, has lessened the side-effects that used to occur. It is clinically efficacious in the conditions outlined in Table 11.11. In depression certain clinical features are said to be predictors of a good response, which include sudden onset, diurnal variation, retardation, weight loss, early waking, pyknic body build, somatic delusions and guilt. Although many schizophrenic patients do not get benefit from this form of treatment, some do, particularly where paranoid excitement and tension are part of the clinical state, or where catatonic features are noted. Patients with anxiety neurosis, personality disorders, and depersonalization, in the absence of depression, do badly. Occasionally it is used in the management of mania, delirium, and chronic pain syndromes, in the latter particularly where an affective element is present. In Parkinson's disease with depression that has become unresponsive to chemotherapy, ECT may be helpful, and in epilepsia partialis continua it may bring the attack to an end.

Table 11.11. Indications for electro-convulsive therapy

Depressive illness	Especially:	Primary depression
		Bipolar affective illness
Schizophrenia	Only:	Catatonic states
		Paranoid excitement
		With accompanying affective symptoms

The mechanism of action of ECT is not understood. Ottosson[566] studied the effect of shortening the duration of the epileptic discharge in ECT with lidocaine, and reported that the antidepressant effect was related directly to the seizure activity. He also noted that memory disturbances were related more to the amount of the electric current administered. Increased turnover of monoamines has been reported in animals following electro-shock administration, and the urinary excretion of MHPG has been shown to increase during a course of ECT, reaching highest levels after treatment has stopped, and being associated in some patients with the development of hypomanic symptoms.[567]

Contraindications are few, but include the presence of an intracranial tumour, and a recent cerebrovascular accident. In that a large increase in CSF pressure occurs during seizure discharge, ECT is best avoided in conditions where raised intracranial pressure may be suspected.

Unilateral non-dominant ECT has been shown in a number of studies to produce as good a clinical effect as bilateral ECT, but to be accompanied by earlier immediate recovery, and less associated with side-effects such as confusion and memory deficits.[568]

Reported side-effects include transient confusion, with memory disturbance characterized by a short retrograde amnesia and a longer post-ECT amnesia. This may persist for several weeks after a course of treatment, although permanent deficits in memory have not been demonstrated. Some studies have actually shown an improvement in memory following ECT, and in these cases the impairment of memory was probably a symptom of the depression, and the results due to the relief of the depression. Verbal learning has been shown to be affected more by ECT to the dominant hemisphere, while non-dominant ECT impairs non-verbal and visuo-spatial abilities. A retrospective survey of delayed retention and remote memory in patients who had received unilateral and bilateral ECT 6 to 9 months previously compared with a control group, indicated no impairment on psychological testing, although the patients who had received bilateral ECT more often actually rated their memory as being impaired.[569] Other side-effects include headaches, nausea, and ataxia, and major hazards are those related to the anaesthesia. The risk of death is negligible, although older patients with cerebrovascular and cardio-vascular disease are more prone than young healthy patients. Fractures, which used to be a major complication, are now rarely seen.

Treatment with ECT is never started following the first consultation unless the patient has all the positive indications of a response to ECT and is actively suicidal, and usually a trial of psychotropic medication is made first. A course of ECT is 6–12 treatments and these, with rare exceptions, are given once or twice weekly. Occasionally maintenance ECT is given fortnightly or monthly to patients who continually relapse.

Psychosurgery

Following the experiments of Fulton and Jacobsen[570] on chimpanzees, which demonstrated marked changes in affective responses after removal of the frontal lobes, Moniz[571] in 1936 carried out the first frontal leucotomies in patients. The technique was fully developed by Freeman and Watts,[572] who defined the standard leucotomy, operating through lateral burr-holes in the temporal region. A cutting instrument was inserted and swept in an arc dividing a large amount of white matter. Later post-mortem studies showed considerable variation in the site of the lesions, although the great bulk of the fibres cut belonged to the thalamo-frontal radiation. The mortality of this operation was around 6% and morbidity was high, side-effects including haemorrhage, epilepsy, incontinence, weight gain, hypersomnia and personality disorder. Modifications of leucotomy were therefore introduced.[573] These included rostral leucotomy, prefrontal leucotomy, and bimedial leucotomy, in which less cerebral tissue was destroyed, and the target area was the lower medial quadrant of the frontal lobe. Following such operations, dramatic initial benefit was often seen, up to 70% of patients being improved at 6 weeks. Birley[574] reported a follow-up study of 106 cases operated on by modified leucotomy, a mean interval of 5 years after surgery, and noted a 75% overall improvement rate, the best results being seen with obsessional and recurrent affective disorders. Severe adverse personality change was noted in 6% of patients. In other series, adverse effects have been reported in up to 60% of patients, although for some leucotomy is reported as 'a decisive event', bringing about improvement after a long history of psychiatric disability.[573,]

More recently the development of stereotactic techniques has enabled small lesions to be placed accurately within the brain, especially target areas within the limbic system. In stereotactic tractotomy,[576] lesions are placed beneath the head of the caudate nucleus. In limbic leucotomy, small lesions are placed in the lower medial quadrant of the frontal lobe, and in the anterior cingulate gyrus. Prior to making the lesion, electrical stimulation is undertaken to identify physiologically active pathways. When such areas are stimulated, changes in respiratory rate, blood pressure and other autonomic responses are noted, and these sites are chosen for destruction. Mitchell-Heggs et al.[577] have recently followed up 66 patients who had this operation: 73% were improved at 6 weeks, and 76% at 16 months. The best results were seen in obsessional neurosis, anxiety and depression although six out of seven schizophrenics also responded. Changes occurred gradually, and improvement continued for up to 1 year. Patients with good premorbid personalities did better than those with poor adjustment in their social and work life before the operation. The adverse effects of this operation were few, with confusion, headache, laziness, and loss of sphincter control being reported immediately post-operatively, and tending to clear within a few weeks. There was no mortality and little change in personality recorded, which stands in marked contrast to the results of the freehand operations.

The indications for psychosurgery have been clearly laid down by Schurr,[578] and Kelly.[573] The type of person considered is likely to have had severe psychiatric illness, be potentially suicidal, and have been ill for an average of 10 years. They will have failed to respond to all alternative forms of therapy. The best responses are noted in patients suffering from depression and obsessional neurosis, with good premorbid personalities, from a stable home environment. Although patients with schizophrenia are said to do poorly with psychosurgery, some respond well to limbic leucotomy, showing a reduction in the number of psychotic episodes, and subsequently a reduced need for phenothiazines. Psychopathy is an absolute contraindication, and patients who are addicted to drug or alcohol are not suitable. The presence of organic brain damage including dementia is also a contraindication although increased age itself is not.

A number of other psychosurgical operations have been employed. In violent and aggressive behaviour, stereotactic operations on the amygdala, thalamus, and hypothalamus have been carried out. Narabayashi[579] in in particular has emphasized the effectiveness of medial amygdaloid lesions in the relief of behaviour disturbances associated with epilepsy. He emphasised the monoaminergic nature of the lesioned neurones, which project to the stria terminalis. A recent follow-up study of 58 patients, who received stereotactic amygdalotomies 1 to 11 years earlier for uncontrolled seizures, aggressive behaviour or both, indicated few post-operative difficulties. Of patients receiving surgery mainly for seizures, 50% were improved, and in those with conduct disorders without severe seizures, 33% showed improvement specifically in their behaviour. Nine patients had died, mostly due to complications of epilepsy.[580]

Biofeedback

The fundamental principle in biofeedback is to provide the patient with information, visual or otherwise, on the state of his own physiological system. Although it was considered that the autonomic nervous system was not under voluntary control, biofeedback techniques have now demonstrated this not to be the case, and specified responses can be 'reinforced' so that they occur with increasing frequency.

Clinically the use of biofeedback has grown rapidly in the last few years. Claims for success have occurred in a number of disorders, including tension, hypertension, insomnia, migraine, epilepsy, tension headache, pain, behaviour problems, alcoholism, Raynaud's disease, and depression, although to-date very few double-blind control trials have been carried out. In neuropsychiatry the main techniques are either EEG or EMG biofeedback. EMG biofeedback has been successfully employed in helping patients to overcome hemiplegia by direct muscle retraining, and to relieve tension and assist relaxation by encouraging patients to decrease EMG potentials in tense muscles, particularly scalp muscles. It has been shown to be particularly helpful in the management of tension headaches, where patients receive auditory feedback of the activity of their frontalis muscle.[581] EEG biofeedback has been claimed to be of value in epilepsy, particularly feedback of 12–14 c/s activity,[582] although further trials are necessary before it can be accepted as useful therapy. Skin temperature biofeedback, training patients to increase their peripheral temperature by hand warming, has been used successfully in migraine.[583]

Insulin coma therapy

This treatment was introduced by Sakel[584] for the treatment of schizophrenia, but is now rarely used. Coma was induced by the administration of the insulin in gradually increasing doses. Seizures often occurred during hypoglycaemia, and the therapeutic effect may well have been due to this, although patients who seemed unresponsive to ECT sometimes improved with this form of therapy.

Other physical treatments

Narcosis therapy or continuous sleep treatment was used for many years, although has now been supplanted by alternative methods. The principle was to provide sleep for 20 hours a day by the use of hypnotics and tranquillizing medications.[585] Today the psychotropic cocktail employed uses large doses of major tranquillizers, sometimes with methaqualone in addition, which treatment can be combined with ECT if necessary.

In sleep deprivation therapy, patients are either kept awake all night, or selectively deprived of REM sleep. Most likely to benefit are those with moderately severe unipolar or bipolar depressive illness, associated with loss of appetite, early waking, guilt and diurnal variation of symptoms. The treatment is well-tolerated and improvement is often noted the day after deprivation.[586]

References

1. Hunter, R. Psychiatry and Neurology. *Proceedings of the Royal Society of Medicine* **66**, 17–22 (1973).
2. Hunter, R., and MacAlpine, I. *Three Hundred Years of Psychiatry 1535–1860.* Oxford University Press, London (1963).
3. Zilboorg, G. *A History of Medical Psychology.* W. W. Norton & Co., New York (1941).
4. Griesinger, W. *Mental Pathology and Therapeutics.* Translated by C. Lockhart Robertson and J. Rutherford. New Sydenham Society, London (1857).
5. Viets, H.R. Heinrich Erb. *In: The Founders of Neurology.* Ed. Haymaker, W., and Schiller, F. Charles C. Thomas, Springfield (1970).
6. Ellenberger, H.F. *The Discovery of the Unconscious.* Basic Books Inc., New York (1970).
7. Bleuler, E. *Textbook of Psychiatry.* Translated by A. Brill. Macmillan, New York (1923).
8. Nieuwenhuys, R. Aspects of the Morphology of the Striatum. *In: Psychobiology of the Striatum.* Ed. Cools, A.R., Lohman, A.H.M., and van den Berken, J.H.L. pp.1–20. North-Holland Publishing Company, Oxford (1977).
9. Hassler, R. Striatal control of locomotion, intentional actions and of integrating and perceptive activity. *Journal of the Neurological Sciences,* **36**, 187–224 (1978).
10. Moruzzi, G., and Magoun, H.W. Brain-stem reticular formation and activation of the EEG. *Electroencephalography and Clinical Neurophysiology,* **1**, 455–473 (1949).
11. Brodal, A. *Neurological Anatomy in Relation to Clinical Medicine,* 2nd Edition. Oxford University Press, London (1969).
12. Aghajanian, G.K., and Wang, R.Y. Physiology and pharmacology of central serotoninergic neurones. *In: Psychopharmacology: A Generation of Progress.* Ed. Lipton, M.A., Dimascio, A., and Killan, K.F. pp.171–184. Raven Press, New York (1978).
13. Dahlstrom, A., and Fuxe, K. Evidence for the existence of monoamine-containing neurones in the CNS. *Acta Physiologica Scandinavica,* **62**, Suppl. 232 (1964).
14. Curzon, G. Transmitter amines in brain disease. *In: Biochemistry and Neurological Disease.* Ed. Davidson, A.M. pp.168–227. Blackwells, London (1977).
15. Cools, A.R. The influence of neuroleptics on central dopaminergic systems. *In: Neurotransmission and Disturbed Behaviour.* Ed. Van Praag, H.M., and Bruinvels, J. pp.73–95. Bohn Scheltema and Holkema, Utrecht (1977).
16. Stevens, J.R., and Livermore, A. Kindling of the mesolimbic dopamine system: animal model of psychosis. *Neurology,* **28**, 36–46 (1978).

17. Bunney, B.S., and Aghajanian, G.K. Mesolimbic and mesocortical dopaminergic systems: Physiology and pharmacology. *In: Psychopharmacology: A Generation of Progress*. Ed. Lipton, M.A., DiMascio, A., and Killan, K.F. Raven Press, New York (1978).
18. Barchas, J.D., Akil, H., Elliott, G.R., Holman, R.B., and Watson, S.J. Behavioural Neurochemistry — Neuroregulators and behavioural states. *Science*, **200**, 964–973 (1978).
19. Popper, K.R., and Eccles, J.C. *The Self and its Brain*. Springer-Verlag, London (1977).
20. Heath, R.G. Subcortical brain function correlates of psychopathology and epilepsy. *In: Psychopathology and Brain Dysfunction*. Ed. Shagass, C., Gershon, S., and Friedhoff, A.J. pp.51–67. Raven Press, New York (1977).
21. Iversen, S.D. Behaviour after Neostriatal Lesions in Animals. *In: The Neostriatum*. Ed. Divac, I. Pergamon Press, Oxford (To be published).
22. Van Rossum, J.M., Pijnenburg, A.J.J., Cools, A.R., Broekkamp, C.L.E., and Struyker Boudier, H.A.J. Behavioural Pharmacology of the Neostriatum and the Limbic System in: Neuropsychopharmacology. Ed. Bolssier, J.R., Hippins, L., and Pichot, P. pp.505–515 Excerpta Medica, New York (1975).
23. Iversen, S.D. Striatal Function and Stereotyped Behaviour. *In: Psychobiology of the Striatum*. Ed. Cools, A.R., Lohman, R.H.M., and van der Becken, J.H.L. pp.99–118. Elsevier, Holland (1977).
24. Jaspers, K. *General Psychopathology*. Translated by Hoenig, J., and Hamilton, M.W. Manchester University Press, Manchester (1963).
25. Charcot, J.M. *Lectures on the Diseases of the Nervous System*. Translated by G. Sigerson. New Sydenham Society, London (1877).
26. Hamilton, M. *Fish's Clinical Psychopathology*. John Wright & Sons, Bristol (1974).
27. Sedman, G. A phenomenological study of pseudo-hallucinations and related experiences. *Acta Psychiatrica Scandinavica*, **42**, 35–70 (1966).
28. Hare, E.H. A short note on pseudohallucinations. *British Journal of Psychiatry*, **122**, 469–476 (1973).
29. Schneider, K. Primäre und Sekundäre Symptome bei der Schizophrenie. *Fortschritte der Neurologie, Psychiatrie und Ihrer Grenzgebiete*, **25**, 487–590 (1957).
30. Lunn, V. On body hallucinations. *Acta Psychiatrica Scandinavica*, **41**, 387–399 (1965).
31. Schneider, K. The concept of delusion. *In: Themes and Variations in European Psychiatry*. Ed. Hirsch, S.R., and Shepherd, M. pp.33–39 John Wright & Sons, Bristol (1974).
32. Lucas, C.J., Sainsbury, P., and Collins, J.G. A social and clinical study of delusions in schizophrenia. *Journal of Mental Science*, **108**, 747–758 (1962).
33. Fish, F.J. *Schizophrenia*. John Wright & Sons Ltd., Bristol (1962).
34. Kleist, K. Schizophrenic symptoms and cerebral pathology. *Journal of Mental Science*, **106**, 246–254 (1960).
35. Goldstein, K. Functional Disturbances in Brain Damage. *In: American Handbook of Psychiatry*. Ed. Reiser, M.F. Vol. 4, pp.182–207. Basic Books, New York (1965).
36. Critchley, M. The neurology of psychotic speech. *British Journal of Psychiatry*, **110**, 353–364 (1964).
37. Notes on eliciting and recording clinical information. Department of Psychiatry Teaching Committee, Institute of Psychiatry, London. Oxford University Press, London (1973).
38. Plum, F., and Posner, J.B. *The Diagnosis of Stupor and Coma*, 2nd Edition. F. A. Davis Company, Philadelphia (1972).
39. Strub, R.L., and Black, F.W. *The Mental Status Examination in Neurology*. F. A. Davis, Philadelphia (1977).
40. Orm, J.E., Lee, D., and Smith, M.R. Psychological assessments of brain

256

damage and intellectual impairments in psychiatric patients. *British Journal of Social and Clinical Psychology*, **3**, 161–167 (1964).
41. McFie, J. *Assessment of Organic Intellectual Impairment.* Academic Press, London (1975).
42. Lishman, W.A. *Organic Psychiatry.* Blackwell, London (1978).
43. Nelson, H.E., and McKenna, P. The use of current reading ability in the assessment of dementia. *British Journal of Social and Clinical Psychology*, **14**, 259–267 (1975).
44. Reitan, R.M. Psychological deficits resulting from cerebral lesions in man. *In: The Frontal Granular Cortex and Behaviour.* Ed. Warren, J.M. and Akert, K. pp.295–312 McGraw-Hill, London (1964).
45. Raven, J.C. *Progressive Matrices.* H. K. Lewis, London (1938).
46. Walton, D., and Black, D.A. The validity of a psychological test of brain damage. *British Journal of Medical Psychology*, **30**, 270–279 (1957).
47. Kendrick, D.C., Parboosingh, R.C., and Post, F. A synonym learning test for use in elderly psychiatric subjects: a validation study. *British Journal of Social and Clinical Psychology*, **4**, 63–71 (1965).
48. Inglis, J. A paired-associate learning test for use with elderly psychiatric patients. *Journal of Mental Science*, **105**, 440–443 (1959).
49. Graham, F.K., and Kendall, B.S. Memory-for-designs Test: Revised General Manual. *Perceptual and Motor Skills*, **11**, 147–188 (1960).
50. Warrington, E.K. Deficient recognition memory in organic amnesia. *Cortex*, **10**, 289–291 (1974).
51. Milner, B. Some effects of frontal lobectomy in man. *In: The Frontal Granular Cortex and Behaviour.* Ed. Warren, J.M. and Akert, K. pp.313–334. McGraw-Hill, New York (1964).
52. Bannister, D. The nature and measurement of schizophrenic thought disorder. *Journal of Mental Science*, **108**, 825–842 (1962).
53. Beck, A.T., Ward, C.H., Mendelson, U., Mock, J., and Erbough, J. An inventory for measuring depression. *Archives of General Psychiatry*, **4**, 561–571 (1961).
54. Zung, W.W.K. A self-rating depression scale. *Archives of General Psychiatry*, **12**, 63–70 (1965).
55. Hamilton, M. A rating scale for depression. *Journal of Neurology, Neurosurgery and Psychiatry*, **23**, 56–61 (1960).
56. Schwab, J.J., Bialow, M.R., and Holger, C.G. A comparison of two rating scales for depression. *Journal of Clinical Psychology*, **23**, 94–96 (1967).
57. Brown, G.L., and Zung, W.W.K. Depression scales: Self or physician rating? A validation of certain clinically observable phenomena. *Comprehensive Psychiatry*, **13**, 361–367 (1972).
58. Hamilton, M. The assessment of anxiety states by rating. *British Journal of Medical Psychology*, **32**, 50–55 (1959).
59. Spielberger, C.D. The measurement of state and trait anxiety: conceptual and methodological issues. *In: Emotions — their Parameters and Measurement.* Ed. Levi, L. pp.713–725. Raven Press, New York (1975).
60. Goldberg, D.P., Cooper, B., Eastwood, M.R., Kedward, H.B., and Shepherd, M. A standardised Psychiatric Interview for use in community surveys. *British Journal of Preventative and Social Medicine*, **24**, 18–23 (1970).
61. Overall, J.E., and Goreham, D.R. The brief psychiatric rating scale. *Psychological Reports*, **10**, 799–812 (1962).
62. McNair, D.M., and Lorr, M. An analysis of mood in neurotics. *Journal of Abnormal and Social Psychology*, **69**, 620–627 (1964).
63. Wing, J.K., Cooper, J.E., and Sartorius, N. *Measurement and Classification of Psychiatric Symptoms.* Cambridge University Press, Cambridge (1974).
64. Shapiro, M.B., Litman, G.K., Nias, D.K.B., and Hendry, E.R. A clinician's approach to experimental research. *Journal of Clinical Psychology*, **29**, 165–169 (1973).

65. Eysenck, H.J., and Eysenck, S.B.J. *Manual of the EPI*. University of London Press, London (1964).
66. Cooper, J. The Leyton Obsessional Inventory. *Psychological Medicine*, **1**, 48–64 (1970).
67. Foulds, G.A. *Personality and Personal Illness*. Tavistock Publications, London (1965).
68. Clare, A. *Psychiatry in Dissent*. Tavistock Publications, London (1976).
69. Fish, F.J. *An Outline of Psychiatry*. John Wright & Sons Ltd, Bristol (1968).
70. I.S.C.D. *A Glossary of Mental Disorders*. H.M.S.O., London (1968).
71. Kernberg, O. Borderline personality organisation. *Journal of the American Psychoanalytic Association,* **15**, 641–685 (1967).
72. Shields, J. *Monozygotic Twins brought up apart and brought up together*. Oxford University Press, London (1962).
73. Hill, J.D.N. EEG in episodic psychotic and psychopathic behaviour: A classification of data. *Electroencephalography and Clinical Neurophysiology*, **4**, 419–471 (1952).
74. Harper, M.A. The significance of an abnormal EEG in psychopathic personalities. *Australia and New Zealand Journal of Psychiatry*, **6**, 215–224 (1972).
75. Williams, D. Neural factors to habitual aggression. *Brain*, **92**, 503–520 (1969).
76. Fenton, G.W., Fenwick, P.B.C., Ferguson, W., and Lam, C.T. The contingent negative variation in antisocial behaviour: A pilot study of Broadmoor patients. *British Journal of Psychiatry*, **132**, 368–377 (1978).
77. Money, J. Human behaviour cytogenetics: review of psychopathology in three syndromes — 47 XXY : 47 XYY : 45 X. *Journal of Sex Research*, **11**, 181–200 (1975).
78. Kringlen, E. Obsessional neurotics. *British Journal of Psychiatry*, **111**, 709–722 (1965).
79. Lewis, A.J. *Inquiries in Psychiatry — Clinical and Social Investigations*. Science House Inc., New York (1967).
80. Perris, C. A study of bipolar (manic-depressive) and unipolar recurrent depressive psychoses. *Acta Psychiatrica Scandinavica*, **42**, Suppl. 194 (1966).
81. Kretschmer, E. The sensitive delusion of reference. *In: Themes and Variations in European Psychiatry*. Ed. Hirsch, S.R., and Shepherd, M. John Wright & Sons, Bristol (1974).
82. Askevold, F. Predictive value of neuropathic traits. *Acta Psychiatrica Scandinavica*, **56**, 32–38 (1977).
83. Sims, A., and Prior, P. The pattern of mortality in severe neuroses. *British Journal of Psychiatry*, **133**, 299–305 (1978).
84. Stengel, E. A study of some clinical aspects of the relationship between obsessional neurosis and psychotic reaction types. *Journal of Mental Science*, **91**, 166–187 (1945).
85. Sacks, O. *Awakenings*. Duckworth, London (1973).
86. Tuke, D. H. *A Dictionary of Psychological Medicine*. J. and A. Churchill, London (1892).
87. Kendell, R.E. The classification of depressions. A review of contemporary confusion. *British Journal of Psychiatry*, **129**, 15–28 (1976).
88. Paykel, E.S., Prusoff, B., and Klerman, G.L. The endogenous-neurotic continuum in depression. *Journal of Psychiatric Research*, **8**, 73–90 (1971).
89. West, E.D., and Dally, P.J. Effect of iproniazid in depressive syndromes. *British Medical Journal*, **1**, 1491–1494 (1959).
90. Shaw, D.M., Camps, F.E., and Eccleston, E. 5-hydroxytryptamine in the hindbrains of depressive suicides. *British Journal of Psychiatry*, **113**, 1407–1411 (1967).
91. Van Praag, H.M. New evidence of serotonin deficient depressions. *Neuropsychobiology*, **3**, 56–63 (1977).
92. Coppen, A., Eccleston, E.G., and Peet, M. Total and free tryptophan concentration in the plasma of depressive patients. *Lancet*, **ii**, 60–63 (1973).

258

93. Åsberg, M., Träskman, L., and Thören, P. 5-HIAA in the cerebrospinal fluid. *Archives of General Psychiatry*, **33**, 1193-1197 (1976).
94. Bridges, P.K., Bartlett, J.R., Sepping, P., Kantamaneni, B.D., and Curzon, G. Precursors and metabolites of 5-Hydroxytryptamine and dopamine in the ventricular CSF of psychiatric patients. *Psychological Medicine*, **6**, 399-405 (1976).
95. Schildkraut, J.J. Depressions and biogenic amines. *In: American Handbook of Psychiatry*, Vol. **6**. Ed. Hanburg, D.A., and Brodie, K.H. Basic Books, New York (1975).
96. Wyatt, R.J., Portnoy, B., and Kupfer, D.J. Resting plasma catecholamine concentrations in patients with depression and anxiety. *Archives of General Psychiatry*, **24**, 65-70 (1971).
97. Bunney, W.E. The switch process in manic-depressive psychosis. *Annals of Internal Medicine*, **87**, 319-335 (1977).
98. Bunney, W.E., Davis, J.M., Weilmalherbe, H., and Smith, E.R. Biochemical changes in psychotic depression. High norepinephrine levels in psychotic vs neurotic depression. *Archives of General Psychiatry*, **16**, 448-460 (1967).
99. Maas, J.W. Biogenic amines and depression. *Archives of General Psychiatry*, **32**, 1357-1361 (1975).
100. Van Praag, H.M. Significance of biochemical parameters in the diagnosis, treatment and prevention of depressive disorders. *Biological Psychiatry*, **12**, 101-131 (1977).
101. Hill, O.W. Child bereavement and adult psychiatric disturbance. *Journal of Psychosomatic Research*, **16**, 357-360 (1972).
102. Birtchnell, J. Psychiatric breakdown following recent parent death. *British Journal of Medical Psychology*, **48**, 379-390 (1975).
103. Paykel, E.S., Myers, J.K., Dienelt, M.N., Klerman, G.L., Lindenthal, J.L., and Pepper, M.P. Life events and depression. *Archives of General Psychiatry*, **21**, 753-760 (1969).
104. Richards, D.H. A post-hysterectomy syndrome. *Lancet*, **ii**, 983-986 (1974).
105. Whitlock, F.A., and Evans, L.E.J. Drugs and depression. *Drugs*, **15**, 53-71 (1978).
106. Cutting, J.C., Clare, A.W., and Mann, A.H. Cycloid psychosis: An investigation of the diagnostic concept. *Psychological Medicine*, **8**, 637-648 (1978).
107. Slater, E., and Roth, M. *Clinical Psychiatry*, 3rd Edition. Baillière, Tindall and Cassell, London (1969).
108. Kety, S.S., Rosenthal, D., Wender, P.H., and Schlusinger, F. Mental illness in the biological and adoptive families of adopted schizophrenics. *American Journal of Psychiatry*, **128**, 302-306 (1971).
109. Hirsch, S.R., and Leff, J.P. Parental abnormalities of verbal communication in the transmission of schizophrenia. *Psychological Medicine*, **1**, 118-127 (1971).
110. Fuller Torrey, E., and Peterson, M.R. Schizophrenia and the limbic system. *Lancet*, **ii**, 942-946 (1974).
111. Smythes, J.R. Recent progress in schizophrenia research. *Lancet*, **ii**, 136-139 (1976).
112. Snyder, S.H., Banerjee, S.P., Yamamura, H.I., and Greenberg, D. Drugs, neurotransmitters and schizophrenia. *Science*, **184**, 1243-1253 (1974).
113. Van Praag, H.M., and Korf, J. Neuroleptics, catecholamines and psychoses. A study of their interrelations. *American Journal of Psychiatry*, **132**, 593-597 (1975).
114. Iversen, L. Neuroleptics and brain dopaminergic systems. *In: Symposium on Neuroleptics and Schizophrenia*. Ed. Simister, J.M. pp.5-15, Lundbeck Ltd, England (1979).
115. Owen, F., Cross, A.J., Crow, T.J., Longden, A., Poulter, M., and Riley, G.J. Increased dopamine-receptor sensitivity in schizophrenia. *Lancet*, **ii**, 223-225 (1978).
116. Domschke, W., Dickschas, A., and Mitznegg, P. CSF β-endorphin in schizophrenia. *Lancet*, **i**, 1024 (1979).

117. Verhoeven, W.M.A., Van Praag, H.M., Botter, P.A., Sunier, A., Van Ree, J.M., and De Wied, D. (Des-Tyr)-γ-endorphin in schizophrenia. *Lancet*, **i**, 1046-7 (1978).

118. Johnstone, E.C., Crow, T.J., Frith, C.D., Stevens, M., Kreel, L., and Husband, J. The dementia of dementia praecox. *Acta Psychiatrica Scandinavica*, **57**, 305-324 (1978).

119. Stevens, J.R. Disturbances of ocular movements and blinking in schizophrenia. *Journal of Neurology, Neurosurgery and Psychiatry*, **41**, 1024-1030 (1978).

120. Bleuler, M. A 23-year longitudinal study of 208 schizophrenics and impressions in regard to the nature of schizophrenia. *In: The Transmission of Schizophrenia*. Eds. Rosenthal, D., and Kety, S.S. Oxford, Pergamon (1968).

121. Stephens, J.H. Long-term course and prognosis in schizophrenia. *Seminars in Psychiatry*, **2**, 464-485 (1970).

122. Brown, G.W., Monck, E.M., Carstairs, G.M., and Wing, J.K. Influence of family life on the course of schizophrenic illness. *British Journal of Preventative and Social Medicine*, **16**, 55-68 (1962).

123. Vaughan, C.E., and Leff, J.P. The influence of family and social factors on the course of psychiatric illness. *British Journal of Psychiatry*, **129**, 125-137 (1976).

124. Creer, C., and Wing, J. Living with a schizophrenic patient. *British Journal of Hospital Medicine*, **14**, 73-82 (1975).

125. Kasanin, J. The acute schizoaffective psychoses. *American Journal of Psychiatry*, **13**, 97-126 (1933).

126. Procci, W.R. Schizoaffective psychosis: fact or fiction. *Archives of General Psychiatry*, **33**, 1167-1178 (1976).

127. Balint, M. *The Doctor, his Patient and the Illness*. International Universities Press Inc., New York (1957).

128. Schiff, S.K., and Pilot, M.L. An approach to psychiatric consultation in the general hospital. *Archives of General Psychiatry*, **1**, 349-357 (1959).

129. Meyer, E., and Mendelson, M. Psychiatric consultations with patients on medical and surgical wards: patterns and process. *Psychiatry*, **24**, 197-220 (1961).

130. Lipowski, Z.J. Review of consultation psychiatry and psychosomatic medicine. I. General principles. *Psychosomatic Medicine*, **29**, 153-171 (1967).

131. Knights, E.B., and Folstein, M.F. Unsuspected emotional and cognitive disturbance in medical patients. *Annals of Internal Medicine*, **87**, 723-724 (1977).

132. Kirk, C., and Saunders, M. Primary psychiatric illness in a neurological outpatient department in North East England. *Acta Psychiatrica Scandinavica*, **56**, 294-302 (1977).

133. De Paulo, J.R., and Folstein, M.F. Psychiatric disturbances in neurological patients: Detection, recognition and hospital course. *Annals of Neurology*, **4**, 225-228 (1978).

134. Lipowski, Z.J., and Kiriakos, R.Z. Borderlands between neurology and psychiatry: Observations in a neurological hospital. *Psychiatry in Medicine*, **3**, 131-147 (1972).

135. Schilder, P. *Contributions to Developmental Neuropsychiatry*. Ed. Bender, L. Tavistock Publications, London (1964).

136. Imboden, J.B. Psychosocial determinants of recovery. *Advances in Psychosomatic Medicine*, **8**, 142-155 (1972).

137. Kahana, R.J., and Bibring, G.L. Personality Types in Medical Management. *In: Psychiatry and Medical Practice in a General Hospital*. Ed. Zinberg, E.N. pp.108-122. International Universities Press, New York (1964).

138. Lipowski, Z.J. Review of consultation psychiatry and psychosomatic medicine. II. Clinical aspects. *Psychosomatic Medicine*, **29**, 201-212 (1967).

139. Wilson-Barnett, J. *Stress in Hospital*. Churchill Livingstone, Edinburgh (1979).

140. Rahe, R.H. Life stress and illness. *In: Consultation-Liaison Psychiatry*. Ed. Pasnau, R.P. pp.115-122 Grune and Stratton, New York (1975).

260

141. Lindemann, E. Symptomatology and management of acute grief. *American Journal of Psychiatry*, **101**, 141–148 (1944).
142. Parkes, C.M. Effects of bereavement on physical and mental health — a study of the medical records of widows. *British Medical Journal*, **2**, 274–279 (1964).
143. Engel, G.L. A life setting conducive to illness. *Annals of Internal Medicine*, **69**, 293–300 (1968).
144. Latimer, P. Psychophysiologic Disorders: A Critical Appraisal of Concept and Theory Illustrated with reference to the Irritable Bowel Syndrome. *Psychological Medicine*, **9**, 71–90 (1979).
145. Bartrop, R.W., Lazarus, L., Luckhurst, E., Kiloh, L., and Penny, R. Depressed lymphocyte function after bereavement. *Lancet*, **i**, 834–836 (1977).
146. Mechanic, D. *Medical Sociology. A Selective View*. The Free Press, New York (1968).
147. Pilowsky, I. The diagnosis of abnormal illness behaviour. *Australia and New Zealand Journal of Psychiatry*, **5**, 136–138 (1971).
148. Pilowsky, I. Dimensions of abnormal illness behaviour. *Australia and New Zealand Journal of Psychiatry*, **9**, 141–147 (1975).
149. Pilowsky, I. The classification of abnormal illness behaviour. *British Journal of Medical Psychology*, **51**, 131–137 (1977).
150. Zborowski, M. *People in Pain*. Jossey-Bass, San Francisco (1969).
151. Breuer, J., and Freud, S. Studies on Hysteria. *In: Complete Psychological Works of Freud*. Vol. 2, pp.1893–1895. Hogarth Press, London (1955).
152. Engel, G. L. Conversion symptoms. *In: Signs and Symptoms*. Ed. MacBryde and Blacklow. 5th Edition, pp.650–668. Pitman Medical, London (1970).
153. Pilowsky, I. Dimensions of hypochondriasis. *British Journal of Psychiatry*, **113**, 89–93 (1967).
154. Veith, I. *Hysteria: The History of a Disease*. University of Chicago Press, Chicago (1965).
155. Merskey, H. *The Analysis of Hysteria*. Baillière Tindall and Co., London (1979).
156. Chodoff, P., and Lyons, H. Hysteria, the hysterical personality and 'hysterical' conversion. *American Journal of Psychiatry*, **114**, 734–740 (1958).
157. Lazare, A., Klerman, G.L., and Armor, D.J. Oral, obsessive and hysterical personality patterns. *Archives of General Psychiatry*, **14**, 624–630 (1966).
158. Ljungberg, L. Hysteria: A clinical, prognostic and genetic study. *Acta Psychiatrica et Neurologica Scandinavica*, **32**, Suppl. 112 (1957).
159. Merskey, H., and Trimble, M.R. Personality, sexual adjustment and brain lesions in patients with conversion symptoms. *American Journal of Psychiatry*, **136**, 179–182 (1979).
160. Gowers, W.R. *A Manual of Diseases of the Nervous System*, 2nd Edition. Churchill, London (1893).
161. Whitlock, F.A. The aetiology of hysteria. *Acta Psychiatrica Scandinavica*, **43**, 144–162 (1967).
162. Merskey, H., and Buhrich, N.A. Hysteria and organic brain disease. *British Journal of Medical Psychology*, **48**, 359–366 (1975).
163. Slater, E., and Glithero, E. A follow-up of patients diagnosed as suffering from hysteria. *Journal of Psychosomatic Research*, **9**, 9–13 (1965).
164. Tissenbaum, M.J., Harter, H.M., and Friedman, A.P. Organic neurological syndromes diagnosed as functional disorders. *Journal of the American Medical Association*, **147**, 1519–1521 (1951).
165. Winokur, G., and Leonard, C. Sexual life in patients with hysteria. *Diseases of the Nervous System*, **24**, 337–343 (1963).
166. Stefanis, C., Markidis, M., and Christodoulou, G. Observations on the evolution of hysterical symptomatology. *British Journal of Psychiatry*, **128**, 269–275 (1976).

167. Head, H. An address on the diagnosis of hysteria. *British Medical Journal*, 1, 827–829 (1922).
168. Ziegler, D.K. Neurological disease and hysteria — the differential diagnosis. *International Journal of Neuropsychiatry*, 3, 388–395 (1967).
169. Slater, E. Diagnosis of 'hysteria'. *British Medical Journal*, 1, 1395–1399 (1965).
170. Carter, A.B. The prognosis of certain hysterical symptoms. *British Medical Journal*, 1, 1076–1079 (1949).
171. Guze, S.B., and Perley, M.J. Observations on the natural history of hysteria. *American Journal of Psychiatry*, 119, 960–965 (1963).
172. Lewis, A. The Survival of hysteria. *Psychological Medicine*, 5, 9–12 (1975).
173. Ziegler, D.G., and Paul, N. On natural history of hysteria in women. *Diseases of the Nervous System*, 15, 301–306 (1954).
174. Schilder, P. *Brain and Personality*. International Universities Press, New York (1951).
175. Chodoff, P. The diagnosis of hysteria: An overview. *American Journal of Psychiatry*, 131, 1073–1078 (1974).
176. Ludwig, A.M. Hysteria — a neurobiological theory. *Archives of General Psychiatry*, 27, 771–777 (1972).
177. Walters, A. Psychogenic regional sensory and motor disorders alias hysteria. *Canadian Psychiatric Association Journal*, 14, 573–589 (1969).
178. Purtell, J.J., Robins, E., and Cohen, M.E. Observations on clinical aspects of hysteria. *Journal of the American Medical Association*, 146, 902–909 (1951).
179. Cloninger, C.R., and Guze, S.B., Hysteria and parental psychiatric illness. *Psychological Medicine*, 5, 27–31 (1975).
180. Scallett, A., Cloninger, R., and Othmer, E. The management of chronic hysteria: a review and a double-blind trial of electrosleep and other relaxation methods. *Diseases of the Nervous System*, 37, 347–353 (1976).
181. Kenyon, F.E. Hypochondriacal states. *British Journal of Psychiatry*, 129, 1–14 (1976).
182. Asher, R. Munchausen's syndrome. *Lancet*, i, 339–341 (1951).
183. Snowdon, J., Solomons, R., and Druce, H. Feigned bereavement: twelve cases. *British Journal of Psychiatry*, 133, 15–19 (1978).
184. Bursten, B. On Munchausen's syndrome. *Archives of General Psychiatry*, 13, 261–268 (1965).
185. Hawkings, J.R., Jones, K.S., Sim, M., and Tibbetts, R.W. Deliberate disability. *British Medical Journal*, 1, 361–367 (1956).
186. Lancet Leading Article. Factitious hypoglycaemia. *Lancet*, i, 1293 (1978).
187. Lipowski, Z.J. Organic Brain Syndromes: Overview and Classification. *In: Psychiatric Aspects of Neurological Disease*. Ed. Benson, D.F., and Blumer, D. pp.11–34. Grune and Stratton, London (1975).
188. Bleuler, M. Acute mental concomitants of physical diseases. *In: Psychiatric Aspects of Neurological Disease*. Ed. Benson, D.F., and Blumer, D. pp.37–61. Grune and Stratton, London (1975).
189. Stengel, E. The organic confusional state and the organic dementias. *British Journal of Hospital Medicine*, 1-2, 719–724 (1969).
190. Lipowski, Z.J. Delirium, clouding of consciousness and confusion. *Journal of Nervous and Mental Disease*, 145, 227–255 (1967).
191. Engel, G.L., and Romano, J. Delirium: A syndrome of cerebral insufficiency. *Chronic Diseases*, 9, 260–277 (1959).
192. Bleuler, M. Psychiatry of cerebral diseases. *British Medical Journal*, ii, 1233–1238 (1951).
193. Victor, M., and Hope, J.M. The phenomenon of auditory hallucinations in chronic alcoholism. A critical evaluation of the status of alcoholic hallucinations. *Journal of Nervous and Mental Disease*, 126, 451–481 (1958).

194. Jacobsen, C.F. Studies of cerebral functions in primates. *Comparative Psychology and Psychiatry*, **33**, 558-559 (1935).
195. Luria, A.R. *The Working Brain. An Introduction to Neuropsychology*. Translated by Haigh, B. Basic Books, New York (1973).
196. Blumer, D., and Benson, D.F. Personality changes with frontal and temporal lobe lesions. *In: Psychiatric Aspects of Neurologic Disease*. Ed. Benson, D.F., and Blumer, D. pp.151-169. Grune and Stratton, London (1975).
197. Hecaen, H., and Albert, M.L. Disorders of mental functioning related to frontal pathology. *In: Psychiatric Aspects of Neurological Disease*. Ed. Benson, D.F., and Blumer, D. pp.137-149. Grune and Stratton, London (1975).
198. Teuber, H.L. The riddle of frontal lobe function in man. *In: The Frontal Granular Cortex and Behaviour*. Ed. Warren, J.M. and Akert, K. pp.410-444. McGraw-Hill, New York (1964).
199. Goldstein, K. The mental changes due to frontal lobe damage. *Journal of Psychology*, **17**, 187-208 (1944).
200. Waxman, S.G., and Geschwind, N. The interictal behaviour syndrome of temporal lobe epilepsy. *Archives of General Psychiatry*, **32**, 1580-1586 (1975).
201. Lishman, W.A. Brain damage in relation to psychiatric disability after head injury. *British Journal of Psychiatry*, **114**, 373-410 (1968).
202. Klüver, H., and Bucy, P.C. Psychic blindness and other symptoms following bilateral temporal lobectomy in Rhesus monkeys. *American Journal of Physiology*, **119**, 352-353 (1937).
203. Benson, D.F., and Geschwind, N. The aphasias and related disturbances. *In: Clinical Neurology*, Vol. 1, Ed. Baker, A.B., and Baker, L.H. pp.1861-1887. Harper and Row, Hagerstown (1971).
204. Malamud, N. Organic Brain Disease mistaken for Psychiatric Disorder: A Clinicopathologic Study. *In: Psychiatric Aspects of Neurological Disease*. Ed. Benson, D.F., and Blumer, D. pp.287-305. Grune and Stratton, New York (1975).
205. Williams, D. Man's temporal lobe. *Brain*, **91**, 639-654 (1968).
206. Tulving, E. Episodic and semantic memory. *In: Organisation of Memory*. Ed. Tulving, E., and Donaldson, W. Academic Press, New York (1972).
207. Hyden, H. Biochemical approaches to learning and memory. *In: Beyond Reductionism*. Ed. Koestler, A., and Smythies, J.R. pp.85-103. Hutchinson, London (1969).
208. Young, J.Z. *Programmes of the Brain*. Oxford University Press, London (1978).
209. Luria, A.R. *The Neuropsychology of Memory*. Winston and Sons, Washington (1976).
210. Korsakoff, S.S. Etude médico-psychologique sur une forme des maladies de mémoire. *Revue Philosophique*, **28**, 501-530 (1889).
211. Symonds, C.P. Disorders of memory. *Brain*, **89**, 625-644 (1966).
212. Victor, M., Adams, R.D., and Collins, G.H. *The Wernicke-Korsakoff Syndrome*. Blackwell Scientific Publications, Oxford (1971).
213. Mercer, B., Wapner, W., Gardner, H., and Benson, D.F. A study of confabulation. *Archives of Neurology*, **34**, 429-433 (1977).
214. Warrington, E.K., and Weiskrantz, L. An analysis of short-term and long-term memory defects in man. *In: The Physiological Basis of Memory*. Ed. Deutch, J.A. pp.365-395. Academic Press, New York (1973).
215. Cutting, J. Patterns of performance in amnesic subjects. *Journal of Neurology, Neurosurgery and Psychiatry*, **41**, 278-282 (1978).
216. Butters, N., and Cermak, L.S. Neuropsychological studies of alcoholic Korsakoff patients. *In: Empirical Studies of Alcoholism*. Ed. Goldstein and Neuringer. pp.153-193. Ballinger, Cambridge (1976).
217. L'Hermitte, F., and Signoret, J.L. Analyse neuropsychologique et differenciation des syndromes amnesiques. *Revue Neurologique*, **126**, 161-178 (1972).

218. Brierley, J.B. Neuropathology of amnesic states. *In: Amnesia*, 2nd Edition. Ed. Whitty, C.W.M., and Zangwill, O.L. pp.199-223. Butterworths, London (1977).

219. Warrington, E.K., Logue, V., and Pratt, R.T.C. The anatomical localisation of selective impairment of auditory verbal short-term memory. *Neuropsychologia*, **9**, 377-387 (1971).

220. Croft, P.B., Heathfield, K.W.G., and Swash, M. Differential diagnosis of transient amnesias. *British Medical Journal*, **4**, 593-596 (1973).

221. Sternberg, D.E., and Jarvik, M.E. Memory functions in depression. *Archives of General Psychiatry*, **33**, 219-224 (1976).

222. Lishman, W.A. Selective factors in memory: Part 2 — Affective disorder. *Psychological Medicine*, **2**, 248-253 (1972).

223. Stengel, E. On the aetiology of fugue states. *Journal of Mental Science*, **87**, 572-599 (1941).

224. Pratt, R.T.C. Psychogenic loss of memory. *In: Amnesia*. Ed. Whitty, C.W.M., and Zanwill, O.L. pp.224-232. Butterworths, London (1977).

225. Kennedy, A., and Neville, J. Sudden loss of memory. *British Medical Journal*, **2**, 428-433 (1957).

226. Butler, R.B., and Benson, D.F. Aphasia: A clinical-anatomical correlation. *British Journal of Hospital Medicine*, **12**, 211-217 (1974).

227. Brown, J.W. The neural organisation of language. Aphasia and neuropsychiatry. *In: American Handbook of Psychiatry*, Vol. 4. Ed. Reiser, M.F. pp.244-278. Basic Books, New York (1975).

228. Geschwind, N. Disconnection syndromes in animals and man. *Brain*, **88**, 237-294, 585-644 (1965).

229. Benson, D.F. Psychiatric aspects of aphasia. *British Journal of Psychiatry*, **123**, 555-566 (1973).

230. Sparks, R., Helms, N., and Albert, M. Aphasia rehabilitation resulting from melodic intonation therapy. *Cortex*, **10**, 303-316 (1974).

231. Warrington, E.K. Constructional apraxia. *In: Handbook of Clinical Neurology*. Ed. Vinken, P.J., and Bruyn, G.W. Vol. 4, pp.67-83. North-Holland Publishing Company, Amsterdam (1969).

232. Brain, W.R. *Speech disorders: Aphasia, Apraxia and Agnosia*. Butterworths, London (1965).

233. Bay, E. Disturbances of visual perception and their examination. *Brain*, **76**, 515-550 (1953).

234. Critchley, M. The problem of visual agnosia. *Journal of the Neurological Sciences*, **1**, 274-290 (1964).

235. Weinstein, E.A., and Kahn, R.L. *Denial of Illness. Symbolic and Physiological Aspects*. Thomas, Springfield, Ill. (1955).

236. Stengel, E. Loss of spatial orientation, constructional apraxia and Gerstmann's syndrome. *Journal of Mental Science*, **90**, 753-760 (1944).

237. Benson, D.F., and Geschwind, N. Developmental Gerstmann syndrome. *Neurology*, **20**, 293-298 (1970).

238. Gardiner, H. *The Shattered Mind*. Vintage Books, New York (1974).

239. Lance, J.W. Simple formed hallucinations confined to the area of a specific visual field defect. *Brain*, **99**, 719-734 (1976).

240. Hess, W.R. *The Biology of Mind*. Translated by Von Bonin, G. University of Chicago Press, London (1964).

241. Brain, W.R., and Walton, J.N. *Brain's Diseases of the Nervous System*. Oxford University Press, London (1969).

242. Riese, W. *Principles of Neurology*. Smith Ely Jelliffe Trust, New York (1950).

243. Zangwill, O.L. The cerebral localisation of psychological function. *Advancement of Science*, **1963**, 335-344.

244. Pearce, J., and Miller, E. *Clinical Aspects of Dementia*. Ballière Tindall, London (1973).

264

245. Kay, D.W.K., Foster, E.M., McKechnie, A.A., and Roth, M. Mental illness and hospital use in the elderly: A random sample followed up. *Comprehensive Psychiatry*, **11**, 26–35 (1970).
246. Marsden, C.D., and Harrison, M.G.H. Outcome of investigation of patients with presenile dementia. *British Medical Journal*, **2**, 249–251 (1972).
247. Ron, M.A., Toone, B.K., Garralda, M.E., and Lishman, W.A. Diagnostic accuracy in presenile dementia. *British Journal of Psychiatry*, **134**, 161–168 (1979).
248. Gordon, E.B., and Sim, M. The electroencephalogram in presenile dementia. *Journal of Neurology, Neurosurgery and Psychiatry*, **30**, 285–291 (1967).
249. Bowen, D.M., Smith, C.B., White, P., and Davison, A.N. Neurotransmitter-related enzymes and indices of hypoxia in senile dementia and other abiotrophies. *Brain*, **99**, 459–496 (1976).
250. Perry, E.K., Perry, R.H., Blessed, G., and Tomlinson, B.E. Necropsy evidence of central cholinergic deficits in senile dementia. *Lancet*, **i**, 189 (1977).
251. Ghoneim, M.M., and Mewaldt, S.P. Studies on human memory. The interactions of diazepam, scopolamine and physostigmine. *Psychopharmacology*, **52**, 1–6 (1977).
252. Robertson, E.E., LeRoux, A., and Brown, J.H. The clinical differentiation of Pick's disease. *Journal of Mental Science*, **104**, 1000–1024 (1958).
253. May, W.W. Creutzfeldt–Jacob disease. *Acta Neurologica Scandinavica*, **44**, 1–32 (1968).
254. Nevin, S. On some aspects of cerebral degeneration in later life. *Proceedings of the Royal Society of Medicine*, **60**, 517–526 (1967).
255. Beck, E., Daniel, P.M., Matthews, W.B., Stevens, D.L., Alpers, M.P., Asher, D.M., Gajdusek, D.C., and Gibbs, C.J. Creutzfeldt–Jacob Disease — The neuropathology of a transmission experiment. *Brain*, **92**, 699–716 (1969).
256. Bernoulli, C., Siegfried, J., Baumgartner, G., Regli, F., Rabinowicz, T., Gajdusek, D.C., and Gibbs, C.J. Danger of accidental person-to-person transmission of Creutzfeldt–Jacob disease by surgery. *Lancet*, **i**, 478–479 (1977).
257. Gajdusek, D.C. Unconventional viruses. *In: Human Diseases Caused by Viruses*. Ed. Rothschild, H., Allison, F., and Howe, C. pp.233–258. Oxford University Press, New York (1978).
258. O'Brien, M.D., and Mallett, B.L. Cerebral cortex perfusion rates in dementia. *Journal of Neurology, Neurosurgery and Psychiatry*, **33**, 497–501 (1970).
259. Hachinski, V.C., Lassen, N.A., and Marshall, J. Multi-infarct dementia. *Lancet*, **ii**, 207–209 (1974).
260. Corsellis, J.A.N. The pathology of dementia. *British Journal of Hospital Medicine*, **2**, 695–702 (1969).
261. Tomlinson, B.E., Blessed, G., and Roth, M. Observations on the brains of demented old people. *Journal of the Neurological Sciences*, **11**, 205–242 (1970).
262. Botwinick, J., and Birren, J.E. Differential decline in the Wechsler Bellevue Subtests in the senile psychoses. *Journal of Gerontology*, **6**, 365–368 (1951).
263. Sourander, P., and Sjogren, H. *Ciba Symposium: Alzheimer's Disease and Related Conditions*. Ed. Wolstenholme, G. and O'Connor, M. pp.11–36. Churchill, London (1970).
264. Bowen, D.M., Spillane, J.A., Curzon, G., Meier-Ruge, W., White, P., Goodhardt, M.J., Iwangoff, P., and Davison, A.N. Accelerated ageing or selective neuronal loss as an important cause of dementia. *Lancet*, **i**, 11–14 (1979).
265. Benson, D.F. The hydrocephalic dementias. *In: Psychiatric Aspects of Neurological Disease*. Ed. Benson, D.F., and Blumer, D. pp.83–97. Grune and Stratton, New York (1975).
266. Adams, R.D., Fisher, C.M., Hakim, S., Ojemann, R., and Sweet, W.H. Symptomatic occult hydrocephalus with 'normal' CSF pressure. A treatable syndrome. *New England Journal of Medicine*, **273**, 117–126 (1965).
267. Symon, L., Dorsch, N.W.C., and Stephens, R.J. Pressure waves in so-called low pressure hydrocephalus. *Lancet*, **ii**, 1291–1292 (1972).

268. Ron, M.A., Acker, W., and Lishman, W.A. Dementia in chronic alcoholism. *In: Biological Psychiatry Today.* Ed. Obiols, J., Ballús, E., Gonzáles Monclús, E., and Pujol, J. pp.1446–1450. Elsevier North Holland, Amsterdam (1979).

269. Catterall, R.D. Neurosyphilis. *British Journal of Hospital Medicine,* **17**, 585–604 (1977).

270. Luxon, L., Lees, A.J., and Greenwood, R.J. Neurosyphilis today. *Lancet,* **i**, 90–93 (1979).

271. Albert, M.L., Feldman, R.G., and Willis, A.L. The 'Subcortical Dementia' of progressive nuclear palsy. *Journal of Neurology, Neurosurgery and Psychiatry,* **37**, 121–130 (1974).

272. Post, F. Dementia, depression and pseudodementia. *In: Psychiatric Aspects of Neurological Disease.* Ed. Benson, D.F., and Blumer, D. pp.99–120. Grune and Stratton, London (1975).

273. Whitlock, F.A. The Ganser syndrome. *British Journal of Psychiatry,* **113**, 19–29 (1967).

274. Anderson, E.W., Trethowan, W.H., and Kenna, J.C. An experimental investigation of simulation and pseudodementia. *Acta Psychiatrica et Neurologica Scandinavica, Suppl. 132, Vol.* **34**, 1–42 (1959).

275. Chierichetti, S.M., Ferrari, P., Sala, P., Vibelli, C., and Pietrzykowski, A. Effects of amantidine on mental status of elderly patients: A double blind comparison with placebo. *Current Therapeutic Research,* **22**, 158–165 (1977).

276. Lewis, C., Ballinger, B., and Presly, A.S. Trial of L-dopa in senile dementia. *British Medical Journal,* **1**, 550–551 (1978).

277. Field, J.H. *Epidemiology of Head Injuries in England and Wales.* H.M.S.O., London (1976).

278. Whitty, C.W.M., and Zangwill, O. Traumatic amnesia. *In: Amnesia,* 2nd Edition. Ed. Whitty, C.W.M. and Zangwill, O.L. pp.118–135. Butterworths, London (1977).

279. Teasdale, G., and Jennett, B. Assessment of coma and impaired consciousness. *Lancet,* **ii**, 81–84 (1974).

280. Miller, H., and Stern, G. The long-term prognosis of severe head injury. *Lancet,* **i**, 225–229 (1965).

281. Fahy, T.J., Irving, M.H., and Millac, P. Severe head injuries. *Lancet,* **ii**, 475–479 (1967).

282. Jennett, B., and Knill-Jones, R.P. Predicting outcome after head injury. *Journal of the Royal College of Physicians,* **9**, 231–237 (1975).

283. Hillbom, E. After effects of brain injuries. *Acta Psychiatrica Neurologica Scandinavica,* **35**, Suppl. 142 (1960).

284. Shaffer, D. Psychiatric aspects of brain injury in childhood: a review. *Development Medicine and Child Neurology,* **15**, 211–220 (1973).

285. Shaffer, D., Chadwick, O., and Rutter, M. Psychiatric outcome of localised head injury in children. *In: Outcome of Severe Damage to the C.N.S.* Ciba Foundation Symposium No. 34, pp.191–213. Elsevier, Amsterdam (1975).

286. Courville, C.B. *Commotio Cerebri.* San Lucas Press, Los Angeles (1953).

287. Lidvall, H.F., Linderoth, B., and Norlin, B. Causes of the post-concussional syndrome. *Acta Neurologica Scandinavica,* **50**, Suppl. 56 (1974).

288. Taylor, A.R., and Bell, T.K. Slowing of the cerebral circulation after concussional head injury. *Lancet,* **ii**, 178–180 (1966).

289. Toglia, J.V. Acute flexion-extension injury of the neck. *Neurology,* **26**, 808–814 (1976).

290. Denny-Brown, D., and Russell, W.R. Experimental cerebral concussion. *Brain,* **64**, 93–164 (1941).

291. Groat, R.A., and Simmons, J.Q. Loss of nerve cells in experimental cerebral concussion. *Journal of Neuropathology and Experimental Neurology,* **9**, 150–163 (1950).

292. Oppenheimer, D.R. Microscopic lesions in the brain following head injury.

Journal of Neurology, Neurosurgery and Psychiatry, **31**, 299–306 (1968).
293. Gronwall, D., and Wrightson, P. Delayed recovery of intellectual function after minor head injury. *Lancet*, **ii**, 605–609 (1974).
294. Pudenz, R.H., and Sheldon, C.H. The lucite calvarium — a method for direct observation of the brain. *Journal of Neurosurgery*, **3**, 487–505 (1946).
295. Brill, N.Q., and Beebe, G.W. Follow-up study of psychoneuroses. *American Journal of Psychiatry*, **108**, 417–425 (1951).
296. Symonds, C.P. The human response to flying stress. *British Medical Journal*, **2**, 703–740 (1943).
297. Symonds, C.P., and Russell, W.R. Accidental head injuries. Prognosis in 'service' patients. *Lancet*, **i**, 7–10 (1943).
298. Lewis, A.J. Discussion on the differential diagnosis and treatment of post-concussional states. *Proceedings of the Royal Society of Medicine*, **25**, 607–608 (1942).
299. Guttman, E. Late effects of closed head injuries: psychiatric observations. *Journal of Mental Science*, **92**, 1–18 (1946).
300. Dencker, S.J. A follow-up study of 128 closed head injuries in twins using co-twins as controls. *Acta Psychiatrica Scandinavica*, **33**, Suppl. 123 (1958).
301. Slater, E. The neurotic constitution. *Journal of Neurology and Psychiatry*, **6**, 1–16 (1943).
302. Ferenczi, S., Abraham, K., Simmel, E., and Jones, E. *Psychoanalysis and the War Neuroses*. G. E. Stehert and Co., New York (1921).
303. Trimble, M.R. *Compensation Neurosis*. (Wiley and Sons in Preparation).
304. Collie, J. *Malingering and Feigned Sickness*. Edward Arnold, London (1917).
305. Miller, H. Accident neurosis. *British Medical Journal*, **1**, 919–925, 992–998 (1961).
306. Hurst, A.F. *Medical Diseases of War*. Edward Arnold, London (1940).
307. Kamman, G.R. Traumatic neurosis, compensation neurosis or attitude pathosis? *Archives of Neurology and Psychiatry*, **65**, 593–603 (1951).
308. Good, R. Malingering. *British Medical Journal*, **2**, 359–362 (1942).
309. Russell, W.R. Cerebral involvement in head injury. *Brain*, **55**, 549–603 (1932).
310. Balla, J.I., and Moraitis, S. Knights in armour: A follow-up study of injuries after legal settlement. *Medical Journal of Australia*, **2**, 355–361 (1970).
311. Merskey, H., and Woodforde, J.M. Psychiatric sequelae of minor head injury. *Brain*, **95**, 521–528 (1972).
312. Stengel, E. Borderlands of neurology and psychiatry. *Recent Progress in Psychiatry*, **11**, 1–32 (1949).
313. London, P.S. Some observations of the course of events after severe injury of the head. *Annals of the Royal College of Surgeons*, **41**, 460–479 (1967).
314. Roberts, A.H. Long-term prognosis of severe accidental head injury. *Proceedings of the Royal Society of Medicine*, **69**, 137–141 (1975).
315. Panting, A., and Merry, P.H. Long-term rehabilitation of severe head injuries — social and medical support for the patient's family. *Injury*, **2**, 33–37 (1970).
316. Bond, M.R. Assessment of psychosocial outcome after severe head injury. *In: Outcome of Severe Damage to the Central Nervous System*. CIBA Foundation Symposium 34. pp.141–155. Elsevier, Amsterdam. (1975).
317. Folstein, M.F., Maiberger, R., and McHugh, P.R. Mood disorder as a specific complication of stroke. *Journal of Neurology, Neurosurgery and Psychiatry*, **40**, 1018–1020 (1977).
318. Davison, K., and Bagley, C.R. Schizophrenia-like psychoses associated with organic disorders of the central nervous system: Review of the literature. *In: Current Problems in Neuropsychiatry*. British Journal of Psychiatry, Special Publ. No. 4 Ed. Herrington, R.N. Headley Brothers, Kent (1969).
319. Ecker, A. Emotional stress before strokes: A preliminary report of 20 cases. *Annals of Internal Medicine*, **40**, 49–56 (1954).

320. Adler, R., MacRitchie, K., and Engel, G.L. Psychologic processes and ischaemic stroke. *Psychosomatic Medicine*, 33, 1–29 (1971).
321. Richardson, A. Subarachnoid haemorrhage. *British Medical Journal*, 4, 89–92 (1969).
322. Penrose, R.J.J. Life events before subarachnoid haemorrhage. *Journal of Psychosomatic Research*, 16, 329–333 (1972).
323. Storey, P.B. The precipitation of subarachnoid haemorrhage. *Journal of Psychosomatic Research*, 13, 175–182 (1969).
324. Storey, P.B. Brain damage and personality change after subarachnoid haemorrhage. *British Journal of Psychiatry*, 117, 129–142 (1970).
325. Logue, V., Durward, M., Pratt, R.T.C., Piercy, M., and Nixon, W.L.B. The quality of survival after rupture of an anterior cerebral aneurysm. *British Journal of Psychiatry*, 114, 137–160 (1968).
326. Hurwitz, L.J., and Adams, G.F. Rehabilitation of hemiplegia: Indices of assessment and prognosis. *British Medical Journal*, 1, 94–98 (1972).
327. Adams, G.F., and Hurwitz, L.J. Mental barriers to recovery from strokes. *Lancet*, ii, 533–537 (1963).
328. Marquardsen, J. The natural history of acute cerebrovascular disease. *Acta Neurologica Scandinavica*, 45, Suppl. 38 (1969).
329. Koenig, H. Dementia associated with the benign form of multiple sclerosis. *Transactions of the American Neurological Association*, 93, 227–231 (1968).
330. McDonald, W.I., and Halliday, A.M. Diagnosis and classification of multiple sclerosis. *British Medical Bulletin*, 33, 4–9 (1977).
331. Jasper, H., Bickford, R., and Magnus, O. The electroencephalogram in multiple sclerosis. *In: Multiple Sclerosis and the Demyelinating Diseases*. ARNMD Research Publication Vol. 28 pp.421–427. Williams & Wilkins, Baltimore (1950).
332. Surridge, D. An investigation into some psychiatric aspects of multiple sclerosis. *British Journal of Psychiatry*, 155, 749–764 (1969).
333. Cottrell, S.S., and Wilson, S.A.K. The affective symptomatology of disseminated sclerosis. *Journal of Neurology and Psychopathology*, 7, 1–30 (1926).
334. Brain, W.R. Disseminated sclerosis. *Quarterly Journal of Medicine*, 23, 343–391 (1930).
335. Pratt, R.T.C. An investigation of the psychiatric aspects of disseminated sclerosis. *Journal of Neurology, Neurosurgery and Psychiatry*, 14, 326–336 (1951).
336. Bergin, J.D. Rapidly progressing dementia in disseminated sclerosis. *Journal of Neurology, Neurosurgery and Psychiatry*, 20, 285–292 (1957).
337. Kahana, E., Liebowitz, U., and Atter, M. Cerebral multiple sclerosis. *Neurology*, 21, 1179–1185 (1971).
338. Young, A.C., Saunders, J., and Ponsford, J.R. Mental change as an early feature of multiple sclerosis. *Journal of Neurology, Neurosurgery and Psychiatry*, 39, 1008–1013 (1976).
339. Rudge, P. Multiple sclerosis — some recent developments. *Health Trends*, 8, 97–100 (1976).
340. Belin, J., Petter, N., Smith, A.D., Thompson, R.H.S., and Zilkha, K.J. Linoleate metabolism in multiple sclerosis. *Journal of Neurology, Neurosurgery and Psychiatry*, 34, 25–29 (1971).
341. Paulley, J.W. The psychological management of multiple sclerosis. *The Practitioner*, 218, 100–105 (1977).
342. Lancet leading article. Psychotherapy for multiple sclerosis. *Lancet*, i, 541 (1978).
343. Corbett, J., Harris, R., Taylor, E., and Trimble, M.R. Progressive disintegrative psychosis of childhood. *Journal of Childhood Psychology and Psychiatry*, 18, 211–219 (1977).
344. Merskey, H., and Spear, F.G. *Pain: Psychological and Psychiatric Aspects*. Baillière, Tindall and Cassell, London (1967).

345. Melzack, R., and Wall, P.D. Pain mechanism: a new theory. *Science*, **150**, 971–978 (1965).
346. Melzack, R., and Loeser, J.D. Phantom body pain in paraplegics: Evidence for a central 'pattern generating mechanism' for pain. *Pain*, **4**, 195–210 (1978).
347. Akil, H., and Liebeskind, J.C. Monoaminergic mechanisms of stimulation-produced analgesia. *Brain Research*, **94**, 279–296 (1975).
348. Stengel, E. Pain and the psychiatrist. *British Journal of Psychiatry*, **111**, 795–802 (1965).
349. Sternbach, R.A. *Pain Patients*. Academic Press, New York (1974).
350. Merskey, H. Psychiatric patients with persistent pain. *Journal of Psychosomatic Research*, **9**, 299–309 (1965).
351. Pilowsky, I., Chapman, C.R., and Bonica, J.J. Pain, depression and illness behaviour in a pain clinic population. *Pain*, **4**, 183–192 (1977).
352. Bond, M.R., and Pearson, I.B. Psychological aspects of pain in women with advanced cancer of the cervix. *Journal of Psychosomatic Research*, **13**, 13–19 (1969).
353. Woodforde, J.M., and Merskey, H. Personality traits of patients with chronic pain. *Journal of Psychosomatic Research*, **16**, 167–172 (1972).
354. Sternbach, R.A., Wolf, S.R., Murphy, R.W., and Akeson, W.H. Traits of pain patients: the low back 'loser'. *Psychosomatics*, **14**, 226–229 (1973).
355. Sternbach, R.A., and Timmermans, G. Personality changes associated with the reduction of pain. *Pain*, **1**, 177–181 (1975).
356. Pilowsky, I., and Spence, N.D. Is illness behaviour related to chronicity in patients with intractable pain? *Pain*, **2**, 167–173 (1976).
357. Engel, G.L. 'Psychogenic' pain and the pain-prone patient. *American Journal of Medicine*, **26**, 899–918 (1959).
358. Penman, J. Pain as an old friend. *Lancet*, **i**, 633–636 (1954).
359. Pilowsky, I., and Spence, N.D. Illness behaviour syndromes associated with intractable pain. *Pain*, **2**, 61–71 (1976).
360. Szasz, T.S. *Pain and Pleasure*. Basic Books Inc., New York (1957).
361. Guzman, F., and Lim, R.K.S. The mechanism of action of the non-narcotic analgesics. *Medical Clinics of North America*, **52**, 3–14 (1968).
362. Lee, R., and Spencer, P.S.J. Antidepressants and pain: A review of the pharmacological data supporting the use of certain tricyclics in chronic pain. *Journal of International Medical Research*, **5**, 146–156 (1977).
363. Merskey, H., and Hester, R.A. The treatment of chronic pain with psychotropic drugs. *Postgraduate Medical Journal*, **48**, 594–598 (1972).
364. Glynn, C.J. Electrical stimulation for pain relief. *British Journal of Hospital Medicine*, Equipment Suppl., 184–189 (1977).
365. Illingworth, R.D. The surgical treatment of pain. *British Journal of Hospital Medicine*, **9**, 589–592 (1973).
366. Schürmann, K. Surgical treatment. *In: Pain, Clinical and Experimental Perspectives*. Ed. Weisenberg, M.P. pp.261–274. C. V. Mosby, St Louis (1975).
367. Elithorn, A., Glithero, E., and Slater, E. Leucotomy for pain. *Journal of Neurology, Neurosurgery and Psychiatry*, **21**, 249–261 (1958).
368. Mandel, M.R. Electroconvulsive therapy for chronic pain associated with depression. *American Journal of Psychiatry*, **132**, 632–636 (1975).
369. Pilowsky, I. The psychiatrist and the pain clinic. *American Journal of Psychiatry*, **133**, 752–756 (1976).
370. Wolff, H.G. *Headache and Other Pain*. Oxford University Press, New York (1963).
371. Lippman, C.W. Certain hallucinations peculiar to migraine. *Journal of Nervous and Mental Diseases*, **116**, 346–351 (1952).
372. Crisp, A.H., McGuinness, B., Kalucy, R.S., Ralph, P.C., and Harris, G. Some clinical, social and psychological characteristics of migraine subjects in the general population. *Postgraduate Medical Journal*, **53**, 691–697 (1977).

373. Lance, J.W. *The Mechanism and Management of Headache.* Butterworths, London (1973).
374. Wilkinson, M.I.P. Migraine. *Pharmaceutical Medicine*, **1**, 188–193 (1979).
375. Graham, J.R. Cluster headache. *In: Pathogenesis and Treatment of Headache.* Ed. Appenzeller, O. pp.49–68. Spectrum Publications, New York (1976).
376. Martin, M.J., Rome, H.P., and Swenson, W.M. Muscle contraction headache: a psychiatric review. *Research and Clinical Studies in Headache*, **1**, 184–217 (1967).
377. Martin, M.J. Tension headache — a psychiatric study. *Headache*, **6**, 47–54 (1966).
378. Kudrow, L. Tension headache. *In: Pathogenesis and Treatment of Headache.* Ed. Appenzeller, O. pp.81–92. Spectrum Publications, New York (1976).
379. Harris, M. Psychosomatic disorders of the mouth and face. *Practitioner*, **214**, 372–379 (1975).
380. Rushton, J.G., Gibilisco, J.A., and Goldstein, N.P. Atypical facial pain. *Journal of the American Medical Association*, **171**, 545–548 (1959).
381. Lance, J.W. Headaches related to sexual activity. *Journal of Neurology, Neurosurgery and Psychiatry*, **39**, 1226–1230 (1976).
382. Wolkind, S.N., and Forrest, A.J. Low back pain: a psychiatric investigation. *Postgraduate Medical Journal*, **48**, 76–79 (1972).
383. Gilles, L. The management of the painful amputation stump and a new theory for the phantom phenomena. *British Journal of Surgery*, **51**, 87–95 (1964).
384. Critchley, M. *The Divine Banquet of the Brain and Other Essays.* Raven Press, New York (1979).
385. Critchley, M. Congenital indifference to pain. *Annals of Internal Medicine*, **45**, 737–747 (1956).
386. Schilder, P. *The Image and Appearance of the Human Body.* Kegan, Paul, Trench, Trubner *et al.*, London (1935).
387. Jackson, J.H. *Selected Writings of John Hughlings Jackson.* Ed. Taylor, J. Hodder & Stoughton, London (1931-2).
388. Williams, D. Modern views on the classification of epilepsy. *British Medical Journal*, **1**, 661–663 (1958).
389. Gastaut, H. Clinical and electroencephalographical classification of epileptic seizures. *Epilepsia*, **10**, Suppl., 1–28 (1969).
390. Fenton, G.W. Epilepsy and automatism. *British Journal of Hospital Medicine*, **7**, 57–64 (1972).
391. Penry, J.K., and Dreifuss, F.E. Automatisms associated with the absence of petit mal epilepsy. *Archives of Neurology*, **21**, 142–149 (1969).
392. Corbett, J.A., Harris, R., and Robinson, R.G. Epilepsy. *In: Mental Retardation and Developmental Disabilities.* Ed. Wortis, J. Vol. 7, pp.79–111. Brunner Mazel, New York (1975).
393. Meldrum, B.S. Neuropathology and pathopsysiology. *In: A Textbook of Epilepsy.* Ed. Laidlaw, J.P., and Richens, A. pp.314–354. Churchill Livingstone, London (1976).
394. Chadwick, D., Harris, R., Jenner, P., Reynolds, E.H., and Marsden, C.D. Manipulation of brain serotonin in the treatment of myoclonus. *Lancet*, **ii**, 435–436 (1975).
395. Trimble, M.R. The relationship between epilepsy and schizophrenia: a biochemical hypothesis. *Biological Psychiatry*, **12**, 299–304 (1977).
396. Betts, T.A. A follow-up study of a cohort of patients with epilepsy admitted to psychiatric care in an English city. *In: Epilepsy. Proceedings of the Hans Berger Centenary Symposium.* Ed. Harris, P., and Mawdsley, C. pp.326–338. Churchill Livingstone, London (1974).
397. Henry, J.A., and Woodruff, Q.H.A. A diagnostic sign in states of apparent unconsciousness. *Lancet*, **ii**, 920–921 (1978).
398. Bowden, A.N., Gilliatt, R.W., and Willison, R.G. The place of EEG telemetry and closed circuit television in the diagnosis and management of

270

epileptic patients. *Proceedings of the Royal Society of Medicine*, **68**, 246–248 (1975).

399. Trimble, M.R. Prolactin in epilepsy and hysteria. *British Medical Journal*, **4**, 1682 (1978).
400. Guerrant, J., Anderson, W.W., Fischer, A., Weinstein, M.R., Jaros, R.M., and Deskins, A. *Personality in Epilepsy*. Thomas, Springfield (1962).
401. Henderson, P. Epilepsy in school children. *British Journal of Preventative and Social Medicine*, **7**, 9–13 (1953).
402. Pond, D.A., and Bidwell, B.H. A survey of epilepsy in fourteen general practices: II. Social and psychological aspects. *Epilepsia*, **1**, 285–299 (1959).
403. Juul-Jensen, P. Epilepsy: A clinical and social analysis of 1020 adult patients with epileptic seizures. *Acta Neurologica Scandinavica*, **40**, Suppl. 15, 1–148 (1964).
404. Gudmundsson, G. Epilepsy in Iceland. *Acta Neurologica Scandinavica*, Suppl. 25 (1966).
405. Rutter, M., Graham, P., and Yule, W. A neuropsychiatric study in childhood. *In: Clinics in the Developmental Medicine* No. 35. Spastics International Press, Heinemann, London (1970).
406. Mellor, D.H., Lowit, I., and Hall, D.J. Are epileptic children behaviourally different from other children? *In: Epilepsy: Proceedings of the Hans Berger Centenary Symposium*. Eds. Harris, P., and Maudsley, C. pp.313–316. Churchill Livingstone, London (1973).
407. Pond, D.A. Psychiatric aspects of epilepsy in children. *Journal of Medical Science*, **98**, 404–410 (1952).
408. Tizard, B. The personality of epileptics: a discussion of the evidence. *Psychological Bulletin*, **59**, 196–210 (1962).
409. Standage, K.F., and Fenton, G.W. Psychiatric symptom profiles of patients with epilepsy. A controlled investigation. *Psychological Medicine*, **5**, 152–160 (1975).
410. Small, J., Hayden, M., and Small, I. Further psychiatric investigations of patients with temporal and non-temporal lobe epilepsy. *American Journal of Psychiatry*, **123**, 303–310 (1966).
411. Stevens, J.R. Interictal clinical manifestations of complex partial seizures. *In: Advances in Neurology*. Ed. Penry, J.K., and Daly, D.D. Vol. 11, pp.85–107. Raven Press, New York (1975).
412. Hill, J.D.N. Psychiatric aspects of epilepsy. *Medical Press*, **229**, 473–475 (1953).
413. Ervin, F., Epstein, A.W., and King, H.E. Behaviour of epileptic and non-epileptic patients with 'temporal spikes'. *Archives of Neurology and Psychiatry*, **74**, 488–497 (1955).
414. Ounstead, C., Lindsay, J., and Norman, R. Biological factors in temporal lobe epilepsy. *Clinics in Developmental Medicine No. 22*. William Heinemann, London (1966).
415. Stores, G. Behaviour disturbance and type of epilepsy in children attending ordinary schools. *In: Epilepsy. The Eighth Internation Symposium*. Ed. Penry, J.K. pp.245–249. Raven Press, New York (1977).
416. Rodin, E.A., Katz, M., and Lennox, K. Differences between patients with temporal lobe seizures and those with other forms of epileptic attacks. *Epilepsia*, **17**, 313–320 (1976).
417. Bear, D.M., and Fedio, P. Quantitative analysis of interictal behaviour in temporal lobe epilepsy. *Archives of Neurology*, **34**, 454–467 (1977).
418. Tempkin, O. *The Falling Sickness*. Johns Hopkins Press, Baltimore (1971).
419. Slater, E., and Beard, A.W. The schizophrenia-like psychoses of epilepsy. *British Journal of Psychiatry*, **109**, 95–112 (1963).
420. Landolt, H. Serial electroencephalographic investigations during psychotic episodes in epileptic patients and during schizophrenic attacks. *In: Lectures on Epilepsy*. Ed. Lorentz de Haas, A.M. pp.91–133. Elsevier, London (1958).

421. Dongier, S. Statistical study of clinical and electroencephalographic manifestations of 536 psychotic episodes occurring in 516 epileptics between clinical seizures. *Epilepsia*, **1**, 117–142 (1959).
422. Yde, A., Edel, L., and Faurbye, A. On the relation between schizophrenia, epilepsy and induced convulsions. *Acta Psychiatrica Scandinavica*, **16**, 325–388 (1941).
423. Gruhle, H. Wahn Uber den bei Epilepsie. *Zeitschrift fur die Gesamte, Neurologie und Psychiatrie*, **154**, 395–399 (1936).
424. Pond, D.A. Psychiatric aspects of epilepsy. *Journal of the Indian Medical Profession*, **3**, 1441–1451 (1957).
425. Rodin, E.A., DeJong, R.N., Waggoner, R.W., Basu, K., and Bagchi, B.K. Relationship between certain forms of psychomotor epilepsy and 'schizophrenia'. *Archives of Neurology and Psychiatry*, **77**, 449–463 (1957).
426. Beard, A.W., and Slater, E. The schizophrenia-like psychoses of epilepsy. *Proceedings of the Royal Society of Medicine*, **55**, 311–316 (1962).
427. Flor-Henry, P. Psychosis and temporal lobe epilepsy. *Epilepsia*, **10**, 363–395 (1969).
428. Bruens, J.H. Psychosis in epilepsy. *Psychiatria, Neurologia & Neurochirurgia*, **74**, 175–192 (1971).
429. Trimble, M.R., and Meldrum, B.S. Monoamines, epilepsy and schizophrenia. *In: Biological Psychiatry Today*. Ed. Obiols, J., Ballús, C. and González Monclús, E. et al. pp.470–475. Elsevier North Holland, Amsterdam (1979).
430. Symonds, C.P. The schizophrenic-like psychoses of epilepsy (discussion). *Proceedings of the Royal Society of Medicine*, **55**, 311 (1962).
431. Hill, J.D.N. Psychiatry. *In: Electroencephalography — A Symposium on its Various Aspects*. Ed. Hill, D., and Parr, G. pp.319–363. MacDonald, London (1950).
432. Lennox, W.G., and Lennox, M.A. *Epilepsy and Related Disorders*. J. A. Churchill, London (1960).
433. Trimble, M.R. Anticonvulsant drugs, behaviour and cognitive abilities. *In: Current Developments in Psychopharmacology*. Ed. Essman, W.B., and Valzelli, L. (In the Press) (1980).
434. Trimble, M.R., and Reynolds, E.H. Anticonvulsant drugs and mental symptoms: a review. *Psychological Medicine*, **6**, 169–178 (1976).
435. Taylor, D.C. Sexual behaviour and temporal lobe epilepsy. *Archives of Neurology*, **21**, 510–516 (1969).
436. Blumer, D., and Walker, A.E. The neural basis of sexual behaviour. *In: Psychiatric Aspects of Neurological Disease*. Ed. Benson, D.F., and Blumer, D. pp.199–217. Grune & Stratton, London (1975).
437. Mitchell, W., Falconer, M.A., and Hill, D. Epilepsy with fetishism relieved by temporal lobectomy. *Lancet*, **ii**, 626–630 (1954).
438. Hunter, R., Logue, V., and McMenemy, W.H. Temporal lobe epilepsy supervening on long-standing transvestism and fetishism. *Epilepsia*, **4** 60–65 (1963).
439. Richens, A. *Drug Treatment of Epilepsy*. Henry Kimpton, London (1976).
440. Chadwick, D., Jenner, P., and Reynolds, E.H. Amines, anticonvulsants and epilepsy. *Lancet*, **i**, 473–476 (1975).
441. Reynolds, E.H. Chronic anti-epileptic toxicity. A review. *Epilepsia*, **16**, 319–352 (1975).
442. Reynolds, E.H. Drug treatment of epilepsy. *Lancet*, **ii**, 721–725 (1978).
443. Loughnan, P.M., Gold, H., and Vance, J.C. Phenytoin teratogenicity in man. *Lancet*, **i**, 70–72 (1973).
444. Shorvon, S.D., Chadwick, D., Galbraith, A.W., and Reynolds, E.H. One drug for epilepsy. *British Medical Journal*, **1**, 474–476 (1978).

445. Trimble, M.R. Non-MAOI antidepressants and epilepsy. *Epilepsia*, **19**, 241–250 (1978).
446. Taylor, D.C., and Falconer, M.A. Clinical, socio-economic and psychological changes after temporal lobectomy for epilepsy. *British Journal of Psychiatry*, **114**, 1247–1261 (1968).
447. Falconer, M.A. Reversibility by temporal-lobe resection of the behavioural abnormalities of temporal lobe epilepsy. *New England Journal of Medicine*, **289**, 451–455 (1973).
448. Tavriger, R. Some parental theories about the causes of epilepsy. *Epilepsia*, **7**, 339–343 (1966).
449. Fenton, G.W. Clinical disorders of sleep. *British Journal of Hospital Medicine*, **14**, 120–145 (1975).
450. Jouvet, M. Paradoxical sleep — a study of its nature and mechanisms. *In: Sleep Mechanisms*. Ed. Akert, K., Bally, C., and Schade, J.P. pp.20–57. Elsevier, London (1965).
451. Von Economo, C. Sleep as a problem of localisation. *Journal of Nervous and Mental Disease*, **7**, 249–259 (1930).
452. Akert, K. The anatomical substrate of sleep. *In: Sleep Mechanisms*. Ed. Akert, K., Bally, C., and Schade, J.P. pp.9–19. Elsevier, London (1965).
453. Parkes, J.D. The sleepy patient. *Lancet*, **i**, 990–993 (1977).
454. Hunter, R., Blackwood, W., and Bull, J. Three cases of frontal meningiomas presenting psychiatrically. *British Medical Journal*, **3**, 9–16 (1968).
455. Pond, D.A. Narcolepsy: a brief critical review and study of eight cases. *Journal of Mental Science*, **98**, 595–604 (1952).
456. Smith, C. Psychosomatic aspects of narcolepsy. *Journal of Mental Science*, **104**, 593–607 (1958).
457. Sours, J. Narcolepsy and other disturbances in sleep-walking rhythm: a study of 115 cases with review of the literature. *Journal of Nervous and Mental Diseases*, **137**, 525–542 (1963).
458. Roy, A. Psychiatric aspects of narcolepsy. *British Journal of Psychiatry*, **128**, 562–565 (1976).
459. Parkes, J.D., Fenton, G., Struthers, G., Curzon, G., Kantameneni, B.A., Buxton, B.H., and Record, C. Narcolepsy and cataplexy. Clinical findings, treatment and cerebrospinal fluid findings. *Quarterly Journal of Medicine*, **43**, 525–536 (1974).
460. Critchley, M., Periodic 'hypersomnia' and megaphagia in adolescent males. *Brain*, **85**, 627–656 (1962).
461. Billiard, M., Guilleminault, C., and Dement, W. A menstruation-linked periodic hypersomnia. *Neurology*, **25**, 436–443 (1975).
462. Roth, B., Nevsimalova, S., and Rechtschaffen, A. Hypersomnia with 'sleep drunkenness'. *Archives of General Psychiatry*, **26**, 456–462 (1972).
463. Kraepelin, E. *Dementia Praecox and Paraphrenia*. Translated by Barclay, R.M. Livingstone, Edinburgh (1919).
464. Olkon, D.M. *Essentials of Neuropsychiatry*. Henry Kimpton, London (1945).
465. Reiter, P.J. Extrapyramidal motor-disturbances in dementia praecox. *Acta Psychiatrica et Neurologica*, **1**, 287–310 (1926).
466. Jones, M., and Hunter, R. Abnormal movements in patients with chronic psychiatric illness. *In: Psychotropic Drugs and Dysfunctions of the Basal Ganglia*. Proceedings of a workshop held in Bethesda, Maryland. Ed. Crane, G.E., and Gardner, J. pp.53–65. Public Health Service Publication No. 1938. NIMH Bethesda, Md. (1969).
467. Jones, I.H. Observations in schizophrenia stereotypes. *Comprehensive Psychiatry*, **6**, 323–335 (1965).
468. Von Economo, C. *Encephalitis Lethargica — its Sequelae and Treatment*. Translated by Newman, K.O. Oxford University Press, London (1931).

469. Ayd. F.J. A survey of drug induced extrapyramidal reactions. *Journal of the American Medical Assocation*, **175**, 1054–1060 (1961).
470. Korczyn, A.D., and Goldberg, G.J. Extrapyramidal effects of the neuroleptics. *Journal of Neurology, Neurosurgery and Psychiatry*, **39**, 866–869 (1976).
471. Bishop, M.P., Gallant, D.M., and Sykes, T.F. Extrapyramidal side effects and therapeutic response. *Archives of General Psychiatry*, **13**, 155–162 (1965).
472. Gelenberg, A.J., and Mandel, M.R. Catatonic reactions to high potency neuroleptic drugs. *Archives of General Psychiatry*, **34**, 947–950 (1977).
473. Tarsy, D., and Baldessarini, R.J. The tardive dyskinesia syndrome. *In: Clinical Neuropharmacology*. Ed. Klawans, H.L. Vol. 1, pp.29–61. Raven Press, New York (1976).
474. Greenblatt, D.L., Dominick, J. R., and Stotsky, B.A. Phenothiazine-induced dyskinesia in nursing home patients. *Journal of the American Geriatric Society*, **16**, 27–34 (1968).
475. Crane, G.E., and Chase, C. Dyskinesia and neuroleptics. *Archives of General Psychiatry*, **19**, 700–703 (1968).
476. Polizos, P., Engelhardt, D.M., and Hoffman, S.P. CNS consequences of psychotropic drug withdrawal in schizophrenic children. *Psychopharmacology Bulletin*, **9**, 34–35 (1973).
477. Brandon, S., McClelland, H.A., and Protheroe, C. A study of facial dyskinesia in a mental hospital population. *British Journal of Psychiatry,* **118**, 171–184 (1971).
478. Crane, G.E. Persistent dyskinesia. *British Journal of Psychiatry*, **122**, 295–405 (1973).
479. Hunter, R., Blackwood, W., Smith, M.C., and Cummings, J.N. Neuropathological findings in three cases of persistent dyskinesia following phenothiazine medication. *Journal of the Neurological Sciences*, **7**, 763–773 (1968).
480. Christensen, E., Møller, J.E., and Faurbye, A. Neuropathological investigation of 28 brains from patients with dyskinesia. *Acta Psychiatrica Scandinavica*, **46**, 14–23 (1970).
481. Pin, D.K., and Faurbye, A. Concentration of homovanillic acid and 5-hydroxy-indole-acetic-acid in the cerebrospinal fluid after treatment with probenecid in patients with drug-induced tardive dyskinesia. *Acta Psychiatrica Scandinavica*, **46**, 323–326 (1970).
482. Ng, L.K.Y., Gelhard, R.E., Chase, T.N., and McLean, P.D. Drug-induced dyskinesia in monkeys — A pharmacologic model employing 6-hydroxydopamine. *In: Advances in Neurology*. Vol. 1, Huntington's Chorea 1872-1972. Ed. Barbeau, A., Chase, T.N., and Paulson, G.W. pp.651–655. Raven Press, New York (1973).
483. Kazamatzuri, H., Chien, C., and Cole, J.O. Therapeutic approaches to tardive dyskinesia. *Archives of General Psychiatry*, **27**, 491–499 (1972).
484. International Drug Therapy Newsletter. Drug therapies for tardive dyskinesia. Ed. Ayd, F.J. Vol. **13**, pp.37–40. Ayd Medical Communications (1978).
485. Gibson, A.C. Depot injections and tardive dyskinesia. *British Journal of Psychiatry*, **132**, 361–365 (1978).
486. Nashold, B.S. The effect of central tegmental lesions on tardive dyskinesia. *In: Psychotropic Drugs and Dysfunctions of the Basal Ganglia*. Ed. Crane, G.E., and Gardner, R.J. pp.111–116. U.S. Public Health Service Publication No. 1938, Washington, D.C. (1969).
487. Parkinson, J. *An Essay on the Shaking Palsy*. Sherwood, Neely and Jones, London (1817).
488. Warburton, J.W. Depressive symptoms in Parkinson patients referred for thalamotomy. *Journal of Neurology, Neurosurgery and Psychiatry*, **30**, 368–370 (1967).
489. Mindham, R.H.S. Psychiatric symptoms in Parkinsonism. *Journal of Neurology, Neurosurgery and Psychiatry*, **33**, 188–191 (1970).

274

490. Robins, A.H. Depression in patients with Parkinsonism. *British Journal of Psychiatry*, **128**, 141–145 (1976).
491. Mindham, R.H.S. Psychiatric aspects of Parkinson's disease. *British Journal of Hospital Medicine*, **11**, 411–414 (1974).
492. Crow, T.J., Johnstone, E.C., and McClelland, H.A. The coincidence of schizophrenia and Parkinsonism: Some neurochemical implications. *Psychological Medicine*, **6**, 227–233 (1976).
493. Crown, S. Psychosomatic aspects of Parkinsonism. *Journal of Psychosomatic Research*, **15**, 451–459 (1971).
494. Celesia, C.G., and Wanamaker, W.M. Psychiatric disturbances in Parkinson's disease. *Diseases of the Nervous System*, **33**, 577–583 (1972).
495. Talland, G.A. Cognitive function in Parkinson's disease. *Journal of Nervous and Mental Disease*, **135**, 196–205 (1962).
496. Loranger, A.W., Goodell, H., McDowell, F.H., Lee, J.E., and Sweet, R.D. Intellectual impairment in Parkinson's disease. *Brain*, **95**, 405–412 (1972).
497. Riklan, M., Weiner, H., and Diller, L. Somatopsychologic studies in Parkinson's disease. *Journal of Nervous and Mental Diseases*, **129**, 263–272 (1959).
498. Riklan, M. *L-dopa and Parkinsonism*. Charles C. Thomas, Springfield (1973).
499. Shy, G.M., and Drager, G.A. A neurological syndrome associated with orthostatic hypotension. *Archives of Neurology*, **2**, 511–527 (1960).
500. Steele, J.C., Richardson, J.C., and Olszewski, J. Progressive supranuclear palsy. *Archives of Neurology*, **10**, 333–359 (1964).
501. Birkmayer, W., Jellinger, K., and Riederer, P. Striatal and extrastriatal dopaminergic functions. *In: Psychobiology of the Striatum*. Ed. Cools, A.R., Lohman, A.H.M., and Van Den Bercken, J.H.L. pp.141–154. North Amsterdam Publishing Co., Amsterdam (1977).
502. Sandler, M. Is Parkinsonism a dopamine deficiency syndrome? *In: Neurotransmission and Disturbed Behaviour*. Ed. Van Praag, H.M. and Bruinvels, J. pp.150–161. Bohn Scheltema a Holkema, Utrecht (1977).
503. Lees, A.J., Kohout, L.J., Shaw, K.M., Stern, G.M., Elsworth, J.D., Sandler, M., and Youdim, M.B.H. Deprenyl in Parkinson's disease. *Lancet*, **ii**, 791–795 (1977).
504. Marsden, C.D., and Parkes, J.D. 'On-Off' effects in patients with Parkinson's disease on chronic L-dopa therapy. *Lancet*, **i**, 292–296 (1976).
505. Mindham, R.H.S., Marsden, C.D., and Parkes, J.D. Psychiatric symptoms during L-dopa therapy for Parkinson's disease and their relationship to physical disability. *Psychological Medicine*, **6**, 23–33 (1976).
506. O'Brien, C.P., Digiacomo, J.N., Fahn, S., and Schwarz, G.A. Mental effects of high dosage levodopa. *Archives of General Psychiatry*, **24**, 61–64 (1971).
507. Huntington, G. On chorea. *The Medical and Surgical Reporter*, **26**, 317–321 (1872).
508. Brothers, C.R.D. Huntington's chorea in Victoria and Tasmania. *Journal of the Neurological Sciences*, **1**, 405–420 (1964).
509. Minski, L., and Guttman, E. Huntington's chorea: A study of thirty-four families. *Journal of Mental Science*, **84**, 21–96 (1938).
510. Bolt, J.M. Huntington's chorea in the West of Scotland. *British Journal of Psychiatry*, **116**, 259–270 (1970).
511. Dewhurst, K., Oliver, J., Trick, K.L.K., and McKnight, A.L. Neuropsychiatric aspects of Huntington's disease. *Confina Neurologica*, **31**, 258–268 (1969).
512. Heathfield, K.W.G. Huntington's chorea. *Brain*, **90**, 203–232 (1967).
513. James, W.E., Mefford, R.B., and Kimbell, I. Early signs of Huntington's chorea. *Diseases of the Nervous System*, **30**, 556–559 (1969).
514. McHugh, P.R., and Folstein, M.F. Psychiatric syndromes of Huntington's chorea. *In: Psychiatric Aspects of Neurologic Disease*. Ed. Benson, D.F., and Blumer, D. pp.267–285. Grune and Stratton, New York (1975).

515. Oliver, J.E. Huntington's chorea in Northamptonshire. *British Journal of Psychiatry*, **116**, 241–253 (1970).
516. Aminoff, M.J., Marshall, J., Smith, E.M., and Wyke, M.A. Pattern of intellectual impairment in Huntington's chorea. *Psychological Medicine*, **5**, 169–172 (1975).
517. Caine, E.D., Hunt, R.D., Weingartner, H., and Ebert, M.H. Huntington's Dementia. *Archives of General Psychiatry*, **35**, 377–384 (1978).
518. Curzon, G., Gumpert, J., and Sharpe, D. Amine metabolites in the cerebrospinal fluid in Huntington's chorea. *Journal of Neurology, Neurosurgery and Psychiatry*, **35**, 514–519 (1972).
519. Bird, E.D. Biochemical studies on gamma-aminobutyric acid metabolism in Huntington's chorea. *In: Biochemistry and Neurology*. Ed. Bradford, H.F., and Marsden, C.D. pp.83–92. Academic Press, London (1976).
520. Rosenberg, S., Metzig, E., Snider, S.R., Ast, M., and Tobin, D. Detection of presymptomatic carriers of Huntington's chorea. *Neuropsychobiology*, **3**, 144–152 (1977).
521. British Medical Journal (leading article). Predictive tests in Huntington's chorea. *British Medical Journal*, **1**, 528–529 (1978).
522. Wilson, S.A.K. Progressive lenticular degeneration: a familial nervous disease associated with cirrhosis of the liver. *Brain*, **34**, 295–509 (1912).
523. Walshe, J.M. Wilson's disease: its diagnosis and management. *British Journal of Hospital Medicine*, **4**, 91–98 (1970).
524. Denny-Brown, D. *Diseases of the Basal Ganglia and Subthalamic Nuclei*. Oxford University Press, New York (1946).
525. Beard, A.W. The association of hepatolenticular degeneration with schizophrenia. *Acta Psychiatrica et Neurologica Scandinavica*, **34**, 411–428 (1959).
526. Ebaugh, F.G. Neuropsychiatric aspects of chorea in children. *Journal of the American Medical Association*, **87**, 1083–1088 (1926).
527. Aita, J.A. Neurologic manifestations of rheumatic fever. *Postgraduate Medicine*, **54**, 82–86 (1973).
528. Wertheimer, N.M. Rheumatic schizophrenia. *Archives of General Psychiatry*, **4**, 71–88 (1961).
529. Eldridge, R. The torsion dystonias: Literature review and genetic and clinical studies. *Neurology*, **20**, 1–78 (1970).
530. Marsden, C.D., Harrison, M.J.G., and Bundey, S. Natural history of idiopathic torsion dystonia. *In: Advances in Neurology*. Ed. Eldridge, R., and John, S. Vol. **14**, pp.177–186. Raven Press, New York (1976).
531. Marsden, C.D. Dystonia: the spectrum of the disease. *In: The Basal Ganglia*. Ed. Yahr, M.D. pp.351–367. Raven Press, New York (1976).
532. Riklan, M., Cullinan, T., and Cooper, I.S. Psychological studies in dystonia musculorum deformans. *In: Advances in Neurology*. Ed. Eldridge, R., and Fahn, S. Vol. 14, pp.189–200. Raven Press, New York (1976).
533. Tibbetts, R.W. Spasmodic torticollis. *Journal of Psychosomatic Research*, **15**, 461–469 (1971).
534. Cockburn, J.J. Spasmodic torticollis: a psychogenic condition? *Journal of Psychosomatic Research*, **15**, 471–477 (1971).
535. Meares, R. Features which distinguish groups of spasmodic torticollis. *Journal of Psychosomatic Research*, **15**, 1–12 (1971).
536. Crisp, A.H., and Moldofsky, H. A psychosomatic study of writer's cramp. *British Journal of Psychiatry*, **111**, 841–858 (1965).
537. Bindman, E., and Tibbetts, R.W. Writer's cramp — a rational approach to treatment. *British Journal of Psychiatry*, **131**, 143–148 (1977).
538. Marsden, C.D. Blepharospasm-oromandibular dystonia syndrome (Breughel's syndrome). *Journal of Neurology, Neurosurgery and Psychiatry*, **39**, 1204–1209 (1976).

276

539. Gilles de la Tourette, G. Étude sur une affection nerveuse caractérisée par de l'incoordination motrice accompagnée d'l'echolalie et de coprolalie. *Archives of Neurology*, **9**, 19-42, 158-200 (1885).

540. Shapiro, A.K., Shapiro, E.S., Bruun, R.D., and Sweet, R.D. *Gilles de la Tourette Syndrome.* Raven Press, New York (1978).

541. Shapiro, A.K., Shapiro, E.S., and Wayne, H.L. The symptomatology and diagnosis of Gilles de la Tourette syndrome. *Journal of American Academy of Child Psychiatry*, **12**, 702-723 (1973).

542. Yap, P.M. Mental diseases peculiar to certain cultures: a survey of comparative psychiatry. *Journal of Mental Science*, **97**, 313-327 (1951).

543. Corbett, J.A. The nature of tics and Gilles de la Tourette's syndrome. *Journal of Psychosomatic Research*, **15**, 403-409 (1971).

544. Corbett, J.A., Matthews, A.M., Connell, P.H., and Shapiro, D.A. Tics and Gilles de la Tourette's syndrome. A follow-up study and critical review. *British Journal of Psychiatry*, **115**, 1229-1241 (1969).

545. Bruun, R.D., Shapiro, A.K., Wayne, H., and Solomon, G.E. A follow-up of 78 patients with Gilles de la Tourette syndrome. *American Journal of Psychiatry*, **133**, 944-947 (1976).

546. Johnstone, E.C., and Marsh, W. Acetylator status and response to phenelzine in depressed patients. *Lancet*, **i**, 567-570 (1973).

547. Davis, J.M., and Janowsky, D.S. Recent advances in the treatment of depression. *British Journal of Hospital Medicine*, **11**, 219-228 (1974).

548. Tyrer, P. Towards a rational therapy with monoamine oxidase inhibitors. *British Journal of Psychiatry*, **128**, 354-360 (1976).

549. Sethna, E.R. A study of refractory cases of depressive illness and their response to combined antidepressant treatment. *British Journal of Psychiatry*, **124**, 265-272 (1974).

550. Horn, A.S. The interaction of tricyclic antidepressants with the biogenic amine uptake systems in the central nervous system. *Postgraduate Medical Journal*, **52**, Suppl. 3, 25-30 (1976).

551. Burrows, G.D., Vohra, J., Hunt, D., Sloman, J.G., Scoggins, B.A., and Davies, B. Cardiac effects of different tricyclic antidepressant drugs. *British Journal of Psychiatry*, **129** 335-341 (1976).

552. Hughes, I.E., and Radwan, S. Cardiotoxicity of antidepressants. *In: Biological Psychiatry Today*. Ed. Obiols, J., Ballús, C., Gonzales Monclús, *et al.* pp.837-842. Elsevier, North Holland (1979).

553. Scoggins, B.A., and Maguire, K.P. Measurement of tricyclic antidepressant drugs in plasma. *In: Handbook of Studies on Depression*. Ed. Burrows, G.D. pp.157-171. Excerpta Medica, Amsterdam (1977).

554. Carney, M.W.P., and Sheffield, B.F. Comparison of antipsychotic depot injections in the maintenancne treatment of schizophrenia. *British Journal of Psychiatry*, **129**, 476-481 (1976).

555. Alarcon, R., and Carney, M.W.P. Severe depressive mood changes following slow release intramuscular fluphenazine injection. *British Medical Journal*, **3**, 564-567 (1969).

556. Riding, J., and Munro, A. Pimozide in the treatment of monosymptomatic hypochondriacal psychosis. *Acta Psychiatrica Scandinavica*, **52**, 23-30 (1975).

557. Möhler, H., and Okada, T. The benzodiazepine receptor in normal and pathological human brain. *British Journal of Psychiatry*, **133**, 261-268 (1978).

558. Haefely, W.E. Central actions of benzodiazepines. General introduction. *British Journal of Psychiatry*, **133**, 231-238 (1978).

559. Alexander, R.W., Davis, J.N., and Lefrowitz, R.J. Direct identification and characterisation of β-adrenergic receptors in the rat brain. *Nature*, **258**, 437 (1975).

560. Tyrer, P.J., and Lader, M.H. Response to propranolol and diazepam in somatic and psychic anxiety. *British Medical Journal*, **2**, 14–16 (1974).
561. Bonn, J.A., Turner, P., and Hicks, D.C. β-adrenergic receptor blockade with practolol in the treatment of anxiety. *Lancet*, **i**, 814–815 (1972).
562. Yorkston, N.J., Zaki, S.A., Malik, M.K.U., Morrison, R.C., and Havard, C.W.H. Propranolol in the control of schizophrenic symptoms. *British Medical Journal*, **4**, 633–635 (1974).
563. Sheard, M.H., Marini, J.L., Bridges, C.I., and Wagner, E. The effect of lithium on impulsive aggressive behaviour in man. *American Journal of Psychiatry*, **133**, 1409–1413 (1976).
564. Ghose, K. Lithium salts: Therapeutic and unwanted effects. *British Journal of Hospital Medicine*, **18**, 578–583 (1977).
565. Von Meduna, L. *Die Konvulsiontherapie der schizophrenie*. Halle, Marburg (1937).
566. Ottosson, J.D. Experimental studies in the mode of action of electroconvulsive therapy. *Acta Psychiatrica Scandinavica*, **35**, Suppl. 145, 5–235 (1960).
567. Schildkraut, J.J., and Draskoczy, P.R. Electroconvulsive shock and norepinephrine turnover. *In: Psychobiology of Convulsive Therapy*. Ed. Fink, M., Kety, S., McGaugh, J., and Williams, T.A.J. Wiley, London (1974).
568. Halliday, A.M., Davison, K., Brown, M.W., and Kreeger, L.C. A comparison of the effects on depression and memory of bilateral ECT and unilateral ECT to the dominant and non-dominant hemispheres. *British Journal of Psychiatry*, **114**, 997–1012 (1968).
569. Squire, L.R., and Chance, P.M. Memory functions six to nine months after E.C.T. *Archives of General Psychiatry*, **32**, 1557–1564 (1975).
570. Fulton, J.F., and Jacobsen, C.G. The functions of the frontal lobes, a comparative study in monkeys, chimpanzees and men. *Advances in Modern Biology*, **4**, 113–123 (1935).
571. Moniz, E. *Tentatives Operatoires dans le traitement de certaines psychoses*. Masson, Paris (1936).
572. Freeman, W., and Watts, J.W. Psychosurgery during 1936–1946. *Archives of Neurology and Psychiatry*, **58**, 417–425 (1947).
573. Kelly, D. Neurosurgical treatment of psychiatric disorders. *In: Recent Advances in Clinical Psychiatry*, No. 2. Ed. Granville-Grossmann, K. pp.227–261. Churchill-Livingstone, Edinburgh (1976).
574. Birley, J.L.T. Modified leucotomy: A review of 106 cases. *British Journal of Psychiatry,* **110** 211–221 (1964).
575. Post, F., Rees, W.L., and Schurr, P.H. An evaluation of medial leucotomy. *British Journal of Psychiatry*, **114**, 1223–1246 (1968).
576. Knight, G. Further observations from an experience of 660 cases of stereotactic tractotomy. *Postgraduate Medical Journal*, **49**, 845–854 (1973).
577. Mitchell-Heggs, N., Kelly, D., and Richardson, A. Stereotactic limbic leucotomy: a follow-up at 16 months. *British Journal of Psychiatry*, **128**, 226–240 (1976).
578. Schurr, P.H. Psychosurgery. *British Journal of Hospital Medicine*, **10**, 53–60 (1973).
579. Narabayashi, H. Stereotactic Amygdalotomy for Behavioural Disorders of Epileptic Aetiology. *In: Excerpta Medica International Congress Series No. 274*. pp.175–184. Excerpta Medica, Amsterdam (1971).
580. Small, I.F., Heimburger, R.F., Small, J.G., Milstein, V., and Moore, D.F. Follow-up of stereotaxic amygdalotomy for seizure and behaviour disorders. *Biological Psychiatry*, **12**, 401–411 (1977).
581. Budzynski, T.H., Stoyva, J.M., and Adler, C.S. EMG biofeedback and tension headache: A controlled outcome study. *Psychosomatic Medicine*, **35**, 484–496 (1978).

582. Sterman, M.B. Neurophysiological and clinical studies of sensorimotor EEG biofeedback training: some effects on epilepsy. *In: Biofeedback: Behavioural Medicine*. Ed. Birk, L. Grune and Stratton, New York (1973).

583. Turin, A., and Johnson, W.G. Biofeedback therapy for migraine headaches. *Archives of General Psychiatry*, **33**, 517–519 (1976).

584. Sakel, M. The pharmacological shock treatment of schizophrenia. *Nervous and Mental Diseases Monograph Series No. 62*. Nervous and Mental Diseases Publications Co., New York (1938).

585. Sargant, W., and Slater, E. *An Introduction to Physical Methods of Treatment in Psychiatry*, 3rd Edition. E. and S. Livingstone, London (1954).

586. Bhanji, S., and Roy, G.A. The treatment of psychotic depression by sleep deprivation: a replication study. *British Journal of Psychiatry*, **127**, 222–226 (1975).

Index

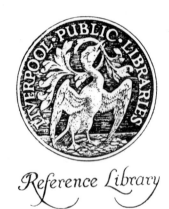